Small Animal Surgical Nursing

FOURTH EDITION

Small Animal Surgical Nursing

Marianne Tear, MS, LVT
Educational Coordinator
Tear Consulting, LLC
Chesterfield, MI
United States of America

ELSEVIER

Elsevier
3251 Riverport Lane
St. Louis, Missouri 63043

SMALL ANIMAL SURGICAL NURSING, FOURTH EDITION   ISBN: 978-0-323-75913-7

Notice

Previous editions copyrighted 2017, 2012, and 2006.

Library of Congress Control Number: 2020951839

Senior Content Strategist: Brandi Graham
Senior Content Development Manager: Luke Held
Senior Content Development Specialist: Maria Broeker
Publishing Services Manager: Deepthi Unni
Project Manager: Sri Vidhya Shankar
Design Direction: Margaret Reid

Printed in India

Last digit is the print number: 9 8 7 6 5 4 3

CONTRIBUTORS

Paige Allen, MS, RVT
Academic Advisor
Veterinary Nursing
Purdue University
West Lafayette, Indiana

Susan Burcham, DVM
Medical Director
Moore Veterinary Hospital
St. Clair Shores, Michigan

Marianne Tear, MS, LVT
Educational Coordinator
Tear Consulting, LLC
Chesterfield, Michigan

Megan Terry, LVT
Field Support Representative
IDEXX Laboratories
Westbrook, Maine

Ann Wortinger, BIS, LVT, VTS (ECC)(SAIM)(Nutrition), Elite FFCP
Education
Ashworth College
Scranton, Pennsylvania

ACKNOWLEDGMENTS

Without the dedication and knowledge base of the amazing contributors this textbook would not be possible! I cannot thank you enough for all your hard work and perfectionism. You all rock.

Thank you to my students – your eagerness and passion for this crazy profession keep me motivated and energized.

To my fellow veterinary professionals and educators – you are a crazy amazing bunch. I count myself blessed to be part of this community.

And finally, thank you to my amazing husband. I know I am not the easiest to get along with during this process, but you somehow managed. Thank you for holding the family together while I get lost during this process.

Each time I am asked to work on the new edition of this text I am equal parts honored and overwhelmed. The task always seems daunting – how to make something I utilize almost daily, better, and more meaningful to students and instructors. Thankfully, my colleagues are always willing to give input, both positive and negative, to share how they utilize the text and to give suggestions on what they would like to see moving forward. I love this profession and its willingness to work together and help each other.

Students are also very willing to give input on what they like and don't like about a textbook. That information also helps shape changes that are incorporated. If they don't read it, it's useless

This edition was laid out to make life less taxing for instructors and students. Chapters from the previous editions have been separated to allow for more ease of assignment if you will. Whole chapters rather than specific page numbers should be able to be assigned. And instructors can more easily, I hope, move through the book in the order that works best for them. This should also help cut down on students having to figure out where on a specific page to stop reading….

A quote my husband is fond of goes something like "In the time of adversity, you don't rise to the challenge, you fall to your level of training." While surgery is not necessarily adversity, it can be challenging and stressful. My hope is that this textbook can be used as a training manual.

CONTENTS

Preoperative Room Considerations

Marianne Tear

LEARNING OBJECTIVES

After completion of this chapter, the reader will be able to:
- Explain the ideal layout of a surgery suite and adjacent areas.
- Differentiate between nonmovable (permanent) and movable equipment in a surgery room.
- Explain the cleaning of the equipment located in the surgery room.
- List examples of equipment used perioperatively in veterinary surgery.

KEY TERMS

Aseptic
Positive pressure ventilation
Suction

One of the most challenging and rewarding activities that a technician can participate in is surgery. The technician is responsible for many different activities during the surgery, and it is imperative that careful preparation takes place every time to ensure successful outcomes.

For elective (non–life-threatening) procedures, facilities should be properly prepared. Preparations include the room, but are not limited to, the equipment, and the instruments.

LAYOUT OF THE SURGERY SUITE

The American Animal Hospital Association (AAHA) recommends three distinct, separate areas for a surgical facility: the preparation area, the scrub area, and the surgery room. Although AAHA certification is not a legal requirement for veterinary facilities, a surgical facility should strive to create the safest environment for the patient. In addition, some state licensing boards have specific requirements regarding surgical facilities that a veterinary hospital must meet to pass inspection and to receive authorization to offer surgery.

Preparation Area

The preparation area should be adjacent to but separate from the surgery room. This prep room can be used for patient preparation (e.g., clipping and initial scrub) and the storage of surgical supplies. The surgeon can use the preparation area to scrub and gown for surgery if a separate scrub area is not available. It is ideal to have a separate anesthesia machine for the prep room so that cross-contamination does not occur when the machine is moved from one room to another. Procedures that are considered clean but not sterile or procedures that are classified as dirty should be done in the prep area. Procedures such as abscessed wound care, debridement of old wounds, and treatment of impacted anal sacs are often defined as dirty. Feline neuters and, although controversial, declaw procedures, tail docking, and dewclaw removal are considered clean, not sterile, procedures.

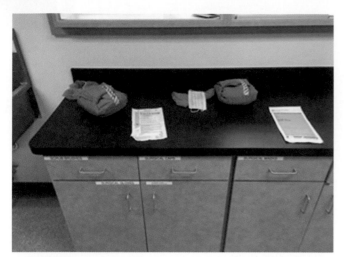

Fig. 1.1 Gowning table. Note the absence of clutter on the table and the sufficient space to allow two people to gown and glove simultaneously (the sink is to the left).

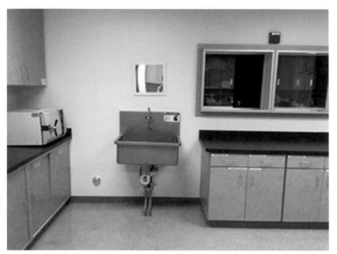

Fig. 1.2 Dual-purpose area with scrub sink, autoclave, and gowning area.

Scrub Area

The scrub area may be a small area with the scrub sink, autoclave, and room to put on gown and gloves (Fig. 1.1). This is a transitional area where the veterinarian and technician can prepare to move into the surgery room. Adding the autoclave to the space makes it a dual-purpose area that works well for personnel, because the counter area is not in use for pack preparation while the surgeon and assistant are gowning and gloving for surgery (Fig. 1.2).

Surgery Room

The surgery room is a separate room that should be used only for surgery. The surgery room should be easy to clean and be closed off from the rest of the hospital. Closing the door minimizes traffic, maximizes cleanliness, and helps ensure that the surgery room is used only for **aseptic** (free from contamination) procedures. The surgery room should be a dedicated room reserved for aseptic surgical procedures; it should not be used for other types of procedures that may introduce bacteria into the room. The surgery room should be large enough that personnel can easily

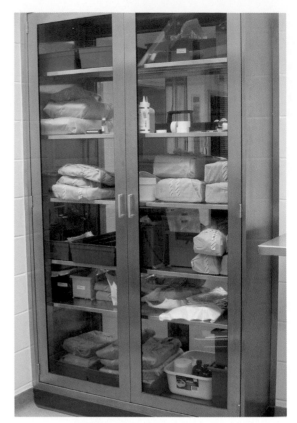

Fig. 1.3 Storage cabinet.

move around the surgery table without contaminating the surgical field or the surgeon. Cabinets should be constructed of nonporous material. The cabinets that hold sterile supplies should have doors that can be closed to protect the packs and other supplies from dust, debris, and other contaminants (Fig. 1.3).

The surgery room should also be free of clutter and items that may collect dust or harbor bacteria. Only required surgical equipment should be kept in the surgery suite; extra intravenous (IV) poles and anesthetic machines should not be stored in this area. It should have a door that can be closed, and this door should be opened only when necessary to limit the amount of traffic and air flow in and out of the room.

If possible, the air pressure should be greater in the surgery room to reduce the influx of bacteria from the rest of the veterinary facility. The increased air pressure, **positive pressure ventilation,** pushes air out of the surgical suite, reducing the influx of bacteria from the rest of the facility.

EQUIPMENT CLEANING

Different types of equipment are located in a surgery room. Some equipment is nonmovable (i.e., permanently affixed), and some is movable. Cleaning of these pieces of equipment varies according to their use and design.

Nonmovable (Permanent) Equipment

Permanent items are pieces of equipment that are attached to the floor, wall, or ceiling in the surgery room. These pieces are usually not moved from the room because of their weight or the physical difficulty of moving them. These items should be wiped down daily before surgery with a cloth dampened with disinfectant to remove any dust that may have accumulated. The surgery room should never be dry dusted because this may aerosolize the dust and bacteria. Nonmovable pieces of equipment include the following:

- Surgery lights (Fig. 1.4)
- Surgery table (Fig. 1.5)
- Radiographic view box

Movable Equipment

Movable pieces of equipment can be transported to other areas of the hospital. Although movable items should not leave the surgery room, they are required to serve a dual purpose in many veterinary facilities and are moved to other areas of the hospital. If these items must be moved, they must be cleaned and disinfected thoroughly before being returned to the surgery room. Movable equipment items include the following:

- Anesthesia machine (Fig. 1.6)
- Monitoring equipment:
  - Electrocardiogram (ECG) machine (Fig. 1.7)
  - Blood pressure (BP) cuffs and monitors
  - Airway tubes and monitors
- Heating pads
- IV drip stand (or IV pole)
- Instrument table, Mayo stand (Fig. 1.8)

- Suction unit
- Cautery unit
- Kick bucket (Fig. 1.9)

General Cleaning Instructions

All equipment should be wiped daily before surgery with the appropriate cleaning or disinfecting solution. It is important to follow the manufacturer's instructions because improper cleaning or use of inappropriate solutions may damage the equipment. The

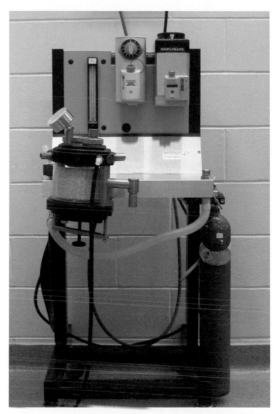

Fig. 1.6 Anesthesia machine.

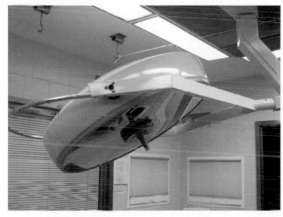

Fig. 1.4 Surgery light. Note that the shiny surface of the lamp is dust free.

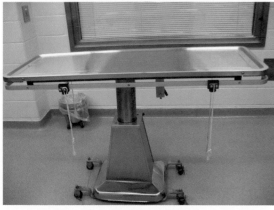

Fig. 1.5 Surgery table.

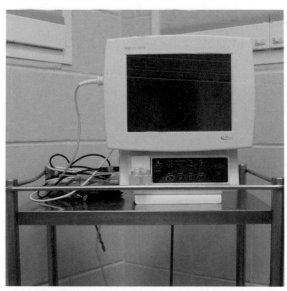

Fig. 1.7 Electrocardiography (ECG) monitor.

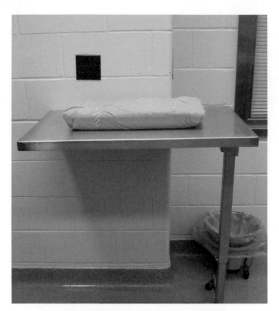

Fig. 1.8 Mayo stand or instrument table.

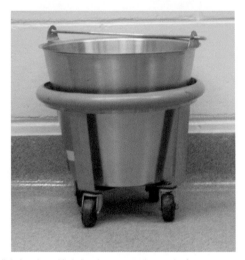

Fig. 1.9 Kick bucket. Kick buckets are cleaned after every surgery and prepared with a new plastic liner before every surgery.

Centers for Disease Control and Prevention (CDC) states that the manufacturers of medical equipment should provide care and maintenance instructions that are specific to the equipment. This information should include the equipment's compatibility with chemical germicides, whether it can be immersed for cleaning, and how it should be decontaminated (see Appendix B).

PERIOPERATIVE EQUIPMENT

Many pieces of equipment besides surgical instruments are critical to the success of a surgical procedure. Whether related to providing patient comfort, assisting the surgeon, or monitoring anesthesia, each item is an integral part of the process.

Patient Warming Devices

Circulating warm-water blankets are commonly used with surgical patients and critically ill patients. The circulating warm-water

blanket is a good way to provide a heated surface on which the patient can lie during surgery (Fig. 1.10). The heated surface helps prevent the loss of body heat to a cold metal surface, thereby diminishing the hypothermia that so often occurs during surgery. Water blankets are available in a variety of sizes, and some are considered disposable. Unless damaged by a patient, water blankets can be used repeatedly. A cat's claw, a misplaced towel clamp, or even a set of teeth can easily puncture holes in the water blanket, making it unusable. Single puncture holes or small tears can be repaired with use of a vinyl patch kit in some cases, but more often the best solution is disposing of the blanket. To prevent thermal burns, a patient should never be placed directly on the heated blanket; a towel or large drape should be placed between the heated surface and the patient's body.

One alternative to constantly replacing the water blanket is using a hard heated pad (Fig. 1.11). This pad, made of acrylic plastic glass (Plexiglas), operates on the same principle as the disposable pad and connects to many currently available circulating water pumps. The hard heated pad also is available in a variety of sizes. The main advantage to this style of heating system is the pad itself, because the acrylic plastic glass is puncture

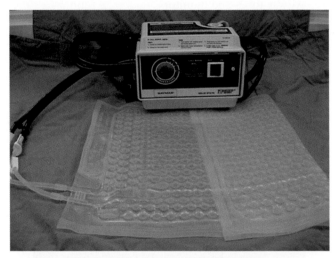

Fig. 1.10 Circulating warm-water blanket.

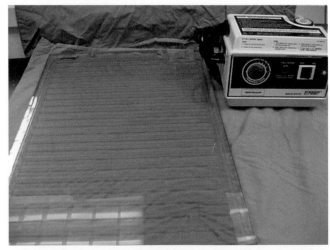

Fig. 1.11 Hard pad for circulating warm water.

proof. As with the heated water blanket, a barrier should be placed between the patient and the heated surface to prevent burns.

A device available for thermoregulation is a Hot Dog Warming Controller and Blanket (Augustine Temperature Management, Eden Prairie, MN; Fig. 1.12). This system uses electricity to warm the pad but does not pose the same threat for thermal burns as a traditional heating pad pose. The Hot Dog Blanket has a sensor in the pad to regulate the heat generated. The pads are not puncture proof but are not harmed if punctured by a cat claw or other penetrating object. Pads are available in a variety of sizes, and cleanup is easily accomplished by spraying the pads with any commonly used disinfectant.

Another option for thermoregulation of the surgical patient is the use of forced warm air (Fig. 1.13). One example is the Bair Hugger (Arizant Inc., Eden Prairie, MN). The pad is placed around the patient, then inflated with warm air. A variety of pads are available to best suit the size of the patient. The constant flow of warm air that envelops the patient is very effective at maintaining or increasing its body temperature. Although expensive, this pad is a viable alternative or addition to a circulating warm-water blanket. The pad is not puncture proof, but there is less risk of puncture because the pad is not placed near the animal until the patient is anesthetized. The Bair Hugger is most often used postoperatively to prevent the forced air from causing contamination during surgery.

Surgical Lights

The lights used in the surgery room can make a huge difference for the surgeon. Adequate lighting is imperative. Many brands and styles of lights are available. Single-beam lights that have a mechanism for a wide lateral as well as a vertical range of motion are desirable. Ceiling- or wall-mounted lights are a much better choice than the standing floor models. If installed in the

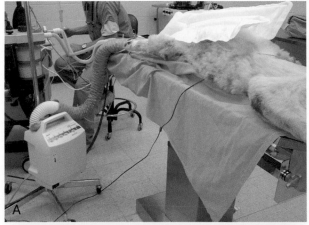
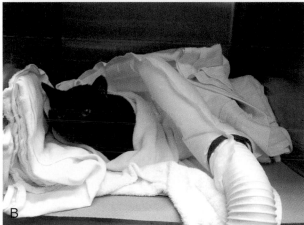

Fig. 1.13 A, Forced hot-air unit being used on a surgery patient. B, Forced hot-air unit being used on a recovering patient.

ceiling, the lights are out of the way and easily manipulated. Removable light handles that can be autoclaved are a helpful feature because once wrapped and sterilized, the handles can be aseptically opened and placed on the sterile field (Fig. 1.14). The surgeon or surgical technician can then place the handles on the lights, allowing either person to adjust the lights directly (Fig. 1.15).

Surgery Table

It is also important to have a quality surgery table. Many different types are available depending on the size of the surgery room and financial constraints. A tabletop can be a solid surface or can be designed in a split-surface style. The solid-top model is generally less expensive but can be more difficult to work with because fluids pool on the tabletop and collect on the patient (Fig. 1.16). The split-top table has the double advantage of (1) a tray under the space in the table to collect any fluid that may run off the surgical field and (2) the ability to be adjusted to help maintain the patient (especially large, deep-chested dogs) in dorsal recumbency (Fig. 1.17).

Another available feature in surgery tables is the incorporation of a heated tabletop. This heated surface aids in thermoregulation and eliminates the need for a circulating-water blanket under the patient. Surgery tables should also have the capability to be raised and lowered and to tilt in one direction.

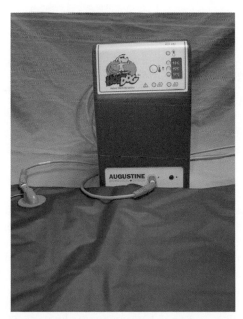

Fig. 1.12 Hot Dog Warming Controller and Blanket (Augustine Temperature Management, Eden Prairie, MN).

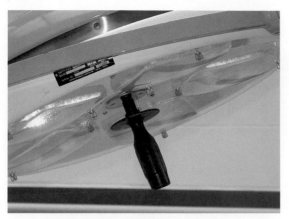

Fig. 1.14 Removable, sterilizable surgery light handles.

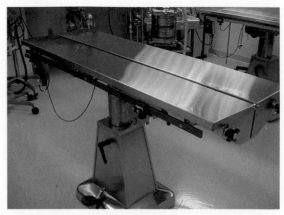

Fig. 1.17 Split-top, heated surgery table.

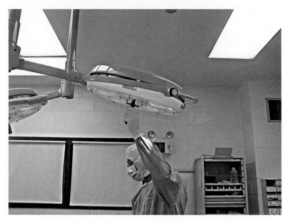

Fig. 1.15 The surgeon is able to manipulate and position the lights as needed if the handles have been sterilized.

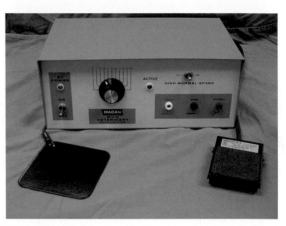

Fig. 1.18 Basic cautery unit with ground plate (*left*) and foot pedal (*right*).

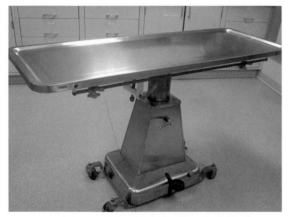

Fig. 1.16 Solid-top, adjustable surgery table.

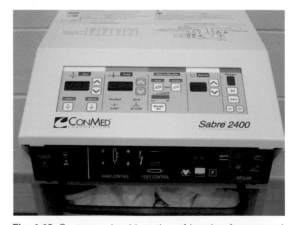

Fig. 1.19 Cautery unit with option of hand or foot control.

Hydraulics or electric power can be employed to accomplish variation in height, whereas manual effort is generally required to tilt the table.

Electrosurgery

The use of electricity, transmitted through a special hand piece to cut or coagulate vessels, is very advantageous in surgery. Hemostasis is vital during surgery, and cautery is an important tool available to accomplish it. Both single-use and reusable

cautery hand pieces are available. A member of the sterile team activates a hand piece by pushing switches or buttons on the hand piece or by stepping on a foot pedal (Figs. 1.18 and 1.19).

Electrosurgery can be either monopolar or bipolar. When monopolar electrosurgery is used, a ground plate must be placed under the patient. When the hand piece is activated, the electric current passes through the patient to the ground plate and then is diverted away from the patient. The ground plate must have sufficient contact with the patient to transmit the current properly to the ground plate. A water- or saline-saturated sponge should be placed on the ground plate between the patient and the plate. Alcohol is never used to saturate the sponge because it may lead to patient burns or even fire. Bipolar electrosurgery utilizes a hand piece that resembles a thumb tissue forceps. As the hand piece is activated, the current passes from one tip to another, and therefore no ground plate is needed.

Monopolar electrosurgery can be used in one of two ways. First, the hand piece can be activated, and the tip of the hand piece can directly touch the tissue or vessel that needs cauterizing (Fig. 1.20). Second, a hemostat can be placed on the tissue or vessel that needs to be cauterized. The hemostat is then elevated off the surgical field so that the only metal touching the patient is the tip of the hemostat. The cautery hand piece tip can then be touched to the hemostat as the hand piece is activated. The metal of the instrument conducts the electric current, therefore cauterizing the tissue held in the clamp (Fig. 1.21). Monopolar hand pieces can also be used with the appropriate tip to make the surgical incision. Although wonderful at keeping bleeding to a minimum, an incision created with an electrosurgery unit takes longer to heal because of the charring of the tissue. Bipolar electrosurgery hand pieces, by design, look like a thumb tissue forceps. They can pick up either tissue or a vessel that needs to be coagulated.

Charred material may build up on the tip of the hand piece, impeding the flow of current. It may be cleaned by scraping with a scalpel blade (away from the sterile field) or by using a commercially available scratch pad.

Suction

Suction can be defined as the ability to remove fluid or air from an area by using either a manual or a mechanical device. Suction can be performed with a syringe, a bulb syringe, or a mechanical pump. For application in surgery, the mechanical pump is commonly used. Suction is an extremely important tool in surgery and if unavailable can make the procedure increasingly more difficult and frustrating for the surgeon. Whether an abdominal, orthopedic, or neurologic procedure is performed, having suction available is essential. For abdominal procedures, suction can be used to remove abdominal fluid in the event of a hemoabdomen or uroabdomen. Abdominal lavage is a common practice after an exploratory procedure, and mechanical suction assists in the removal of the lavage fluid better than any other option. Lavaging a joint, flushing a septic site, and removing bone dust created while drilling screw holes for a fracture repair are examples of how suction is useful in orthopedic surgery.

There are also risks associated with suction, and veterinary personnel must understand these risks to prevent unnecessary trauma to the patient. The vacuum pressure of the suction is easy enough to control with a manual device, but care must be taken to use appropriate levels of vacuum with mechanical devices. In abdominal procedures, if the vacuum level is too high, omentum may become entrapped in the suction tip and may be damaged. A sufficiently strong vacuum that meets the needs of the surgical procedure without being excessive is the goal. Inappropriately low vacuum settings will not adequately suction the fluid and debris on the field and will prove to be frustrating.

Suction Machines

Many different models of suction machine are available. Some models run on electric power; a motor is used to generate the vacuum (Fig. 1.22). Other models require a central vacuum

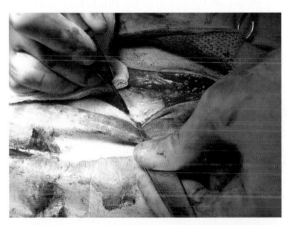

Fig. 1.20 Electrocautery applied directly to the tissue to be cauterized.

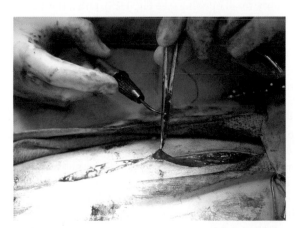

Fig. 1.21 Electrocautery applied indirectly to the tissue to be cauterized through an instrument grasping the tissue.

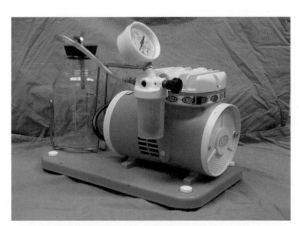

Fig. 1.22 Electric, motorized suction machine.

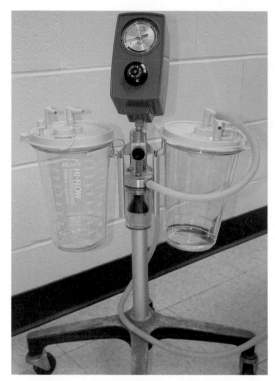

Fig. 1.23 Central vacuum, double-collection suction unit.

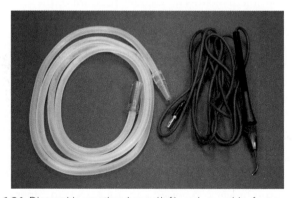

Fig. 1.24 Disposable suction hose (*left*) and reusable foot-operated cautery pencil (*right*).

system to operate (Fig. 1.23). Any type of machine requires some sort of bottle or receptacle for the collected fluid. Older models may still have glass jars, which can be dangerous and easily broken. Plastic bottles or canisters are more desirable. Usually the cover of the bottle has some type of float or safety device that will not allow fluid into the working mechanism of the suction machine if the bottle becomes too full.

In addition to the suction machine, a suction tip and tubing are needed. Suction tubing is available in 6- and 10-foot lengths (Fig. 1.24). The tubing is usually prepackaged and

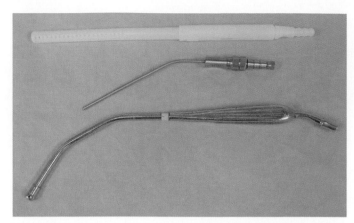

Fig. 1.25 Suction tips. Top to bottom: Poole, Frazier, Yankauer. (From Bassert: McCurnin's Clinical Textbook for Veterinary Technicians, 9th Ed, St. Louis, 2018, Elsevier.)

sterilized for single-time use. After the package is opened onto the sterile field, one end of the tubing is attached to the suction tip (usually sterilized separately), and the other end is dropped off the field to be connected to the nonsterile suction unit. Because of the length of the tubing and the difficulty in cleaning it appropriately, this is one piece of equipment that is truly disposable and should be discarded after surgery. If for some reason the tubing is not used after being opened, it can be resterilized. Ethylene oxide sterilization must be used because this vinyl tubing will not withstand steam sterilization.

Suction Tips

Different designs of suction tips are more appropriate for some procedures than others.

Poole. A Poole suction tip is a two-piece instrument best used to remove large volumes of liquid or fluid (Fig. 1.25). The inner cannula can be used alone or in conjunction with the outer basket. The basket is designed with many holes to remove the liquid quickly without entrapping any tissue.

Frazier/Adson. The Frazier/Adson suction tip is a single tube with a fairly small opening (see Fig. 1.25). Often there is a thumb hole to help control the amount of vacuum. This instrument is often used in orthopedic and neurologic procedures.

Yankauer. The Yankauer suction tip is also a single-tube design, but it is bulkier than the Frazier (see Fig. 1.25). The Yankauer is a general-purpose suction tip.

Plastic Tubing Connector

Some surgeons have concerns that the abrasive metal tip of the Frazier suction tip may be traumatizing to the bone or cartilage during orthopedic procedures. A good alternative is an Argyle Bubble connector (Fig. 1.26). This plastic tubing connector fits securely into the suction hose and is small enough to be efficient and lightweight enough to be easy to use.

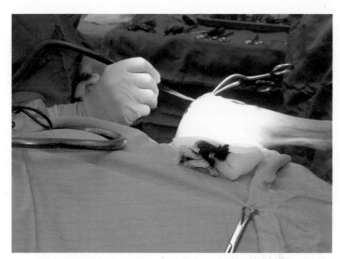

Fig. 1.26 Plastic suction tip for orthopedic procedures.

SETTING UP THE SURGERY SUITE

After the surgery room has been appropriately cleaned for the start of the day, setup of the room may begin. It is most efficient to have a "case card" for each procedure performed by each surgeon. Each case card has listed on it all the supplies and equipment the surgeon will need for the procedure. It is important to minimize the traffic flow in and out of the surgery room, and having most if not all of the supplies in the room will accomplish this goal. Reducing the number of times the veterinary technician has to leave the room to retrieve something is also better time management. It is usually better to be overprepared with supplies in the room than to constantly run out. In operating rooms at human hospitals, everything that enters the room, regardless of whether it is used or not, gets thrown away at the end of the procedure. This is not the case in veterinary surgery rooms. Unused items can be replaced on the storage shelf for use another day.

Types of Packs

A general soft tissue instrument pack will suffice for most surgical procedures, with the exception of ophthalmic surgery. Specialty instruments can be packaged separately or assembled together in a pack, whichever is better for the clinic. Retractors, periosteal elevators, rongeurs, and so on can be packaged individually and opened on an as-needed basis. This arrangement gives flexibility to the surgical schedule, in that if only one instrument is needed, a whole pack does not need to be opened, thus avoiding the down time waiting for the pack to be reprocessed. Larger groups of instruments, such as multiple cardiovascular clamps or bone plating equipment, can be sterilized as a pack. It gives the surgeon the option of having many different instruments available to meet the needs of the

case. Anything not stored in the room needs to be placed in the room before the beginning of surgery. It is important to remember those items not typically thought of as surgical supplies, for instance, urinary catheters, orogastric tubes, and medications. Forethought must be used, depending on the surgical procedure, to ensure that all necessary supplies are available.

Scheduling Surgical Procedures

When reviewing the surgical procedures planned for the day, it is important to remember to schedule them appropriately. A good rule to follow is to schedule cases from cleanest to dirtiest. This means scheduling the surgery that requires the cleanest environment, such as an orthopedic procedure, first. It is also good to take into consideration the difficulty and anticipated length of each procedure. Surgeons and staff will be fresher and more alert in the morning than at 3:00 p.m. More difficult cases should therefore be scheduled earlier in the day. In orthopedic cases, any joint replacement procedure should be scheduled first thing in the morning. In fact, the room should be set up the night before and no traffic allowed into the room until the patient is wheeled in. Subsequent procedures for the day may be scheduled as follows: a metatarsal fracture, a cranial cruciate ligament (CCL) repair, and, finally, a compound radial fracture repair. For soft tissue procedures, any noninfective intrathoracic procedures should go first, followed by clean abdominal, contaminated, and, finally, dirty procedures.

In addition to difficulty, length, and contamination, there are other things to consider when developing the daily schedule. Patient status is paramount in determining the schedule. Some patients may require an earlier time on the schedule even though it conflicts with some of the other parameters. Animals in critical condition that require surgery to survive obviously take precedence. Another consideration should be equipment needs and turnover. Scheduling three procedures back to back that will need the same equipment may not be the best idea. The potential for down time with the patient on the table while the equipment is cleaned and prepared must be considered. All things being equal, procedures that need the same equipment should be spread out throughout the day to allow for reprocessing.

CONCLUSION

Time the veterinary technician spends readying the surgical suite and the necessary equipment before bringing the patient into the surgery room is important. Being ill-prepared will compromise the patient, try the surgeon's patience, and overall prove to be a very inefficient use of time. Taking those few extra moments at the beginning of the day and of each case will ensure a smooth surgical event.

KEY POINTS

1. The surgery suite ideally should consist of a preparation area, a scrub area, and a surgery area.
2. The preparation area should be next to the surgery room and used for patient preparation and the storage of supplies.
3. Surgical procedures classified as dirty should be done in the preparation area, not in the surgery room.
4. The scrub area can also be used as the sterilization area and the place for gowning and gloving.
5. Ideally, the surgery room should be a separate room.
6. There should be minimal, hard-surfaced cabinets in the surgery room, and, if possible, the cabinets should have doors that can be closed to protect items from contaminants.
7. Permanent (nonmovable) equipment consists of surgery lights, surgery table, and radiographic view box.
8. Movable equipment consists of anesthesia machine, monitoring equipment (ECG, BP, airway), heating pads, IV drip stand, instrument table or Mayo stands, suction unit, cautery unit, and kick bucket.
9. All equipment should be damp-wiped daily before surgery.
10. The manufacturer's instructions for cleaning of equipment should always be followed.
11. External warming devices should be employed to help maintain patient body temperature during anesthesia.
12. Cautery can be activated by hand or foot control devices and can be monopolar or bipolar in function.
13. Suction tip styles vary widely and have recommended uses.

REVIEW QUESTIONS

1. AAHA recommends which distinct areas for a surgical facility?
   a. Scrub area, surgical room, recovery room
   b. Preparation area, scrub area, surgical room
   c. Preparation area, scrub area, recovery room
   d. Preparation area, surgical room, recovery room
2. Where are procedures that are considered clean performed?
   a. Scrub area
   b. Exam room
   c. Surgery room
   d. Preparation area
3. Which item is nonmovable surgery equipment?
   a. Surgery table
   b. Instrument table
   c. Anesthesia machine
   d. Blood pressure monitoring
4. It is recommend to place a blanket or towel between a patient and a circulating warm-water blanket to
   a. help maintain asepsis.
   b. prevent damage to the blanket.
   c. add to the warming of the patient.
   d. protect the patient from thermal burns.
5. When warming a surgical patient, which item is contraindicated?
   a. Hard heated pad
   b. Electric heating pad
   c. Forced warm air blanket
   d. Warming controller and blanket
6. When using bipolar electrocautery the surgeon is able to
   a. make a skin incision.
   b. use the tip to touch and directly cauterize a blood vessel.
   c. pick up tissue or blood vessels that need to be coagulated.
   d. touch the tip to a hemostat that will direct the current to tissue for coagulation.
7. Using a mechanical device to remove fluid or air from an area is called
   a. lavage.
   b. suction.
   c. asepsis.
   d. assisted ventilation.
8. Which suction tip has two pieces and is designed to suction a large amount of fluid?
   a. Poole
   b. Yankauer
   c. Frazier/Adson
   d. Argyle Bubble
9. An advantage of using a monopolar electrosurgical unit to make an incision is
   a. better hemostasis.
   b. faster healing time.
   c. no need for ground plate.
   d. less tissue trauma than a surgical blade.
10. In what instance would a clean abdominal surgery precede a noninfective thoracic surgery on the surgery schedule?
11. What are two advantages of having a split-top surgery table?
12. Which type of electrocautery unit does not require a ground plate?
13. List three qualities of a good surgical light.
14. How can suction be used during an orthopedic surgery?
15. What other equipment is needed when a suction machine is used?

BIBLIOGRAPHY

Allen G: Implementing AORN recommended practices for environmental cleaning. *AORN J*, *99*(5): 570–579; quiz 580–582, 2014.

Association of periOperative Registered Nurses: Recommended practices for environmental cleaning in the surgical practice setting, *AORN J*, 76(6): 1071–1076, 2002.

Association of periOperative Registered Nurses (AORN): *Standards, recommended practices, and guidelines: recommended practices for maintaining a sterile field*, Denver, 2004, AORN.

Bassert JM, McCurnin DM, editors: *McCurnin's clinical textbook for veterinary technicians*, ed 8, St Louis, 2014, Saunders.

Centers for Disease Control and Prevention (CDC): *Healthcare Infection Control Practices Advisory Committee (HICPAC: draft guide-*

lines for environmental infection control in healthcare facilities, Washington, DC, 2001, CDC.

Centers for Disease Control and Prevention (CDC): *Healthcare Infection Control Practices Advisory Committee (HICPAC): guideline for disinfection and sterilization in healthcare facilities,* Washington, DC, 2018, CDC.

Fossum, T. W., et al. (2018). *Small animal surgery* (5th ed.). Mosby.

Healthcare Infection Control Practices Advisory Committee: *Meeting summary report, July 2014.* Washington, DC, 2014, U.S. Department of Health and Human Services, Centers for Disease Control and Prevention.

Kennedy J, Bek J, Griffin D: *G1410: selection and use of disinfectants.* Lincoln, 2000, University of Nebraska. https://digitalcommons.unl.edu/cgi/viewcontent.cgi?article=1102&context=extensionhist

Instruments

Paige Allen

LEARNING OBJECTIVES

After completion of this chapter, the reader will be able to:
- Describe the steps used to manufacture surgical instruments.
- List the common surgical instruments used in general, orthopedic, and ophthalmic surgery in veterinary medicine.
- Describe the different styles of suture needles.
- Describe the characteristics of suture material.
- List examples of suture material and their main properties.

KEY TERMS

Absorbable (suture)
Atraumatic
Box lock
Capillarity

Flexibility
Memory (suture)
Serrated
Shank

Swaged
Traumatic

SURGICAL INSTRUMENTS

Surgical instruments are a major investment for the veterinary hospital. It is important that instruments be used for their designed purpose. Improper use can damage or destroy instruments.

Manufacturing

Instruments are generally made of stainless steel, although some disposable models may be made of plastic. The stainless steel used is composed of iron, chromium, and carbon. Martensitic stainless steel has higher carbon content and is generally used for cutting instruments because the potential for hardness during the tempering stage is greater. Austenitic stainless steel has higher chromium content and lower carbon content. This

metal is used for hemostats and needle holders. Austenitic steel is not as hard as martensitic steel, and, as a result, tungsten carbide inserts are often added to the austenitic needle holders to increase their durability.

Components

Veterinary surgery personnel must know the basic parts of surgical instruments to use, clean, and inspect them appropriately (Fig. 2.1).

The first part of the instrument to identify is the jaw or tip. This area can be **traumatic** or **atraumatic** in design, depending on the intended use, and can be straight or curved. The jaw or tip can have serrations, teeth, or flat surfaces. Serrations can be horizontal, vertical, or a combination (e.g., Rochester Carmalt

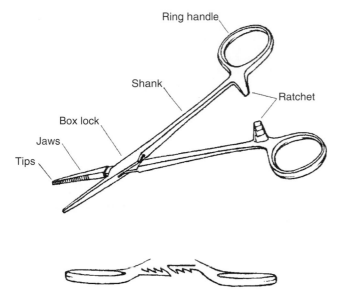

Fig. 2.1 *Top:* Labeled parts of a typical surgical instrument. *Bottom:* End-on view of the ratchet mechanism. The ratchets should be slightly separated when the jaws are closed. (From Auer J, Stick J: *Equine surgery,* ed 4, St Louis, 2011, Saunders.)

hemostatic forceps). The arrangement of the teeth can be 1 × 2, 2 × 3, and so on. Tips with a 1 × 2 configuration have one tooth on one side of the tip and two teeth on the opposite side. The teeth can also be arranged in rows (e.g., Adson Brown thumb tissue forceps). The tips or jaws can easily become damaged. Teeth and serrations of the tips or jaws should be thoroughly evaluated after each use to observe any defects that may have resulted from use. Blades are available on most types of scissors as curved or straight. Some types of scissors also have the option of blades with sharp or blunt tips. In a description or identification of instruments, the blades or tips can provide important information. For example, identifying an instrument as "curved Metzenbaum scissors" defines the shape and type of scissors. Identifying operating scissors as "curved, sharp/blunt (s/b) operating scissors" reveals even more about the instrument.

The second important part of the instrument, the box lock, is present only on instruments with ring handles. The **box lock** is the joint or hinge of the instrument. This area absorbs great stress when the instrument is in use, and therefore the box lock must be inspected carefully to detect any cracks or evidence of degradation.

The third part of the instrument to identify is the **shank** (also referred to as the "shaft"), or body, of the instrument. This part is usually the longest area and determines the instrument's overall length. Instruments may range from 3 to 12 inches in total length depending on the length of the shank.

The ratchet is the next part of the instrument, but it is found only on instruments with ring handles. The ratchet is a device with interlocking teeth that will lock an instrument jaw in a closed position. Degradation of this part of the instrument is usually seen as the inability of the ratchet to remain locked.

Some instruments also have ring handles, which serve as the means for using and controlling the instrument. Proper handling of an instrument with ring handles is achieved by placing the thumb and ring finger in the rings. Neither ring should advance beyond the first knuckle of the finger or thumb. The index finger can rest on the shank to help stabilize the instrument (Fig. 2.2).

General surgical instruments are available in a variety of sizes. Depending on the area of the body on which the surgery will be performed, shorter or longer instruments may make the task easier for the surgeon. For instance, needle holders may be found in sizes ranging from 4 to 12 inches. Thumb tissue forceps are also available in up to 12-inch lengths. Indications for use of the longer instruments include thoracic surgery on a deep-chested dog and an abdominal exploratory procedure on a large dog.

General Surgery Instruments

This section is intended to give an overview of common surgical instruments. It is not intended as a stand-alone, comprehensive list.

Scissors

Many types of scissors are available to the veterinary surgeon (Fig. 2.3). As with all instruments, it is important that scissors be used only for their intended function.

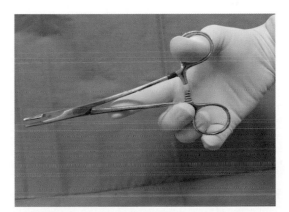

Fig. 2.2 Thumb-ring finger grip for ring-handled instruments.

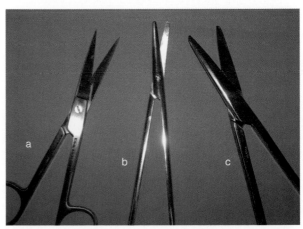

Fig. 2.3 Surgical scissors. (A) Sharp/sharp straight operating scissors. (B) Curved Metzenbaum scissors. (C) Straight Mayo scissors.

Operating scissors. The intended use of operating scissors is to cut only inanimate objects (e.g., suture, paper drapes, and sponges). Their design can be straight or curved, and the blades can be sharp tipped or blunt tipped (Fig. 2.4).

Mayo scissors. The Mayo scissors are used when cutting large muscle masses, cartilage, or any other nondelicate tissue. The blades are thick and approximately one-third the instrument's length. The blades can be straight or curved.

Metzenbaum scissors. The Metzenbaum scissors are used for delicate surgical dissection. The blades are thin, delicate, and approximately one-fourth the instrument's overall length. The shaft is long and thin, and the blades can be straight or curved.

Suture removal scissors. Sometimes called suture scissors, the suture removal scissors usually are not found in the surgery pack but rather are stored in the treatment area or examination room. The suture scissors have one blade in the shape of a hook that cradles the suture to be cut (Fig. 2.5). This instrument is designed to remove external sutures from the skin.

Hemostats

Although there are many types of hemostats, only six styles are typically used in veterinary surgery (Figs. 2.6 and 2.7). As their name implies, hemostats are used to aid in controlling hemostasis in the surgical field. Hemostats can have jaws that are

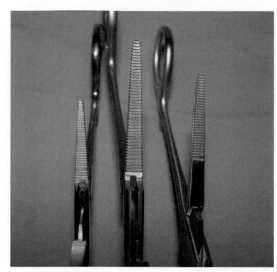

Fig. 2.6 Hemostatic forceps tips. *Left to right:* Halstead mosquito, Crile, Kelly.

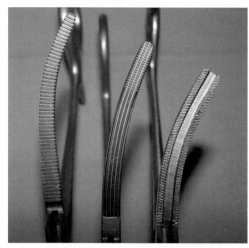

Fig. 2.7 Hemostatic forceps tips. *Left to right:* Rochester-Pean, Rochester-Carmalt, Ferguson Angiotribe.

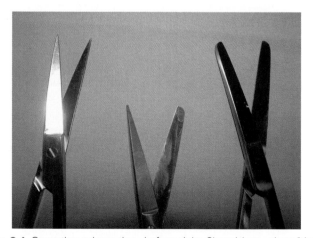

Fig. 2.4 Operating scissor tips. *Left to right:* Sharp/sharp, sharp/blunt, blunt/blunt.

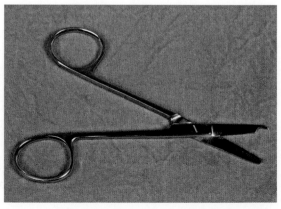

Fig. 2.5 Suture removal scissors.

straight or curved and serrations that are horizontal, vertical, or a combination. Serrations also may be partial or may extend the full length of the jaw.

Halstead mosquito hemostatic forceps. The Halstead hemostat has small jaws with fine horizontal serrations that extend the entire length of the tip. The instrument is generally used to clamp small vessels (e.g., "skin bleeders").

Kelly hemostatic forceps. The Kelly hemostat is larger than the Halstead hemostat. The horizontal serrations are wider and only extend half the length of the jaw. The Kelly hemostat can be used for medium-sized vessels or small tissue masses.

Crile hemostatic forceps. The Crile hemostat is similar to the Kelly hemostat, with the difference being how far the serrations extend along the jaws. The Crile hemostatic forceps has serrations that extend the entire length of the jaw.

Ferguson angiotribe. Although not a true hemostat, the Ferguson angiotribe is an extremely strong forceps that is quite traumatic, with a crushing jaw design that has one raised jaw and one recessed jaw. This clamp can be used on vessels of almost any size and on any tissue that will not need to be viable in the body (e.g., uterine stump).

Rochester-Carmalt hemostatic forceps. The Rochester-Carmalt hemostat is quite different from other hemostats. The instrument has both horizontal and vertical serrations on the jaw near the tip. The result is a checkerboard appearance at the tip of the jaw. This hemostatic forceps is usually about 8 inches long, making it a large instrument, and the jaw is approximately 3½ inches of the total length. It can be used to clamp large vessels or large tissue masses.

Rochester-Pean hemostatic forceps. The Rochester-Pean hemostatic forceps is a large hemostat (usually 8 inches in length) with horizontal serrations the entire length of the jaw. The jaw length is similar to that of the Rochester-Carmalt hemostatic forceps (≈3½ inches). The length is the factor distinguishing it from the Crile hemostatic forceps. This forceps can also be used to clamp large muscle/tissue masses or large vessels.

Needle Holders

Needle holders have very short jaws that have a roughened platform in the tips to allow for a secure grip of the suture needle (Fig. 2.8). As previously mentioned, tungsten inserts may be used in the jaws of needle holders to increase instrument longevity. Needle holders are the only surgical instruments designed with the specific intent of holding metal. Therefore, the needle holder is the only instrument that should be used to hold needles or to place scalpel blades onto scalpel handles.

Derf. The Derf needle holder is small in length and is used with small patients, with special species, and in extraocular ophthalmic procedures (considered too large for intraocular surgery).

Olsen-Hegar. The Olsen-Hegar instrument is different from other needle holders in that it has scissors built into the jaws (Fig. 2.9). This added feature is a time-saving device that allows the suture to be cut without having to reach for another instrument. The main disadvantage to having the scissors as part of this needle holder is that an inexperienced user may inadvertently cut suture material when trying to grasp the needle.

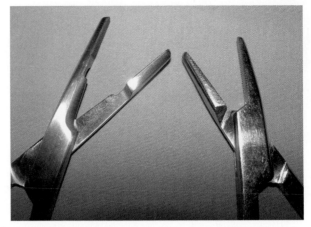

Fig. 2.9 Needle holder tips. *Left:* Olsen-Hegar; *Right:* Mayo-Hegar.

Mayo-Hegar. The Mayo-Hegar needle holder is a commonly used instrument available in a variety of lengths, depending on the surgical procedure and the surgeon's preference (Fig. 2.9).

Scalpels

Scalpel blade handles. Scalpel blade handles are designed to hold scalpel blades for easier and safer use. Scalpel blades numbered 10 through 15 are the most common blades for the No. 3 scalpel handle (Fig. 2.10). Blades numbered 20 through 23 fit on the No. 4 handle (Fig. 2.11). Handles often have units of measurement on them to be used as needed. One such use may be as a reference marker for procedures requiring photographic documentation (e.g., mass removal, foreign body removal). Scalpel handles can be held with a pencil grip, fingertip grip, or palmed grip. The pencil grip, with the index finger on the noncutting edge of the blade, stabilizing the scalpel, allows for a finer, more precise cut due to the angle the blade presents to the skin (Fig. 2.12).

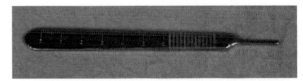

Fig. 2.10 No. 3 scalpel blade handle.

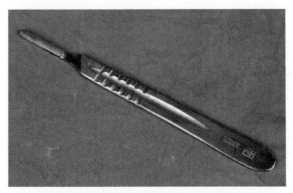

Fig. 2.11 No. 4 scalpel blade handle.

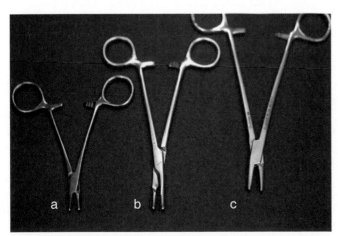

Fig. 2.8 Needle holders. (A) Derf. (B) Olsen-Hegar. (C) Mayo-Hegar. (Photo by John T. Miller.)

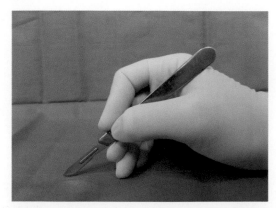

Fig. 2.12 The pencil grip used for holding a scalpel.

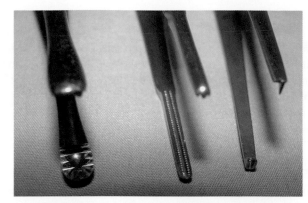

Fig. 2.14 Thumb tissue forceps. *Left to right:* Russian, DeBakey, 1 × 2.

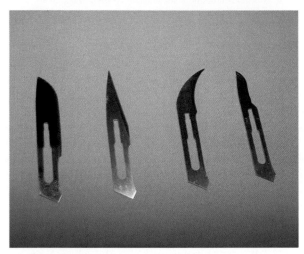

Fig. 2.13 Scalpel blades. *Left to right:* 10, 11, 12, 15.

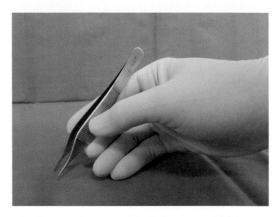

Fig. 2.15 The pencil grip used for holding thumb tissue forceps.

Scalpel blades. The most common scalpel blade used in small animal surgery is the No. 10 (Fig. 2.13). This blade is used primarily for skin incisions. A No. 11 blade is tapered to a pointed shape and is generally used to create a "stab" incision. The No. 12 blade resembles a hook, with the cutting edge on the inside curve, and is often used to declaw a cat. A No. 15 blade has the appearance of a No. 10 blade, but with only half the No. 10's length. The larger scalpel blades (Nos. 20–23) are generally reserved for use in large animal surgery.

Thumb Tissue Forceps

A thumb tissue forceps is an instrument used to grasp and retract tissue on a short-term basis (Fig. 2.14). Instruments in this category resemble a tweezers, but thumb tissue forceps should never be referred to as tweezers. A pencil grip is used to hold this instrument in the nondominant hand (Fig. 2.15). The best control of pressure is achieved when the forceps is held as if it were a pencil. The shaft of a thumb tissue forceps is generally straight, but some designs have unique shapes to the shaft that help distinguish them from others (e.g., Adson, Bayonet). The tips can be toothed, smooth (atraumatic), or fairly traumatic in design.

DeBakey thoracic thumb tissue forceps. Originally designed as a cardiovascular instrument, the DeBakey thoracic thumb tissue forceps is an excellent example of an atraumatic

forceps that should be used only on delicate tissue. The tips have no teeth but rather a ridge or groove design. These forceps are often used in thoracic, vascular, or neurologic procedures.

Tissue thumb forceps. The tissue thumb forceps has a straight shaft and can range in length from 5 to 12 inches. The tips can have 1 × 2 or 3 × 4 teeth.

Russian thumb tissue forceps. The Russian thumb tissue forceps has a very traumatic, bulky tip. This instrument is generally reserved for use on skin or tissue that is being removed from the patient.

Adson thumb tissue forceps. The Adson thumb tissue forceps has a very narrow tip that broadens to a ½-inch-wide shaft. The tips can be of various designs and are described as follows:

Adson dressing. The Adson dressing forceps tip has no teeth but does have flat, atraumatic serrations. This Adson style is generally used as an aid in placing or removing dressings on wounds.

Adson-Brown. The tip of the Adson-Brown instrument has two parallel rows of nine shallow teeth on both tips. A common general surgery tissue forceps, the Adson-Brown forceps can be found in most general instrument packs.

Adson 1 × 2. The tip of the Adson 1 × 2 Adson style has one tooth on one tip and two teeth on the other. The teeth interdigitate to grasp tissue firmly. It can be fairly traumatic if used on delicate tissue or too aggressively.

Allis tissue forceps. The Allis tissue forceps is neither a hemostat nor a thumb tissue forceps. Its intended use of grasping tissue in a fairly traumatic way makes it a unique instrument. This ring-handled instrument has tips that may have teeth configured in a 3 × 4 or 4 × 5 style (Fig. 2.16). Because of its traumatic nature, the Allis tissue forceps is generally used to grasp tough tissue (e.g., linea alba) or tissue being removed from the patient (e.g., tumor, skin).

Retractors

Retractors are instruments used to deflect or retract tissue or other structures away from the surgical field where the surgeon is working. Retractors can be handheld (Fig. 2.17), which requires a member of the surgical team to hold, or self-retaining (Fig. 2.18).

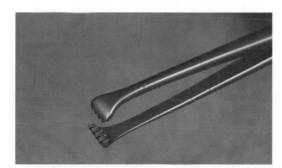

Fig. 2.16 Allis tissue forceps tips. (Photo by John T. Miller.)

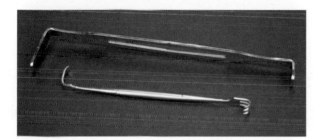

Fig. 2.17 Handheld retractors. *Top:* U.S. Army retractor. *Bottom:* Senn double-ended retractor. (Photo by John T. Miller.)

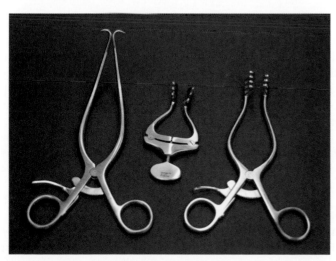

Fig. 2.18 Self-retaining retractors. *Left to right:* Gelpi, Jansen, Weitlaner. (Photo by John T. Miller.)

Handheld retractors

U. S. Army. The U.S. Army handheld retractor is a double-ended retractor with different lengths of blades on either end. It has no teeth on the blades and therefore causes little tissue trauma, other than pressure damage if applied too forcefully to the tissue (Fig. 2.19).

Senn. The Senn retractor is also a double-ended handheld retractor. One end is a narrow, blunt blade, and the other end is a toothed, traumatic end. The teeth can be sharp or blunt, which may affect where it is used.

Self-Retaining Retractors

Gelpi. With its single, sharp-pointed tips, the Gelpi self-retaining retractor is a fairly traumatic instrument. It has limited use in soft tissue surgery but is extremely useful in orthopedic and neurologic surgery.

Weitlaner. The Weitlaner self-retaining retractor has teeth in the jaw that can be blunt or sharp. Although it is used more often in orthopedic surgery, the blunt-toothed version can be used in some soft tissue surgical cases.

Balfour. The Balfour retractor is one of the few self-retaining retractors commonly used in soft tissue surgery (Fig. 2.20). Available in adult and pediatric sizes, it is extremely useful for abdominal procedures. While keeping the abdominal walls in lateral retraction, it also has a third blade for cranial retraction as well. This widespread retraction provides excellent visualization of the abdominal cavity for the surgeon.

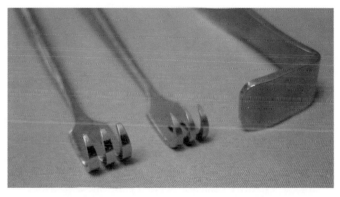

Fig. 2.19 Handheld retractor ends. *Left to right:* Blunt Senn, sharp Senn, U.S. Army.

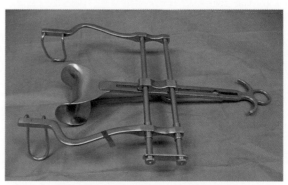

Fig. 2.20 Balfour abdominal retractor.

Towel Clamps

Towel clamps are instruments used to secure the sterile drapes to the patient during surgery or to secure the sterile drapes to one another (Fig. 2.21). Towel clamps may have a penetrating design, which means the tips are sharp and pointed and are intended to pierce the patient's skin to hold the sterile drape in place. They also may have a nonpenetrating style, which is more likely to be used to secure one drape to another.

Backhaus. The most common style of towel clamp, the Backhaus has penetrating tips and is available in 3½- or 5½-inch sizes.

Roeder. The Roeder style is unique in that it has balls on the tips. The balls prevent the towel clamp from being placed too deeply into the tissue.

Jones. A penetrating towel clamp, the Jones is more delicate and lightweight than the other styles. Instead of the usual ratchet and ring handle, the Jones towel clamp has a squeeze-handle mechanism, which makes it convenient to use on smaller patients.

Lorna (Edna). Also known as the Edna nonpenetrating towel clamp, the Lorna, like the Backhaus, is available in 3½- and 5½-inch sizes. The feature of nonpenetrating tips makes this an ideal clamp for securing second-layer drapes, whether cloth or paper, to the ground drapes.

Miscellaneous General Instruments

A few miscellaneous instruments are found in most veterinary surgical packs.

Snook spay hook. Some surgeons use the Snook spay hook to find and exteriorize the uterine horns when performing an ovariohysterectomy on dogs and cats.

Dowling spay retractor. The Dowling spay retractor was designed to assist the solo veterinary surgeon in performing an ovariohysterectomy on a canine or feline patient. By isolating the uterine horn with the retractor, the surgeon has better visualization and stabilization for ligation and excision (Fig. 2.22).

Needle rack. The needle rack is a spring mounted on a metal base designed to store "eyed" free needles during the autoclaving process (Fig. 2.23).

Groove director. The groove director is designed to aid the surgeon in making incisions on the linea alba. This instrument provides a "channel" that the scalpel can follow to avoid accidental incising of abdominal viscera (Fig. 2.24).

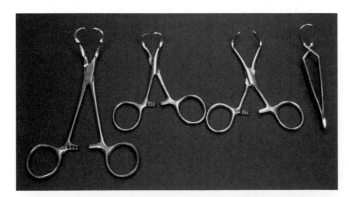

Fig. 2.21 Towel clamps. *Left to right:* Roeder, Backhaus, Lorna, Jones. (Photo by John T. Miller.)

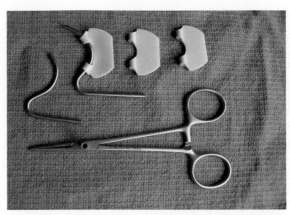

Fig. 2.22 Dowling spay retractor. (U.S. Patent #7722639B2; Brian Dowling, DVM, Elma, WA.) (Photo by Dr. Dowling.)

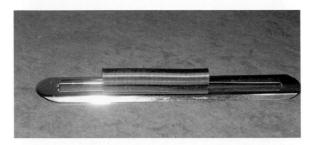

Fig. 2.23 Needle Rack. (Photo by Marianne Tear.)

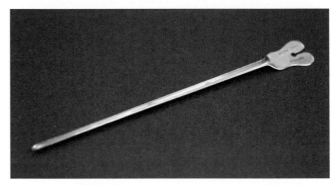

Fig. 2.24 Groove director. (Photo by John T. Miller.)

Staple remover. When skin staples are used instead of suture, a special instrument is required to remove the staples (Fig. 2.25). The staple remover has two "teeth" on one side and one tooth on the other. To use it properly, the two teeth are placed between the staple and the patient; the single tooth then presses into the top of the staple. This arrangement bends the staple, removing the edges from the skin.

Bowls. Some instrument packs include a sterile bowl. The bowls can be used for holding saline for lavage or for storing sharps during the procedure to help keep the instrument table safe and clean (Fig. 2.26).

Soft Tissue Surgery Instruments

Many instruments are available for use in soft tissue surgery. The use of specialized intestinal clamps, thoracic vascular clamps, or thoracic retractors can significantly enhance the efficiency with which the surgeon performs.

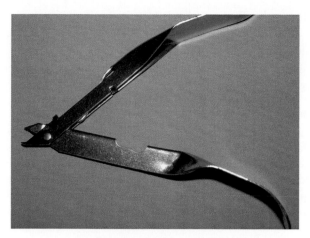

Fig. 2.25 Staple remover.

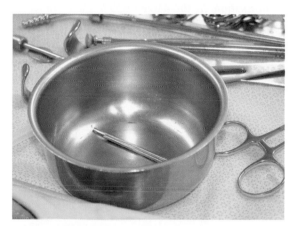

Fig. 2.26 Stainless steel bowl for sharps or saline.

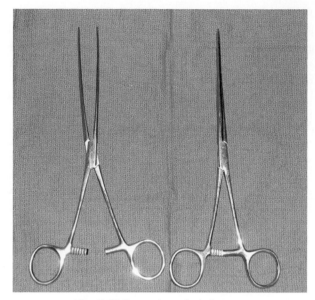

Fig. 2.27 Doyen intestinal clamps.

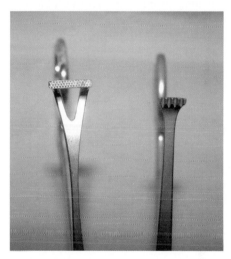

Fig. 2.28 *Left:* Babcock intestinal forceps. *Right:* Allis tissue forceps.

Intestinal Clamps

Intestinal clamps are varied in construction, and the type used in a procedure depends on the intended outcome of the tissue being clamped. Tissue that is not viable or that is being removed can be clamped with a more traumatic clamp, like a Rochester-Carmalt forceps. Tissue that merely needs to be manipulated but will remain in the patient needs to be handled with more care. Intestinal forceps such as Doyen intestinal forceps (Fig. 2.27) and Babcock intestinal forceps allow handling of the delicate tissue without traumatization or compromise of blood flow. Because of similarities in appearance and construction, it is easy to confuse the Babcock intestinal forceps and the Allis tissue forceps (Fig. 2.28). It is the responsibility of the veterinary technician to keep the two forceps separate and to understand the differences between the two very unique instruments.

Thoracic Instrumentation

Retractors. Thoracic surgery requires the use of appropriately designed instrumentation. A Finochietto retractor is designed to retract the thoracic wall. With the adjustable blades and sturdy construction, the Finochietto is the retractor of choice for thoracic surgery. Two sizes are available: large, which is appropriate in patients larger than 10 kg, and small, which is appropriate for patients smaller than 10 kg. Malleable retractors, although handheld, may be of use in thoracic surgery as

well. The wide variety of widths available and the ability to conform the retractor to whatever depth and shape is needed are a benefit. For instance, a wide malleable retractor would be an effective instrument to employ to retract the lungs within the surgical field.

Thoracic forceps. Depending on the procedure being performed, specific thoracic clamps can be very beneficial. Satinsky clamps, Cooley clamps, and 90-degree Mixter forceps are all examples of vascular instrumentation that can make a surgical procedure easier. With different angles of jaws and different tips, these clamps can be used to clamp off vessels in places that are difficult to reach with conventional clamps.

Biopsy Instrumentation

Special instruments have been created for the efficient collection of a tissue biopsy specimen. Depending on the type of tissue to be biopsied (i.e., liver, kidney, bone), different pieces of equipment should be used to encourage the best possible sample.

Punch biopsy. A punch biopsy instrument comes in a variety of sizes (Fig. 2.29). Usually 2-mm, 4-mm, and 6-mm are available. The appropriate size to use depends on the size of the tumor. The intent of the punch biopsy instrument is to collect a core sample from the suspicious tissue. A thumb tissue forceps and a Metzenbaum scissors are also needed when using a punch biopsy.

Needle punch biopsy. Needle punch biopsy instruments are currently manufactured by a variety of companies. Instruments are equipped with either a cutting or core biopsy needle and are available as manual and automatic devices. These instruments take a small piece of tissue (approximately the size of a pencil lead) for microscopic evaluation. Ultrasound-guided biopsies of internal organs, including liver, spleen, kidney, and prostate, are often performed with these instruments. The technique for using these types of biopsy punches is somewhat complicated, and the surgeon and technician must have a thorough understanding of the mechanics of the instrument in order for it to work properly.

Bone biopsy. Bone biopsy specimens are often collected using either a Michele trephine or a Jamshidi biopsy needle. Both these instruments obtain a core sample from the tissue. The Jamshidi needle biopsy yields a smaller sample but is a less invasive procedure. The Michele trephine collects a larger sample of tissue, but higher risks are associated with its use because of the size of the sample.

Orthopedic Surgery Instruments

Many types of orthopedic instruments are available. The instruments described here are the basics needed for orthopedic surgery and provide a starting point for building an orthopedic surgical instrument inventory.

Bone Holders

Bone-holding clamps are designed to hold bone fragments together until permanent fixation can be achieved. Bone holders can have pointed tips, toothed tips, or **serrated** tips (Fig. 2.30). Bone holders are available in a variety of sizes and styles (Fig. 2.31). Depending on the bone that is fractured and the type of fracture, certain styles of bone holders may be better suited than others.

Periosteal Elevators

The periosteal elevator is used to prepare the fractured bone for permanent fixation. As the name implies, the intended use is to elevate the periosteum from the bone so that the implants can be placed. Periosteal elevators are available in many shapes and sizes, with the most popular styles being the Freer elevator (Fig. 2.32), the ASIF (Association for the Study of Internal Fixation) or Synthes elevator (Fig. 2.33), and the Adson elevator.

Bone Rongeurs

Rongeurs have cupped tips with sharp edges and work with a squeezing action of the handles (Fig. 2.34). Rongeurs are used

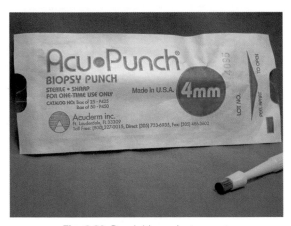

Fig. 2.29 Punch biopsy instrument.

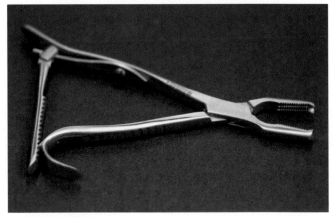

Fig. 2.30 Kerns bone-holding forceps. (Photo by John T. Miller.)

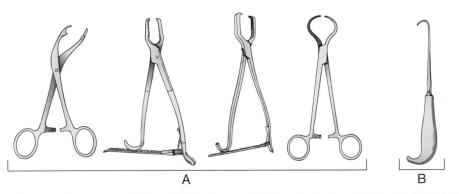

Fig. 2.31 Grasping instruments. (A) Bone-holding forceps. (B) Bone hook. (From Phillips N: *Berry & Kohn's Operating room technique,* ed 11, St Louis, 2007, Mosby.)

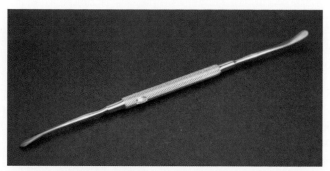

Fig. 2.32 Freer periosteal elevator. (Photo by John T. Miller.)

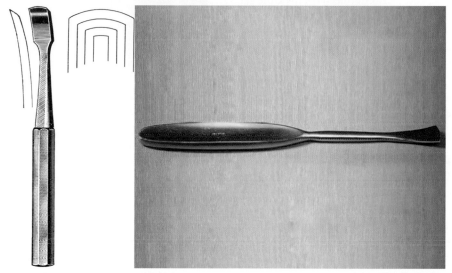

Fig. 2.33 Periosteal elevator. (From Sonsthagen T: *Veterinary instruments and equipment,* ed 2, St Louis, 2011, Elsevier.)

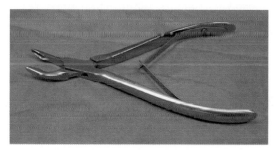

Fig. 2.34 Single-action rongeur.

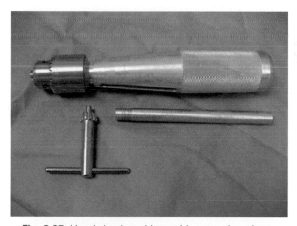

Fig. 2.35 Hand chuck and key with extension piece.

to break up bits and pieces of bone for grafting purposes. Pieces of bone too small to reattach to the patient are broken down into small pieces and packed around the fracture lines to encourage new osteoblast formation and promote healing. Rongeurs can also be used to remove pieces of unnecessary bone.

Bone Cutters

Bone cutters have handles with squeezing and spring action, similar to those of rongeurs. Bone cutters have cutting-edged tips designed to cut through bone and to remove small pieces of bone.

Bone Curettes

Bone curettes are single-handled instruments that have a cupped tip surrounded by sharp edges. They are used to harvest bone graft material or to shape and scrape bony surfaces.

Hand Chuck (Jacob's Chuck)

A hand chuck is designed to hold and drive intramedullary pins for repair of a fracture or for other orthopedic procedures requiring the use of pins (Fig. 2.35). The hand chuck is a manual drill. It can hold wires with sizes from 0.035 inch and up to $^5/_{16}$ inch. The pins are held securely in the hand chuck when the key is used to tighten the chuck. An extension piece is available to protect the surgeon from the pin, which may extend beyond the end of the chuck.

SURGICAL "POWER TOOLS"

Many types of surgical procedures require the use of "power tools." These tools can be powered by compressed nitrogen, batteries, or electricity. Fracture repair requires the use of a power drill to place implants. Neurosurgery requires the use of a specialized drill to remove the vertebral body bone. Even soft tissue surgery sometimes requires power tools. For example, a sternotomy for a thoracic surgery requires a power saw to open the sternum.

Some power devices are sold as individually functioning pieces, whereas others are available in sets that have interchangeable, multifunctional pieces. One available device has a pin driver, sagittal saw, and power drill in one set. This same set is also available in a larger and more powerful size to accommodate larger patients. Other styles of drills are available for use in neurosurgery. These drills have burrs, as opposed to drill bits, that attach to the hand piece to precisely shave or grind away the vertebral body bone. Some power tools are sold with their own sterilizing cases. The manufacturer's recommendations should be consulted for the best way to sterilize specific power tools, such as the Synthes orthopedic drill (Fig. 2.36).

Internal Fixation Implants

Implants can be used for internal fixation of bone fractures, as curative measures for traumatic situations (e.g., tibial plateau leveling osteotomy, cranial cruciate ligament repair), and to correct congenital limb deformities. Many types of implants are available, from pins and orthopedic wire to standard dynamic compression plates and specially designed bone plates. This section describes the basic types of implants and the equipment necessary to use them.

Intramedullary Pins

Intramedullary pins are made of metal and range in size from 1/16 to 1/2 inch (Fig. 2.37). Intramedullary (IM) pins are used to stabilize certain types of fractures or soft tissue in specific orthopedic situations. These pins can be smooth tipped or can have threaded ends. IM pins can be used alone or in conjunction with wire, plates, and screws. Pins can be placed with a hand chuck or a nitrogen air drill or electric drill.

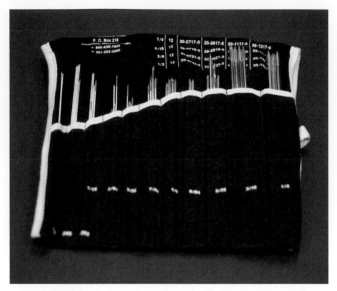

Fig. 2.37 Intramedullary pin set. (Photo by John T. Miller.)

Pin Cutter

A pin cutter is used to cut pins once they have been placed in the patient (Fig. 2.38). Depending on the size of the pin, a squeeze-handle cutter or a bolt cutter may be needed.

Orthopedic Wire

Orthopedic wire is stainless steel wire designed for long-term implantation in a patient (Fig. 2.39). This wire is sized from 16 to 30 gauge; the smaller the number, the larger (thicker) the wire. The most common sizes used in veterinary surgery are 18, 20, and 22 gauge, but the choice depends on the size of the patient, the procedure performed, and the expected stress level of the wound and, therefore, its ability to heal. Wire can be used in conjunction with pins, plates, or screws. Wire twisters are used to secure the wire and are available in many styles (Fig. 2.40). Previously used needle holders are often reserved for the purpose of securing wires as well.

Bone Plates and Screws

Bone plates are stainless steel (except for vertebral plates, which are made of plastic) and are designed to aid in the reduction of fractures and the repair of bone fragments. Plates are available in

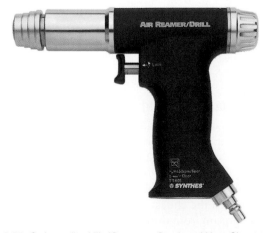

Fig. 2.36 Orthopedic drill. (Courtesy Synthes, West Chester, PA.)

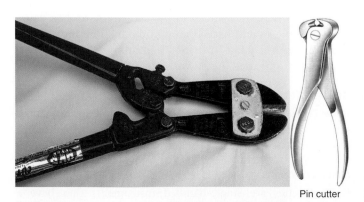

Pin cutter

Fig. 2.38 Pin cutter. (From Sonsthagen TF: *Veterinary instruments and equipment,* ed 3, St Louis, 2014, Mosby.)

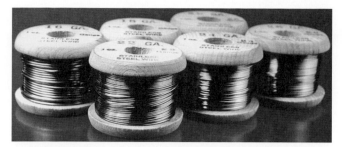

Fig. 2.39 Orthopedic wire. (From Sonsthagen TF: *Veterinary instruments and equipment,* ed 3, St Louis, 2014, Mosby.)

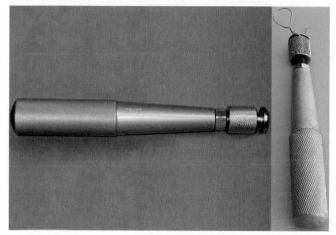

Fig. 2.40 Wire twister. (From Sonsthagen TF: *Veterinary instruments and equipment,* ed 3, St Louis, 2014, Mosby.)

a wide variety of sizes. The size chosen by the surgeon primarily depends on the size of the patient, the particular bone being repaired, and its size. Plates can have different shapes (e.g., straight, T plates, L plates), widths (e.g., 2.0, 2.7, and 3.5 mm), and lengths (e.g., four, five, or six holes). The width number indicates the size of screw that should also be used to secure the plate, and the length is defined by the number of holes available to be filled with screws. Accordingly, the larger the implant, the

more expensive the piece. Bone screws are sized to match the width of the plates. For example, a 3.5-mm plate would have 3.5-mm screws used with it. Bone screws also are sized by length. Screws can be anywhere from 6 to 45 mm long.

Bone plating specialty instrumentation. Many special instruments are needed to place bone plates and screws to hold the plates to the bone. Placement of the screws requires that a hole be drilled with the appropriate size drill bit. After the hole has been made, a depth gauge is used to determine the length of screw that will be needed. After that, a tap is used to prethread the bone so the screw grabs onto the bone more securely. A dedicated screwdriver is then used to place the screw. Other instruments, such as drill sleeves, tap sleeves, and countersinks, are also used to place a screw (Fig. 2.41). Bone plates can be bent and conformed to the shape of the bone by a variety of methods. Either handheld bone plate benders or a tabletop plate bender can be utilized (Fig. 2.42).

External Fixation Implants

External fixation implants (Fig. 2.43) are used, as their name implies, on the external surface of the skin to stabilize fractures. Often they are used for compound fracture repair. Rods, clamps, and sometimes rings are used with this method of stabilization. This type of surgical intervention is quite complicated, and explanation of this technique is well beyond the scope of this text.

Ophthalmic Surgery Instruments

Every veterinary surgical area should have a basic set of ophthalmic instruments available for use (Fig. 2.44). These instruments are extremely delicate and expensive and should be handled with great care. Because of the nature of the tissue for which these instruments are routinely used, the tips are very fine, the shafts tend to be short, and the mechanism of use may be box lock or squeeze handle.

Beaver Blade Handle

The Beaver blade handle is used to hold Beaver scalpel blades (see Fig. 2.44F). Although some ophthalmic procedures can be

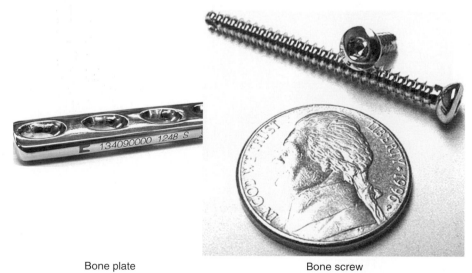

Bone plate   Bone screw

Fig. 2.41 Bone plate and screws. (From Sonsthagen TF: *Veterinary instruments and equipment,* ed 3, St Louis, 2014, Mosby.)

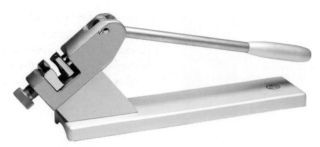

Fig. 2.42 Tabletop plate bender used to bend and form an implant (plate) to the bone surface. (Courtesy Synthes, West Chester, PA.)

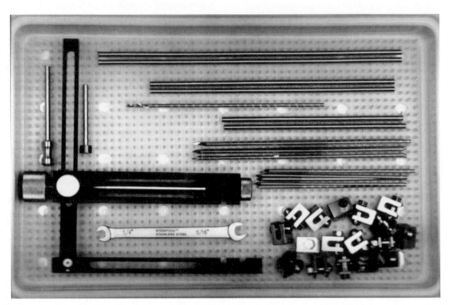

Fig. 2.43 External fixation kit. (From Sonsthagen TF: *Veterinary instruments and equipment*, ed 3, St Louis, 2014, Mosby.)

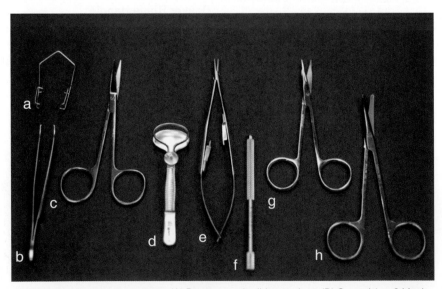

Fig. 2.44 Ophthalmic surgery instruments. (A) Barraquer wire lid speculum. (B) Curved 1 × 2 iris thumb tissue forceps. (C) Straight iris scissors. (D) Chalazion lid speculum. (E) Castroviejo locking needle holder. (F) Beaver blade handle. (G) Stevens tenotomy scissors. (H) Curved baby Metzenbaum scissors. (Photo by John T. Miller.)

performed using a No. 15 scalpel blade on a No. 3 handle, some intraocular procedures may require the use of a beaver blade.

Lid Speculum

An eyelid speculum may or may not be used, depending on the procedure performed. For intraocular procedures, a Barraquer wire speculum is often used to retract the eyelids away from the surgical site (see Fig. 2.44A). For lid procedures, a chalazion lid speculum may be used (see Fig. 2.44D). This instrument is most helpful in the removal of an eyelid tumor.

Lacrimal Cannulas

Both straight and curved lacrimal cannulas are available (Fig. 2.45). These stainless steel cannulas can be used to flush lacrimal ducts. One end of the cannula is adapted to accept a syringe to allow for infusion of solution. The other end is blunt or bulb shaped to permit easy passage into the lacrimal duct.

Thumb Tissue Forceps

Thumb tissue forceps are extremely delicate in design. Their function in ophthalmic surgery is the same as in general surgery. Gentle holding of tissue is imperative because the tips of these instruments are extremely delicate. It is crucial to handle the tissue of the eye and its associated structures in an atraumatic manner to avoid damaging the tissues. Examples of thumb tissue forceps are the iris 1 × 2 (see Fig. 2.44B).

Scissors

The scissors used in ophthalmic surgery may be miniature versions of general surgery instruments, such as the baby Metzenbaum scissors (see Fig. 244H). Others are specially designed and crafted for delicate eye surgery, such as the Castroviejo scissors. Many of the specialty scissors have a squeeze-action operation instead of the more traditional ring-handled mechanism. Two general-purpose utility scissors are typically used in ophthalmology: the Stevens tenotomy scissors (see Fig. 2.44G) and the iris scissors (see Fig. 2.44C). Compared with the Stevens tenotomy scissors, the iris scissors have a slightly longer blade, which tapers at a more constant rate from box lock to tip, as well as sharper points. Both of these scissors can be used to

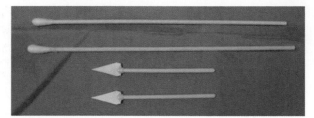

Fig. 2.46 Hemostatic tools for ophthalmic surgery. *Top:* Cotton-tipped applicators. *Bottom:* Weck-Cel surgical spears (Medtronic, Inc., Jacksonville, FL).

cut the extra-fine suture material used in ophthalmic surgery, as well as tissue.

Needle Holders

The type of needle holder used depends on whether the surgical procedure is intraocular or extraocular. Extraocular procedures may be managed with a small (4-inch) Mayo-Hegar or Derf needle holder. Intraocular procedures may require a more delicate instrument, such as a Castroviejo needle holder (see Fig. 2.44E). As with the scissors, the specialty needle holders may have a squeeze-handle mechanism instead of the usual, bulkier ring-handle style.

Miscellaneous Ophthalmic Equipment

Hemostasis for ophthalmic surgery involves different concerns from those in general or orthopedic surgery. The delicate nature of the tissue surrounding the eye requires that materials other than sponges be used to perform hemostasis. For extraocular procedures (e.g., lid tumor, enucleation), regular, radiopaque surgical sponges are appropriate. For intraocular procedures (e.g., corneal laceration, lens luxation), a more delicate device is needed. Cotton-tipped applicators can be sterilized and used, or surgical spears (e.g., Weck Cel cellulose sponge surgical spears, Medtronic, Inc., Jacksonville, FL) are available commercially (Fig. 2.46). The spears have an arrow shape and permit pinpoint control of hemorrhages in a small working area.

SURGICAL NEEDLES

Many sizes and shapes of surgical suture needles are available. The needle point, the needle body, and the needle eye are considered in the categorization of needles (Fig. 2.47).

Needle Point

The needle point helps to determine the type of tissue in which the needle should be used. A taper-point needle has a sharp point that pierces and penetrates tissues without leaving small cuts because the cross section is rounded. The round needle body associated with the taper point is best used in tissue when a sealed suture line is needed, such as for suturing intestine or other hollow organs. Any tissue that should not be traumatized or is not difficult to pass a needle through will tolerate a taper needle.

A taper-cut needle is a combination of a round, tapered body and a reverse cutting point. This type of needle is easily

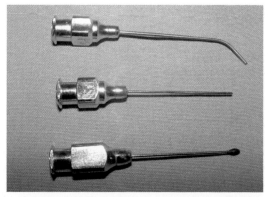

Fig. 2.45 Lacrimal cannulas. *Top to bottom:* Curved blunt, straight blunt, olive tip.

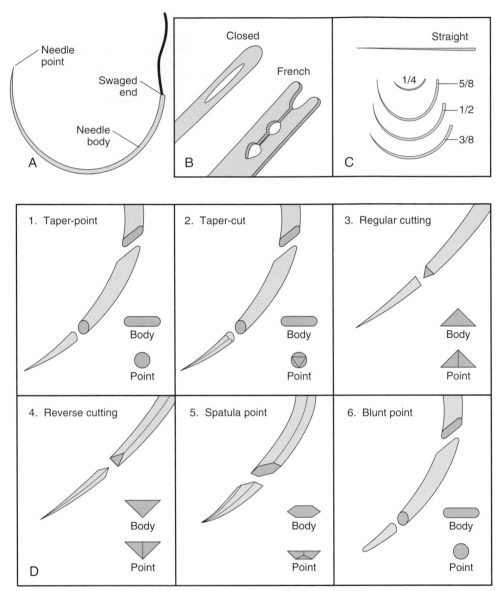

Fig. 2.47 (A) Basic components of a needle. (B) Types of eyed needles. (C) Needle body sizes. (D) Needle body shapes. (From Fossum TW, Hedlund CS, Hulse DA, et al: *Small animal surgery*, ed 4, St Louis, 2013, Mosby.)

used with tough fibrous tissue and some cardiovascular procedures. A reverse cutting needle has three cutting edges on the point—the cross section is triangular, with one of the cutting edges being the outside of the curve—and it maintains that shape in the body and is stronger than the conventional cutting needle.

A cutting-edge needle also has three cutting edges on the point and body, but the third cutting edge is on the inside of the curve. This style of needle may be most traumatic because the cutting edge on the inside of the curve cuts toward the edges of the wound, compromising the strength of the tissue.

Needle Body

The shape of the needle body can also vary widely. Needles can be straight, circular, or curved. Straight needles, sometimes referred to as Keith needles, are available but have limited application in veterinary medicine. One procedure made easier by the

use of a Keith needle is the placement of a purse-string suture in the anus. The straight shape of the needle makes it easier to avoid the anal glands by allowing superficial placement of the suture.

Curved needles can either be full curve, half curve, or double curve. Needles that are double curved have both ends curved in opposite directions. Double-curved needles are generally reserved for use in large animal surgery, especially bovine surgical closures.

Half-curved needles are classified as such because only half the body of the needle is curved. They are rarely used in veterinary surgery.

Full-curved needles have the entire body of the needle involved in the curve. Varying degrees of curvature can be found, based on the portion of a full circle that is involved. For example, a ⅜-circle needle means that if a full circle were divided into eight equal parts, the continuous curve of three of those parts would be this shape. Likewise, a half-circle needle would mean that four continuous parts (or half the circle) would be the shape of the needle. Other common circular needle shapes are ¼ circle and ⅝ circle.

Suture Attachment End

The final portion of the needle is the suture attachment end. Some needles have eyes, which can be single or French style. Single-eyed needles must have the suture material passed through the needle eye. Suture is threaded through the eye from the inside of the curve to the outside. The threading of the needle results in a rather bulky portion of suture that must pass through the tissue, therefore creating excessive tissue drag and damage. The French-eyed needle has one complete eye and one split eye. The suture is passed through the complete eye and then pushed down through the split eye, which securely grips the suture.

The most atraumatic and therefore most common method of suture attachment is with the swaged needle, or eyeless needle. When the suture is manufactured, the needle and suture are attached to each other. With this type of attachment, the tissues undergo minimal damage because the point and diameter of the needle create the hole, and the suture simply follows along without causing further trauma. The ease of use and limited trauma of the eyeless needle make it the first choice of almost all veterinary surgeons.

SUTURE MATERIAL

The purpose of suture material is to hold together wound edges until the wound can withstand the stress of healing without additional support. Some examples of tissue instability that would require suture material are an intentional surgical incision, ligated vessels, and ligament, tendon, or muscle repair. Suture material is available in many forms, sizes, and colors. It is important to understand the terminology used when discussing suture to know the options available and to select the appropriate material for the procedure being performed. Although the technician will not be making the decision about which type of suture to use, he or she must have a working knowledge of the types of suture available (Table 2.1). The veterinary technician who can anticipate the type of suture that may be requested, on the basis of knowledge and experience, will be an invaluable member of the surgical team.

TABLE 2.1	Characteristics of Suture Materials Commonly Used in Veterinary Medicine						
Generic Name	Trade Name	Manufacturer	Suture Characteristics	Reduction in Tensile Strength*	Complete Absorption (Days)	Relative Knot Security†	Tissue Reaction‡
Chromic surgical gut (catgut)	—	—	Absorbable Multifilament	33% at 7 days	60	— Wet	+++
Polyglactin 910	Vicryl and Vicryl Plus	Ethicon	Absorbable Multifilament	25% at 14 days 50% at 21 days;	56–70	++ ++	+ +
	Vicryl Rapide	Ethicon	Absorbable Multifilament	50% at 5 days 100% at 14 days	42	++	+
Polyglycolic acid	Dexon "S" (uncoated) Dexon II (coated)	Covidien	Absorbable Multifilament	35% at 14 days 65% at 21 days	60–90	++	+
Glycolide/lactide polymer	Polysorb	Covidien	Absorbable Multifilament	20% at 14 days 70% at 21 days	60	+++	—
Polydioxanone	PDS II	Ethicon	Absorbable Monofilament	14% at 14 days 31% at 42 days	180	++	+
Polyglyconate	Maxon	Covidien	Absorbable Monofilament	30% at 14 days 45% at 21 days	180	++	+
Poliglecaprone 25	Monocryl	Ethicon	Absorbable Monofilament	40%–50% at 7 days 70%–80% at 14 days	90–120	++	+
Glycomer 631	Biosyn	Covidien	Absorbable Monofilament	25% at 14 days 60% at 21 days	90–110	++	+
Polyglytone 6211	Caprosyn	Covidien	Absorbable Monofilament	40%–50% at 5 days 70%–80% at 10 days	56	+++	+
Silk	Perma-Hand	Ethicon	Nonabsorbable Multifilament	30% at 14 days 50% at 1 year	>2 years	—	+++
Polyester	Mersilene (uncoated) Ethibond (coated) Dacron (uncoated) Ti-Cron (coated)	Ethicon Ethicon Covidien Covidien	Nonabsorbable Multifilament			—	++

Continued

TABLE 2.1	Characteristics of Suture Materials Commonly Used in Veterinary Medicine—cont'd							
Generic Name	Trade Name	Manufacturer	Suture Characteristics	Reduction in Tensile Strength*	Complete Absorption (Days)	Relative Knot Security[†]	Tissue Reaction[‡]	
Polyamide (Nylon)	Ethilon (monofilament) Nurolon (multifilament) Dermalon (monofilament) Surgilon (multifilament)	Ethicon Ethicon Covidien Covidien	Nonabsorbable Monofilament or multifilament	30% at 2 years (monofilament) 75% at 180 days (multifilament)		+	—	
Polypropylene	Prolene Surgilene Fluorofil	Ethicon Covidien Mallinckrodt Veterinary	Nonabsorbable Monofilament			+++	—	
Polybutester	Novafil	Covidien	Nonabsorbable Monofilament			++	—	
Polymerized caprolactam	Supramid Braunamid Vet cassette II	S. Jackson B. Braun Melsungen Ag Mallinckrodt Veterinary	Nonabsorbable Multifilament			++	++ (if coating breaks)	
Stainless steel wire	Flexon (multifilament)	Covidien	Nonabsorbable Monofilament or Multifilament			+++	—	

*Values given are approximate. Actual loss of tensile strength may vary depending on suture and tissue.
[†](−), Poor (<60%); (+), fair (60%–70%); (+ +), good (70%–85%); (+ + +), excellent (>85%).
[‡](−), Minimal to none; (+), mild; (+ +), moderate; (+ + +), severe.
From Fossum TW, Hedlund CS, Hulse DA, et al: *Small animal surgery*, ed 4, St Louis, 2013, Mosby.

Characteristics

Tensile Strength

Tensile strength is the amount of force in psi that the suture can withstand as an untied fiber before it breaks.

Memory

Memory is the ability or tendency of the suture to return to its original packaged form.

Flexibility

Flexibility is the ease with which the suture is manipulated, either by the surgeon or in the tissue. Flexibility is somewhat determined by the diameter size and the material used to make the suture. For example, silk has better flexibility than stainless steel.

Absorbability

Suture can be classified as either nonabsorbable or absorbable. Nonabsorbable suture is not broken down by the body and can remain intact in the body for at least 2 years. Absorbable suture can be broken down by the body through different processes. During phagocytosis, leukocytes, usually neutrophils, are released and travel to the site of concern (incision) to ingest and destroy the microbes or, in the case of suture material, the foreign suture material. Suture material is also absorbed through hydrolysis. The chemical compound in the suture is decomposed as it is exposed to water. Absorption of suture may begin as soon as 7 days after placement, and sutures lose most of their tensile strength within 60 days.

Capillarity

Capillarity describes the ability of the suture to allow microbes to wick (be carried) to the interior of the suture strand. This action can be curtailed if the manufacturer coats the suture at production to decrease the wicking action. Polytetrafluoroethylene (Teflon), wax, paraffin, silicone, and calcium stearate are substances used to coat suture. Generally, multifilament sutures are treated more often for capillarity than monofilament sutures.

Structure

There are two basic structure types of suture: multifilament and monofilament (Fig. 2.48). Multifilament suture, also called braided suture, has two or more strands braided together to form the single strand of suture. Monofilament suture is a single, solid strand of suture material. Monofilament suture material tends to have less tissue drag, or friction, when it is being pulled through the tissues than multifilament suture material.

Knot Security

The ability of suture to hold the knots the surgeon has placed is imperative. Some types of suture materials hold knots better than other types. Usually, braided material has less knot slippage than monofilament suture. Once knots have been formed with the suture, they must stay secure. The slippage of a knot can result in the death of a patient if a knot that was around a major vessel slips, and the patient bleeds to death.

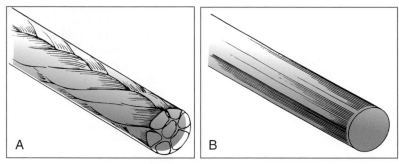

Fig. 2.48 (A) Multifilament suture. (B) Monofilament suture. (From Meeker MH, Rothrock JC: *Alexander's care of the patient in surgery,* ed 12, St Louis, 2003, Mosby.)

Color

Some sutures are dyed during the manufacturing process for easier identification after placement in the tissue. Suture material is available in dyed or undyed styles. Although not as great a concern with veterinary patients as with human patients, suture color should be considered in some cases. For example, if the patient is a black Labrador and both black nylon and blue polypropylene are available for the skin sutures, the blue sutures will be much easier to identify at suture removal in 10 days.

Origin of Material

Suture material is also classified by the origin of the material from which it is made. Natural suture material is a product made from fibers found in nature. Some examples are cotton, silk, and catgut, which is made from sheep intestinal mucosa.

Synthetic material is suture produced with the use of manufactured products. This group includes almost all the remaining suture not previously mentioned (e.g., nylon, polyglactin 910).

Metallic suture is a small category of sutures and is limited to surgical stainless steel suture, which includes suture wire and staples.

The ideal suture material would have no knot slippage, would have high tensile strength, would be absorbable, would cause no tissue reactivity, would be easy to handle, and would be inexpensive. Unfortunately, no one perfect suture material exists, so the surgeon must consider all the characteristics of the material when deciding whether to use it for a particular procedure (Fig. 2.49). In addition to the physical characteristics of the suture material, the surgeon must also consider the following criteria when selecting the suture type and size:

- Patient size
- Area (tissue) of placement (skin vs. hollow organ)
- Strength required
- Healing potential of the tissue
- Importance of cosmetic appearance
- Cost

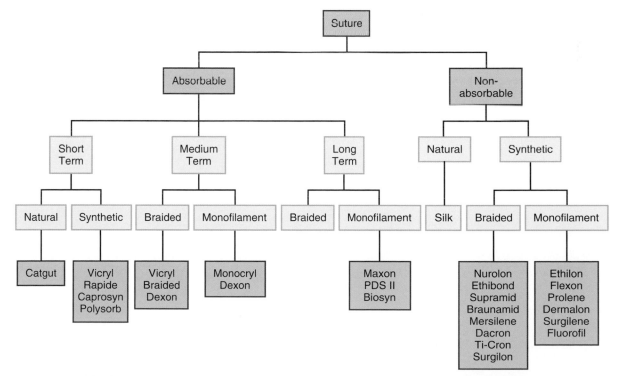

Fig. 2.49 Characteristics of suture used in veterinary medicine. (From Fossum TW, Hedlund CS, Hulse DA, et al: *Small animal surgery,* ed 4, St Louis, 2013, Mosby.)

Sizing

Suture material is classified by size according to the United States Pharmacopeia (USP). The USP uses a numeric scale to denote size from fine to coarse. Suture size is identified by the term *ought*. When sizing suture, the numeral "0" is used to represent "ought" or "zero." The more zeros in a size, the smaller is the suture. For example, "0000" (pronounced "four-ought") is the same as 4-0 (also pronounced "four-ought"). Similarly, "00" is the same as 2-0, which some refer to as "double-ought." Size 5-0 suture material is smaller in diameter (finer) than 3-0 suture. Whole numbers alone can also be used to identify the size of suture (e.g., No. 1, No. 2, No. 3). In the sizing of suture material, whole numbers used alone, that is, without any oughts, increase in size with an increase in the number; the larger the number, the larger the suture. Suture is manufactured in a wide range of sizes, from 11 to 0 to No. 5. Smaller patients and more delicate tissue (ophthalmology or cardiovascular procedures) tend to require the small sizes, whereas the larger sizes are primarily used in large animal surgery (Table 2.2).

Packaging

Most suture material is packaged as single-use items sterilized at the factory by the use of gamma radiation (Figs. 2.50 and 2.51). Suture packaged and sterilized in this manner has a rather long shelf life, which is indicated by an expiration date on the box. Individual suture packs are opened on an as-needed basis, aseptically, onto the surgical field. Exposed but unused suture should not be resterilized but rather saved for use in nonsterile procedures (e.g., necropsy closure). If the inner suture pack was unopened and unused on the sterile field, resterilizing the package may be possible. Under no circumstances should suture be steam sterilized. Any sterilization

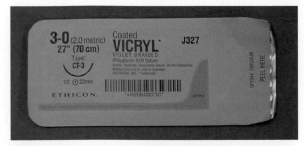

Fig. 2.50 Single-use multifilament, absorbable, synthetic suture.

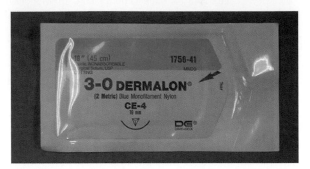

Fig. 2.51 Single-use monofilament, nonabsorbable, synthetic suture.

should be accomplished by the use of an ethylene oxide (EtO) sterilizer.

Another packaging option is to have long lengths (50–100 m) of suture placed on a reel or "cassette" by the manufacturer (Fig. 2.52). Although economically a good idea, this method of storing suture material has a greater potential for contamination than individually packaged products. Also, a knot in the middle of the reel of suture is a common risk and can prove to be a difficult obstacle in removing suture from the cassette.

TABLE 2.2	**Common Suture Size in Veterinary Medicine**			
Synthetic Suture Materials (USP)	**Surgical Gut (USP)**	**Brown and Sharpe Wire Gauge**	**Metric Gauge**	**Actual Size (MM)**
10-0			0.2	0.02
9-0			0.3	0.03
8-0			0.4	0.04
7-0	8-0	41	0.5	0.05
6-0	7-0	38–40	0.7	0.07
5-0	6-0	35	1	0.1
4-0	5-0	32–34	1.5	0.15
3-0	4-0	30	2	0.2
2-0	3-0	28	3	0.3
0	2-0	26	3.5	0.35
1	0	25	4	0.4
2	1	24	5	0.5
3,4	2	22	6	0.6
5	3	20	7	0.7
6	4	19	8	0.8
7		18	9	0.9

USP, United States Pharmacopeia.
From Fossum TW, Hedlund CS, Hulse DA, et al: *Small animal surgery*, ed 4, St Louis, 2013, Mosby.

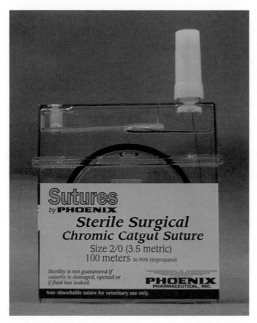

Fig. 2.52 Cassette packaging of monofilament, absorbable, natural suture.

Staples

Internal and external staples are available for use in veterinary surgery and differ dramatically in cost, ease of use, and applicability.

External Staples

Skin staples are stainless steel staples placed perpendicularly to an incision to close the wound (Fig. 2.53A). If a patient has a history of postsurgical incisional licking or tissue reaction to other suture material, external staples may be a good option. Self-contained in a disposable stapling device, the staples can be placed quickly, significantly decreasing anesthesia time. Once placed in the skin, the staples take on a unique shape to inhibit accidental removal. A special staple removal device is required to remove the staples safely and comfortably from the patient at the appropriate time.

Internal Staples

Specific soft tissue cases may benefit from the use of internal stainless steel staples. Internal staples may be most advantageous in certain thoracic cases (e.g., pulmonary resection, excision of tumors in certain locations). Thoracoabdominal (TA) staples are designed to place multiple rows of staples in tissue (Fig. 2.53C). Special staples are also used with gastrointestinal procedures, such as gastrointestinal anastomosis (GIA; Fig. 2.53B) and end-to-end anastomosis (EEA). A number may follow the initials of the staple type to indicate the length of the row of staples. For example, TA 90 is a row of staples 90 mm in length with the TA design. Special staplers are required for each of the different types of staples. Although expensive, these staples can save time in critical cases. The benefit must be weighed against the cost so that these staples are used judiciously.

CONCLUSION

Surgical instruments are an integral part of the veterinary clinic. They represent a significant financial investment. Each has a specific function and should be used accordingly. Having a clear understanding of instruments and their use will help the technician be prepared.

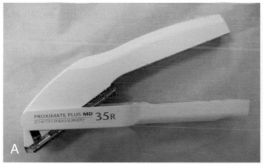
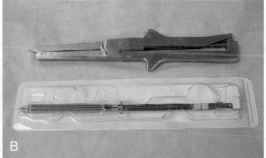
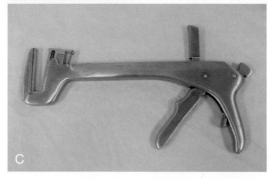

Fig. 2.53 Surgical stapling equipment. (A) Surgical skin stapler applies a single staple with each squeeze of the trigger (staple guns typically hold 25–35 staples). (B) Gastrointestinal anastomosis (GIA) stapler. Staple cartridges are for one-time use and are purchased in presterilized packages. (C) Thoracoabdominal (TA) stapler. Staple cartridges are purchased as for GIA stapler. Shown here with staple cartridge in place. (From Bassert JM, McCurnin DM, editors: *McCurnin's clinical textbook for veterinary technicians,* ed 7, St Louis, 2010, Saunders.)

KEY POINTS

1. Proper use of surgical instruments is vital to maintain the health and usefulness of the instrument.
2. Every instrument needs to be evaluated frequently to assess its ability to function properly.
3. The use of a suture needle is determined by its shape.
4. All the characteristics of suture material should be considered before the decision is made as to the type of material to use in any particular case.

REVIEW QUESTIONS

1. Which surgical instrument has both horizontal and vertical serrations of the jaw?
   a. Kelly hemostatic forceps
   b. Mayo-Hegar needle holders
   c. Rochester-Pean hemostatic forceps
   d. Rochester-Carmalt hemostatic forceps
2. Which part of a ringed instrument locks an instrument in a closed position?
   a. Shank
   b. Ratchet
   c. Box lock
   d. Ring handles
3. The jaw of which instrument has one raised jaw and one recessed jaw?
   a. Ferguson angiotribe
   b. Crile hemostatic forceps
   c. Halsted mosquito hemostatic forceps
   d. Rochester-Carmalt hemostatic forceps
4. Which of these tissue forceps is atraumatic?
   a. Allis tissue forceps
   b. Russian thumb tissue forceps
   c. Adson 1 x 2 thumb tissue forceps
   d. Adson dressing thumb tissue forceps
5. Which is a handheld retractor?
   a. Senn retractor
   b. Gelpi retractor
   c. Balfour retractor
   d. Weitlaner retractor
6. Which type of towel clamp has penetrating tips and a squeeze handle?
   a. Jones
   b. Lorna
   c. Roeder
   d. Backhaus
7. Which needle holders have scissors included in the jaws?
   a. Derf
   b. Olsen-Hegar
   c. Mayo-Hegar
   d. Crile-Wood
8. To properly handle ringed instruments, the digits should be placed in the rings:
   a. Distal to the first knuckle of both the thumb and ring finger.
   b. Proximal to the first knuckle of both the thumb and ring finger.
   c. Distal to the first knuckle of both the thumb and middle finger.
   d. Proximal to the first knuckle of both the thumb and middle finger.
9. Which instrument is used to find and exteriorize the uterine horn during an ovariohysterectomy?
   a. Hand chuck
   b. Snook hook
   c. Groove director
   d. Dowling spay retractor
10. Which forceps are a vascular clamp?
   a. Doyen
   b. Adson 1 x 2
   c. 90-degree Mixter
   d. Rochester-Carmalt
11. A bone biopsy may be taken using which instrument?
   a. Bone cutters
   b. Michele trephine
   c. Periosteal elevator
   d. Needle punch biopsy
12. Which type of needle would be preferred for an intestinal resection and anastomosis?
   a. Taper
   b. Keith
   c. Taper-cutting
   d. Cutting edge
13. Which of the scalpel blade grips allows for better stabilization and a finer, more precise incision?
   a. Fingertip
   b. Pencil
   c. Palmed
   d. Slide
14. A function of the bone rongeurs is to:
   a. Hold and drive intramedullary pins.
   b. Shape and scrape bony surfaces.
   c. Break up pieces of bone for grafting purposes.
   d. Elevate the periosteum from the bone to allow implants to be placed.
15. During production of suture, wax would be used to coat a suture to:
   a. Decrease memory.
   b. Increase flexibility.
   c. Decrease capillarity.
   d. Increase absorbability.
16. Which suture diameter is the largest?
   a. 0
   b. 2-0
   c. 3-0
   d. 5-0

17. What is an advantage of using suture on a reel?
    a. Inexpensive
    b. Knotting of suture in the reel
    c. Less opportunity for contamination
    d. Good option for patients with a history of post-surgical licking
18. Which scissors is designed to be used on delicate tissues?
    a. Mayo
    b. Suture
    c. Operating
    d. Metzenbaum
19. What is an advantage of suture that is dyed?
20. When would a double-curved needle be used?
21. Define swaged needle.

BIBLIOGRAPHY

Bassert JM, McCurnin DM, editors: *McCurnin's clinical textbook for veterinary technicians*, ed 8, St Louis, 2014, Saunders.
Fossum TW: *Small animal surgery*, ed 5, St Louis, 2018, Mosby.

Sonsthagen TF: *Veterinary instruments and equipment: a pocket guide*, ed 3, St Louis, 2014, Mosby.

3

Anesthetic Machine

Paige Allen and Marianne Tear

LEARNING OBJECTIVES

After completion of this chapter, the reader will be able to:
- Describe the function of an anesthesia machine.
- List the individual components of an anesthesia machine.
- Describe the method for performing a leak check of an anesthesia machine.
- Describe the difference between rebreathing and nonrebreathing circuits and the indications for their use.
- Describe how to calculate the size of rebreathing bag to be used.
- Describe the use of different oxygen flow rates and the indications for their use.

KEY TERMS

Atelectasis
Closed system
Open system

Semi-closed system
Semi-open system
Vaporizer

WAGs

ANESTHETIC MACHINE

Anesthesia can be a stressful time for the veterinary technician. However, a thorough understanding of the components of the machine, the flow of gas through the machine, and the options available to deliver the anesthetic gases to the patient can reduce the stress level and can even make surgery a rewarding part of the technician's day.

The primary purpose of an anesthesia machine is to deliver inhalation anesthesia to the patient and then remove the unneeded gases from the patient and the surgery suite. The inhalation anesthetic gas is delivered to the patient through oxygen molecules; oxygen (O_2) is the carrier gas for the anesthetic gas. Another purpose of an anesthesia machine is to deliver oxygen as the sole gas, as in cardiopulmonary resuscitation (CPR). For the anesthesia machine to perform as intended, it must do the following:
1. Deliver O_2 at a controlled rate.
2. Vaporize (turn a liquid into a gas) a designated concentration of liquid anesthetic, mix the anesthetic with oxygen, and deliver the mixture to the patient.
3. Remove exhaled gases from the patient, then dispose of the gases through a scavenging system or recirculate them (after removing the carbon dioxide) to the patient.

The ability of the anesthesia machine to function properly depends on the equipment being in good repair, being properly maintained, and being used appropriately.

Anesthesia machines are configured in many forms, depending on the manufacturer. Well-known producers of anesthesia machines include North American Matrix (Fig. 3.1), Drager (Figs. 3.2 and 3.3), and Ohmeda Medical. Some machines are designed with the simplest intent of delivering inhalation anesthesia (see Figs. 3.1 and 3.2). Other machines may have accessories and the ability to provide automatic ventilation, multiple inhalation gas choices (e.g., isoflurane, sevoflurane), and space for placement and storage of monitoring devices (see Fig. 3.3). Regardless of the machine's appearance, the basic function remains the same.

Components

The anesthesia machine has many components working together to perform its intended function. To best understand

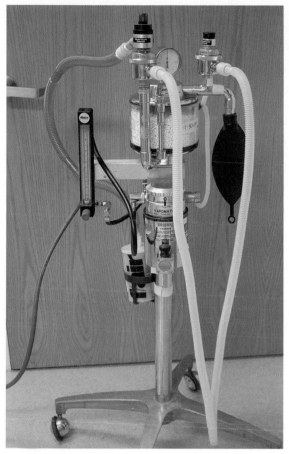

Fig. 3.1 Basic anesthesia machine.

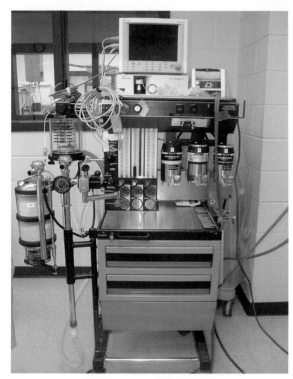

Fig. 3.3 Complex anesthesia machine with multiple vaporizers, storage for monitoring devices, and a ventilator.

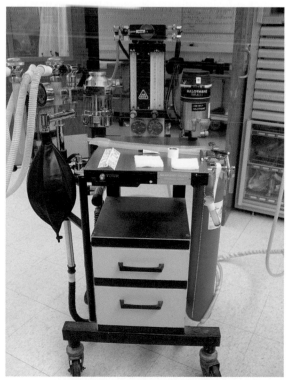

Fig. 3.2 Basic double-vaporizer anesthesia machine.

how the machine works, it is necessary to identify and understand each component. This basic information not only provides a working knowledge of the machine but also assists the technician with troubleshooting problems in the event of a malfunction. Tracing the oxygen flow through the machine allows a view of all the components of the machine.

Oxygen Source

The oxygen source can be a localized cylinder or a large, centrally located source (Fig. 3.4). Cylinders are available in different sizes; the two most common sizes are the E and H tanks. The E tanks are smaller and generally attached to the machine, whereas the H tanks are larger and generally stand alone, away from the anesthesia machine, often chained against a wall. Tanks are color coded for easy recognition (green in the United States, white in Canada) and have a pressure reading of 2200 pounds per square inch (**psi**) when full, regardless of the size. When opening a tank, personnel should remember the rule of "righty tighty, lefty loosey." When turning the valve clockwise (to the right), the tank is being closed; turning the valve counterclockwise (to the left) opens the tank. Using 100% O_2 from an oxygen source is justified because (1) the O_2 acts as a carrier for the vaporized anesthetic gas and delivers it to the patient, and (2) anesthetized patients have a decreased tidal volume, so an increased O_2 concentration will compensate for this decrease.

Yoke

The yoke attaches the E tank, if used, to the anesthetic machine. In addition to allowing the tank to be attached to the machine, the yoke provides additional safety to ensure that the wrong

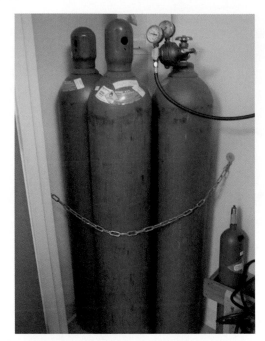

Fig. 3.4 Large H tanks as an oxygen source.

delivery gas is not used. E tanks are equipped with one outlet port and two small pin index holes. On O$_2$ tanks, these line up with the inlet and pins on the yoke. This prevents the accidental use of another gas agent (Fig. 3.5).

Tank Pressure Gauge

Once the O$_2$ tank is turned on, the tank pressure gauge indicates the amount of compressed gas in the tank. The measurement is in pounds per square inch (psi). This gauge should be checked when the tank is first turned on and then frequently throughout

the day. Because oxygen is the carrier for the anesthetic gas, it is imperative that the tank does not run out of oxygen while a patient is under anesthesia.

Pressure-Reducing Valve

The first pressure-reducing valve in the system is found near the oxygen source tank. This valve reduces the pressure leaving the tank and entering the machine to 40 to 50 psi, regardless of the pressure in the tank. The lower pressure gas is carried through the source lines to the anesthesia machine.

Flowmeter

Next in the flow of O$_2$ is the oxygen flowmeter (Fig. 3.6). The flowmeter further reduces the pressure of the gas to 15 psi. This is very close to atmospheric pressure and is well tolerated by patients. The flowmeter regulates how much O$_2$ is entering the system and being delivered to the patient. O$_2$ flow is measured in liters per minute (L/min) or milliliters per minute (mL/min). The O$_2$ flow is regulated by a knob at the bottom of the flowmeter. Personnel must take care to avoid excessive tightening of the knob when turning off the flow. When reading the flowmeter, the float needs to be properly read. Ball floats are read on the scale where the middle of the ball sits on the graduations (Fig. 3.7A). Floats with a point are read at the top of the float (Fig. 3.7B). Graduations on the flowmeter may be in 100-mL increments until the 1-L level, then in 500-mL increments thereafter.

Fast Flush Valve

The fast flush valve, or oxygen flush, is the next component on the machine. On many anesthesia machines the oxygen flush valve is found near the oxygen flowmeter. The fast flush valve allows quick infusion of only oxygen into the breathing circuit.

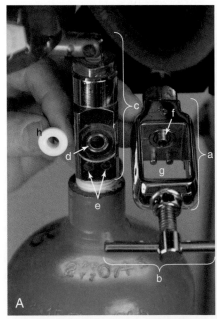
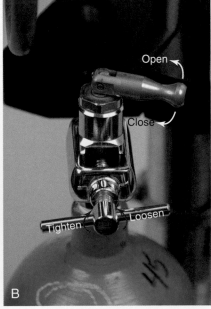

Fig. 3.5 Parts of a size E compressed gas cylinder and yoke. (a), yoke; (b), wing nut; (c), outlet valve; (d), outlet port; (e), pin index safety system holes; (f), nipple of yoke; (g), index pins; (h), nylon washer. (From Lerche T: *Anesthesia and analgesia for veterinary technicians*, ed 5, St Louis, 2017, Mosby.)

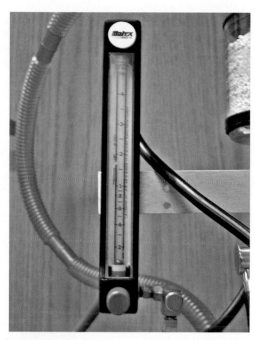

Fig. 3.6 Oxygen flowmeter. Note the graduations for measuring oxygen flow. The float is shown at the bottom of the flowmeter. The fast flush valve is to the right of the regulating knob.

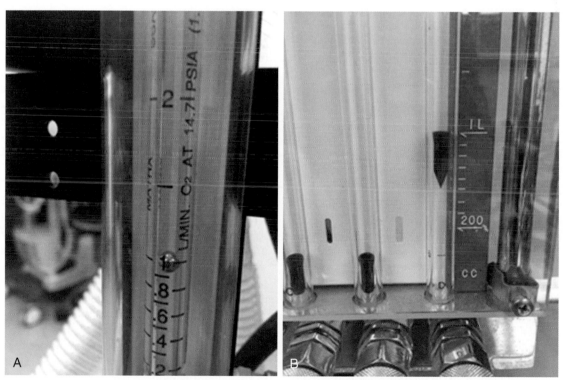

Fig. 3.7 A, Ball float reading 1 L. B, Point float reading 1 L.

This infusion can occur because, with a vaporizer out of the circle, the vaporizer is bypassed with the tubing arrangement of the machine. There is inherent risk in using this flush valve when the patient is connected to the machine. Because the vaporizer is bypassed, the patient receives straight oxygen, which may alter the depth of anesthesia. The fast flush valve should never be used if the pressure relief, or pop-off, valve is closed.

This could lead to a dangerous increase in pressure in the patient's lungs and **atelectasis** (complete or partial collapse of a lobe or the entire lung). The fast flush valve should never be used with a nonrebreathing system for two reasons. First, the pressure of oxygen coming out of the system is too high and may harm the patient. Second, the nonrebreathing systems use such a high oxygen flow that the valve's purpose becomes moot;

the high flows result in oxygen levels similar to those achieved with the fast flush valve.

Vaporizer

The **vaporizer** is usually found next when tracing O_2 flow. Its primary function is to hold liquid anesthetic and to turn that liquid into a gas form that can be delivered to the patient in a controlled manner. The vaporizer inlet is the point where the O_2 enters the vaporizer to carry anesthetic gas molecules to the patient. The vaporizer outlet is the point at which the O_2 and anesthetic gas leave the vaporizer to enter the circuit. Up to this point the O_2 flow has been "out of the circle," assuming the anesthesia machine being used has the vaporizer out of the circle. The "circle," or circuit, is the loop that the gases travel to cycle in and out of the patient when a rebreathing system is used.

Vaporizers are calibrated internally for a specific type of inhalation anesthetic. Only the type of anesthetic for which the machine has been calibrated should be used in the vaporizer. All designs of vaporizers have some style of indicator window at the base of the unit. This window allows determination of the amount of liquid anesthetic remaining in the machine. Once the level reaches one-half to one-quarter remaining, liquid anesthetic should be added to avoid running out during a procedure. Ideally the machine is refilled each evening at the close of business to prevent employee exposure to anesthetic agents. If the vaporizer does need to be filled while the machine is in use, personnel must be sure to turn off the vaporizer before filling it. This action prevents the anesthetic from bubbling out and contaminating the environment with anesthetic fumes. Some vaporizers have two indicator windows, one to show anesthetic level and one to show when to refill. Vaporizers have some type of device to determine the amount of anesthetic being delivered to the system. Depending on the type of vaporizer, this amount is determined as a percentage or just a setting on the dial.

Vaporizers should be serviced annually to ensure a properly functioning mechanism. In the event that a vaporizer needs to be shipped for servicing, it should be drained of any liquid anesthetic to avoid any accidental spill or leaks during shipping. If the machine is tipped, the vaporizer should be serviced to ensure that it is still delivering the correct anesthetic percentage.

Precision vaporizers are the most commonly used. Nonprecision vaporizers may still be available. Nonprecision vaporizers are seen less and less in veterinary medicine with the development of safer inhalant anesthetics that require precision vaporizers. Inhalants used in nonprecision vaporizers are not even available anymore. A nonprecision vaporizer is basically a glass canister that allows liquid anesthetic to vaporize at an uncontrolled rate. The construction of the nonprecision vaporizer does not permit compensation for the three factors discussed in the next section that affect anesthetic vaporization.

Precision Vaporizer

Precision vaporizers (Fig. 3.8) are used with high-vapor-pressure anesthetics and are always found out of the circle. The liquid phase of a high-pressure anesthetic vaporizes easily and quickly and must be delivered in a controlled state. If uncontrolled delivery occurs, the concentration of the drug in the carrier gas could

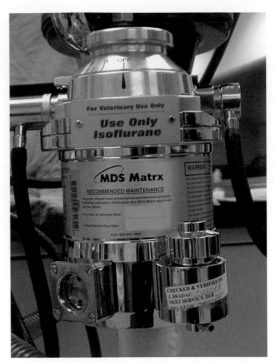

Fig. 3.8 Isoflurane precision vaporizer.

easily become excessive and dangerous. Three factors affect vaporizer function and are compensated for in the precision vaporizer: (1) temperature, (2) gas flow rate, and (3) back pressure. First, if the room temperature is cold, the amount of volatile anesthetic vaporized may be less than the amount indicated on the dial. In a warm room, however, the amount of anesthetic vaporized may be much higher, and therefore a higher level will be delivered to the patient than indicated on the dial setting. The precision vaporizer is constructed with insulation to the liquid anesthetic chamber, so the problems with temperature are eliminated.

The second factor that the precision vaporizer compensates for is the carrier gas flow rate. The O_2 flow rate can affect the amount of vaporized anesthetic delivered to the patient. Extremely high flows (>10 L/min) or extremely low flows (<500 mL/min) are difficult to compensate for, and therefore they should not be used routinely. In a vaporizer that is compensated, the amount of vaporized gas will match the amount indicated on the dial. As the O_2 flow rate is reduced from 300 to 200 to 100 mL/min, the reliability of the dial setting becomes more questionable. Because the flow is reduced, less fresh gas is being delivered. Even though the amount of vaporized gas being sent to the circuit is constant, the amount of gas delivered to the patient is reduced. Vaporizer settings for lower O_2 flow rates need to be adjusted to deliver the amount of anesthetic gas that is actually desired. Newer precision vaporizers compensate for the carrier gas flow and will deliver the amount of anesthetic agent selected on the dial.

The third factor affecting vaporizer function and compensation is **back pressure** (increased pressure in the circuit). Vaporizers exposed to pressurized gas may release additional anesthetic agent, increasing the concentration in the circuit. This occurs when a patient is "bagged." Modern precision vaporizers are designed to adjust for any increase in pressure so that the amount of anesthetic released is not affected.

Precision vaporizers are designed to eliminate or reduce the effect of these three factors on the liquid anesthetic and its vaporization. Precision vaporizers have a dial that shows, in a percent unit, the amount of anesthetic that is being delivered to the circuit.

Unidirectional Inspiratory Valve

The unidirectional inspiratory valve, also called the inspiration valve or inspiratory flutter valve, is a component of anesthesia machines designed to allow movement of gases in only one direction (Fig. 3.9A). It consists of a thin, plastic circular piece (wafer) that moves each time the patient inspires. As the patient inspires, the gases are moved through this valve, then through corrugated tubing, and are delivered via the endotracheal tube to the patient. When the patient inspires, this valve opens, and it closes when the patient exhales, allowing for a one-way or unidirectional flow of gases.

Negative-Pressure Relief Valve

The next part in many anesthesia machines is the negative-pressure relief valve (Fig. 3.9B). This valve is primarily intended as a safety device. If negative pressure is detected in the system, this valve will allow room air to enter the system. Negative pressure may occur, for example, if the oxygen source is empty. Without this safety device, the patient would be without oxygen. The negative-pressure relief valve allows room air into the system, thereby providing 21% O_2 rather than no O_2. Negative pressure may also result if an active scavenging system is being used with the vacuum set too high or if the O_2 flow rate is too low.

Corrugated Breathing Tubing and Y Piece

Gases pass through the tubing as the patient inspires and expires. This corrugated tubing is available in a variety of materials, lengths, and diameters. Although there is no formula to determine the size of tubing to use, shorter tubing with a smaller diameter generally is used for smaller patients, weighing 7 to 20 kg. Larger tubing is used with patients weighing more than 20 kg. It is important to remember that this tubing is not unidirectional; tube ends can be placed on either the inspiratory valve or the expiratory valve. The unidirectional valves determine gas flow direction. The tubes come together at a Y piece that connects to the patient either via the endotracheal tube or mask.

Unidirectional Expiratory Valve

The unidirectional expiratory valve, expiratory flutter valve, functions on the same premise as the inspiratory valve, except it works with expired gases (Fig. 3.9C). As the patient exhales, the gases travel though the corrugated tubing to the unidirectional expiratory valve. As with the inspiratory valve, a wafer of plastic moves as the expired gases pass through the valve. The movement of these two valves may indicate the patient's respiration for the anesthetist.

Adjustable Pressure Relief Valve ("Pop-Off" Valve)

The adjustable pressure relief valve, or pop-off valve, is generally located close to the unidirectional expiratory valve (Fig. 3.9D). The pop-off valve has several functions in the anesthesia machine. First, it can act as a vent. When in the completely open position, the pop-off valve prevents buildup of pressure in the system. This is important because if pressure builds up in the system, the alveoli of the lungs expand and may rupture, leading to atelectasis. Second, the pop-off valve can be used to determine flow rate techniques (e.g., low flow). When varying degrees of "open" are used (i.e., the pop-off valve is partially opened), different O_2 flow rates can be used. Higher flow rates need to be used with a wide-open pop-off valve, and lower flow rates can be used with the valve partially closed or "closed," meaning mostly closed. (The only time the pop-off valve should be completely closed is when "bagging" the patient, and even then it is only temporarily closed because the patient cannot breathe against a closed pop-off valve.) Any level of closure is dangerous because the pressure may build in the system and cause alveolar damage.

Manometer

The manometer is the pressure gauge of the anesthesia machine (Fig. 3.9E). This component only measures the pressure in the system; the manometer does not regulate the pressure. The pressure reading of the system, as indicated by the manometer, is useful information because it gives the anesthetist a good indication of the pressure in the patient's lungs. The unit of measure for the manometer, most commonly, is in centimeters of water (cm H_2O). Some manometers may have a double scale, one in cm H_2O and the other in millimeters of mercury (mm Hg). Personnel must be careful to read the correct scale because the graduations between the units are not the same and therefore display different information. For example, 20 mm Hg of pressure is approximately at the same graduation as 33 cm H_2O, but a reading of 33 cm H_2O is a dangerous pressure for a patient. It is a rare situation that would require the pressure reading on the manometer to exceed 20 cm H_2O, even when bagging the patient. Normal resting pressure, with the pop-off valve

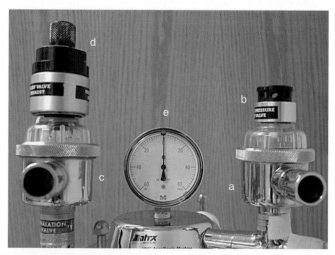

Fig. 3.9 Anesthesia machine components: (a), unidirectional inspiratory valve; (b), negative-pressure relief valve; (c), unidirectional expiratory valve; (d), pop-off valve; (e), manometer.

open, should read 0 cm H$_2$O. The manometer and the pop-off valve have a direct relationship; the more closed the pop-off valve, the higher the pressure reading on the manometer.

Rebreathing Bag (Reservoir Bag)

The rebreathing bag or reservoir bag is a rubber bag that may serve different purposes depending on the circuit with which it is being used. One purpose, when the bag is being used with a rebreathing system, is to allow the patient to rebreathe some of the exhaled gases stored in the rebreathing bag. The level of fullness of the bag adjusts as the gases enter and leave the circuit. The bag deflates as the patient inspires and inflates as the patient expires. This movement may be a good indication of respiratory rate that the anesthetist can monitor. An indirect level of respiratory quality can also be assessed on the basis of how much of the bag is deflated with each breath (i.e., shallow breaths are evident as barely moving the bag).

Another purpose of the rebreathing bag, regardless of the circuit, is to allow manual ventilation of the patient, bagging. Whether as an alveolar expanding sigh or as a resuscitative measure, being able to provide manual ventilation to the patient is essential. When providing artificial ventilation, the first step is to close the pop-off valve. Then the rebreathing bag is squeezed to a pressure no greater than 20 cm H$_2$O on the manometer, and the pop-off valve is immediately opened. It is important to ventilate the patient with as normal a respiratory character as possible. For example, a pattern of longer inspiration and then quick expiration best simulates a normal breath.

With the rebreathing bag storing excess gases and providing backup quantities of gases to be inspired, the proper size bag must be used. One formula to calculate bag size is simple and relies on the tidal volume of the patient (Box 3.1). Tidal volume is calculated as 10 mL/kg of body weight and is the volume of air inhaled during a normal breath at rest. That volume is then multiplied by a factor of 5 to ensure that enough gas will be available for the patient in the event of a full, deep breath. Another formula takes the patient's body weight in pounds and multiplies it by a factor of 30 to determine the correct bag size.

Rebreathing bags are available in several sizes, ranging from 0.25 to 5.0 L for small patients (Fig. 3.10). After calculating the volume needed, the bag is selected. If the calculation does not correspond to a bag size, round up to the next size to ensure the minimum volume required is provided (see Box 3.2 for examples).

Carbon Dioxide Absorber

As the patient exhales, the waste gases pass either to the carbon dioxide (CO$_2$) absorber or to the scavenger. The CO$_2$ absorber is a canister that contains a material made of either barium hydroxide lime (Baralyme, A-M Systems, Everett, WA) or sodium

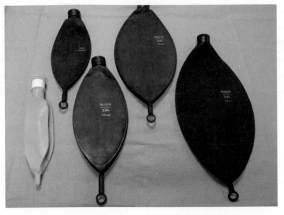

Fig. 3.10 Various rebreathing bags.

> **BOX 3.2   Examples of Rebreathing Bag Calculations**
>
> **Example 1: 40 kg Patient**
>
> 5 × (40 kg × 10 mL/kg) = Volume (mL)
> 5 × 400 mL = Volume (mL)
>
> 2000 mL, or 2 L
> Use a 3-L rebreathing bag because the volume needed is equal to bag size.
> *or*
> 40 kg = 88 lb
> 88 lb × 30 = 2640 mL, or a 3-L bag
>
> **Example 2: 16 kg Patient**
>
> 5 × (16 kg × 10 mL/kg) = Volume (mL)
> 5 × 160 mL = Volume (mL)
>
> 800 mL
> Use a 1 L rebreathing bag because 800 mL is less than 1000 mL (1 L).
> *or*
> 16 kg = 35.2 lb
> 35.2 lb = 1056 mL or a 1-L bag

---

hydroxide lime (Sodasorb, WR Grace, Columbia, MD). The crystals absorb the exhaled CO$_2$, and the resulting chemical reaction produces heat, water, and a color change. The crystals have a pH indicator added to allow for the color change. Once the crystals have undergone the chemical reaction, they are depleted. Fresh crystals are easily crushed, but depleted crystals are very hard and may exhibit a color change from white to violet (Fig. 3.11). When isoflurane is used, the color change may be evident only while the crystals are exposed to the anesthetic gas. Once the vaporizer is turned off, the color will disappear. Crystals should be disposed of and replenished when no more than ⅓ to ½ of the crystals in the canister display a color change. The hours of use should be tracked, rather than using a set time frame of every week or every two weeks, to determine when to replenish the crystals. Crystals should be changed after six to eight hours of use regardless of color change.

When the crystals are replaced, the old material can be disposed of in the regular trash. Local health departments may have other guidelines or ordinances; these can be consulted if disposal options are unclear. New crystals should be added to

---

> **BOX 3.1   Calculation for Size of Rebreathing Bag**
>
> 5 × Tidal volume = Bag size in milliliters (mL)
> Tidal volume calculated as 10 mL/kg of body weight
> *or*
> Body weight in pounds × 30 = Bag size in milliliters (mL)

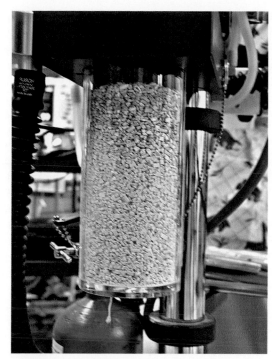

Fig. 3.11 Carbon dioxide (CO$_2$) canister. The machine is in use with a patient attached. Partially depleted crystals are evident by the color change at the top of the canister.

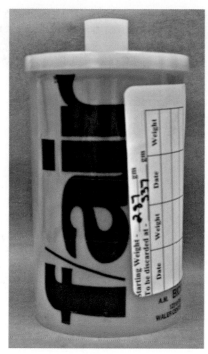

Fig. 3.12 Activated-charcoal scavenger canister for waste anesthetic gas.

the canister in increments, and the canister should be shaken to settle the crystals. About half an inch of air space is left at the top of the canister to allow proper gas flow over the crystals.

Scavenging System

It is important to use some type of system to evacuate waste gases (WAGs) from the anesthesia machine and out of the surgery suite. Two types of scavenging systems are available, active and passive. Active scavenging systems are mechanical devices attached to the anesthesia machine and then connected to a general building source that produces a vacuum to remove the gases. These systems are generally incorporated into the building plans for a new facility. The centrally located vacuum in this system removes the gases from the anesthesia machine and then evacuates the waste out of the building. Anesthesia machines require a local vacuum control on the machine as well as hosing to connect to the central source, similar to the oxygen hose used to connect with the general oxygen source.

Passive scavenging systems rely on gravity to remove the gases from the system. Anesthetic gases are the heaviest of the expired gases and naturally gravitate to the lowest point. Tubing attached to the pop-off valve can carry the anesthetic waste gas either to an activated-charcoal canister attached to the base (Fig. 3.12) or stand of the machine or to an outside wall vent. Wherever the canisters are attached, it is important that they be suspended so that air can circulate through the vents found on the bottom of the canisters. If the canisters are placed on the floor, these vents are effectively plugged. To ensure that the canister is effectively scavenging the waste gases, its use needs to be monitored and documented. The canister should be weighed

with a gram scale before its first use and before being suspended on the machine. After each use, or on a set schedule, the canister should be reweighed, and the weight recorded on the canister. Once the unit has gained 50 grams (g) from the initial weight, it should be disposed of because it will no longer adequately absorb the waste gas. Canisters can be disposed of in the regular trash. Hoses from the pop-off valve that attach to an outside wall vent should be no longer than 20 feet; longer hoses would compromise the system's function. Scavenging to a vent limits the mobility of the anesthesia machine, but this arrangement is appropriate if the machine remains in the same area all the time. Scavenging of waste gas to the floor without any type of collection or evacuation is unsafe and should not be done.

Leak Testing

Properly functioning equipment is extremely important in anesthesia. Technicians are responsible for maintaining equipment and should take this responsibility seriously. In addition to the use of a scavenging system, leak testing the machine aids in reducing or eliminating any gas that may be inappropriately leaving the system. (It is sometimes referred to as a low pressure test because it tests for leaks in the circuit where the pressure has been reduced.) Before every use, the anesthesia machine should be leak tested. If the machine was cleaned or replenished or if hoses or bags were changed, the potential exists for a leak in the system. Box 3.3 outlines the steps for performing a machine leak test. Machine leak tests should be performed only with a rebreathing circuit.

Any area on the machine has the potential for leaking, but some sites are more likely than others to develop leaks. One of the first places to check is the pop-off valve. This valve must be completely closed when doing the leak check. If the pop-off

BOX 3.3   Steps for Performing an Anesthesia Machine Leak Test

1. Connect oxygen hose to oxygen source or turn on local oxygen source.
2. Attach circuit to be used.
3. Check vaporizer for adequate level of liquid anesthetic.
4. Securely occlude patient end of circuit with thumb or palm of hand.
5. Completely close pop-off valve.
6. Depress fast flush valve until a pressure reading of 40 cm H_2O registers on the manometer.
7. Observe needle of manometer for declining movement, which would indicate a leak.
8. If there is no leak, proceed to step 12.
9. If there is a leak, turn on oxygen flow to 200 mL/min.
10. If leak is corrected—indicated by a stable needle on the manometer—no further action is needed. Proceed to step 12.
11. If leak is not corrected, perform machine maintenance to determine location of leak (see text for possible locations of leak). Correct leak.
12. Without removing the occlusion from the patient end of the circuit, open the pop-off valve. The rebreathing bag should deflate.
13. Remove hand or thumb from circuit end.
14. Check scavenging system to ensure that connections are intact.
15. Completely open pop-off valve.

valve is left open, there is no way for pressure to build up in the system. Even if the pop-off valve is only partially closed, a leak will result, so complete closure of this valve is critical. Another common place for leaks is the rebreathing bag or the corrugated hosing. Many of these products are intended as single-use items, but the economics of veterinary medicine often dictate their reuse. Anesthetic gas can degrade the integrity of the rubber in these items, and areas of thinning or microscopic holes can develop. If the leak is isolated to the bag or hoses, these items should be discarded and replaced with new equipment. Another place for a leak is the occluding of the Y piece. If the Y piece is not fully occluded with a finger or the palm of the hand, a leak may persist.

Other, more subtle areas of the anesthesia machine that may leak include the metal rings on the inspiratory and expiratory valves. If removed or loosened for cleaning purposes, the rings may not have been securely replaced and fully tightened. Another place for a leak is the CO_2 absorber. When the canister is removed to replenish the crystals, the tightening mechanism may easily be left a little loose. Finally, all the tubing on the machine is continually exposed to the detrimental effects of anesthetic gas, which may lead to small, barely detectable holes in the tubing.

Regardless of the location of the leak, it needs to be corrected before the machine is used.

Breathing Circuits

The size of the patient determines the breathing circuit that should be used to deliver anesthetic gases. There are two types of circuits: rebreathing and nonrebreathing that can further be subdivided into semi-closed, closed, semi-open, and open depending on the amount of expired gases that are recirculated into the system.

Rebreathing Circuit

The rebreathing circuit is useful because it allows the recirculation of some expired anesthetic gases and permits a lower flow of oxygen because some of the gases are rebreathed. This circuit is used with patients that have a body weight greater than 7 kg. The traditional circuit is two corrugated hoses connected at one end by a Y piece (Fig. 3.13A-B). The hosing can be plastic or rubber, and the Y piece can be plastic or metal. The open end of the tubing is placed on the inspiratory and expiratory valve openings on the anesthesia machine.

An alternative to the traditional rebreathing circuit is the Universal F circuit (SurgiVet, Waukesha, WI) (Fig. 3.14). This circuit is used with patients weighing more than 7 kg and offers some distinct advantages over the traditional circuit. The design of the inspiratory tube inside the expiratory tube allows the inspired gases to be warmed by the expired gases surrounding the tube. The single-tube design is also beneficial in offering

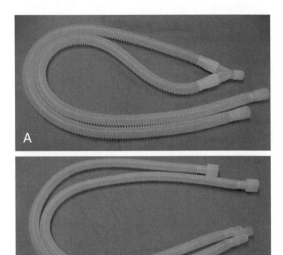

Fig. 3.13 A, Large-diameter rebreathing circuit. B, Small-diameter rebreathing circuit.

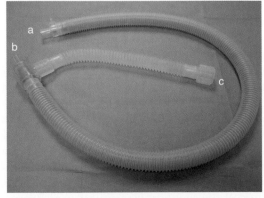

Fig. 3.14 Universal F rebreathing circuit (a), connects to the endotracheal tube; (b), connects to the inspiratory valve; (c), connects to the expiratory valve.

less congestion at the head and mouth. This advantage is especially appreciated during a dental prophylaxis.

The rebreathing circuits can be divided into the semi-closed and **closed systems** based on the amount of exhaled gases that are allowed to reenter the system for rebreathing.

The **semi-closed system** is the most common rebreathing circuit used in veterinary medicine. The pop-off valve is open and allows for the escape of most of the exhaled gas to the scavenger system. There is partial rebreathing of expired gases.

The closed system involves the total rebreathing of expired gases. The pop-off valve is closed or almost closed. The patient rebreathes the expired gases after the CO_2 is removed by the absorber. While the system is economical, has lower flow rate and lower vaporizer settings, and is environmentally safe as WAGs are not released, it can pose dangers for the patient. Because the patient is rebreathing expired gases, there is the possibility of oxygen depletion; because the pop off is closed, there can be a dangerous increase in the pressure in the system. Therefore constant monitoring is required.

Nonrebreathing Circuit

The nonrebreathing circuit is used so that none or very little of the gases are rebreathed. Patients weighing less than 7 kg benefit the most from the use of this circuit because of the low gas resistance. The use of this circuit requires a high flow of oxygen to ensure adequate levels of anesthetic. The CO_2 absorber and pressure manometer are bypassed.

A major advantage of the nonrebreathing system is that it has low resistance for breathing for the patient. Fresh gases are constantly being provided to the patient with minimal effort required of the patient. The design and high flows of the nonrebreathing system allow the gases to be delivered at the endotracheal tube, and the patient merely breathes a normal respiration and takes in fresh, new gases.

Nonbreathing circuits come in several configurations. They are organized using the Mapleson classification system, A-F. These include the Magill circuit, Ayre's T-piece, and Bain coaxial circuit. Fig. 3.15 shows two examples of nonrebreathing circuits.

There are disadvantages to the **semi-open system**. Patients lose moisture and body heat more readily due to the increased oxygen flow rate. There is no conservation of gases and manual ventilation is difficult.

The Bain circuit may be mounted to a device called a universal control arm or Bain Block. This device has a reservoir bag, pop-off valve, and pressure manometer (Fig. 3.16).

Mask and tank induction are other types of nonrebreathing circuits. They are considered **open systems** and do not allow for rebreathing of expired gases. Masks allow for the rapid administration of oxygen and anesthesia to patients that either cannot be intubated or in which intubation may be delayed. Anesthesia chambers are used in induction for patients that are intractable or that would experience extensive stress with handling.

Both open systems have several disadvantages. They do not maintain an open airway and do not protect against aspiration. Additionally chamber induction does not allow for close monitoring of the patient.

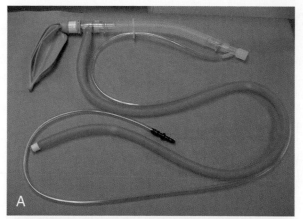
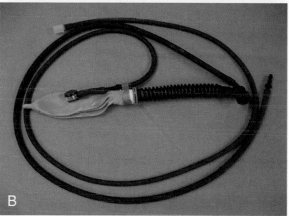

Fig. 3.15 A, Modified Jackson Reese nonrebreathing circuit. B, Modified Mapleson nonrebreathing circuit.

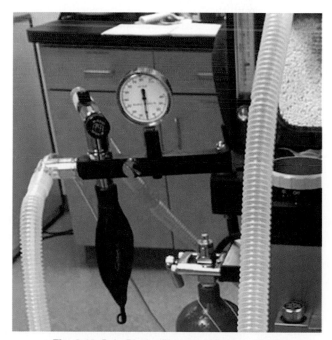

Fig. 3.16 Bain Block. (Photo by Marianne Tear)

OXYGEN FLOW RATES

Depending on the type of breathing circuit and patient needs, appropriate O_2 flow rates should be employed. Providing adequate oxygen to the patient is critical, but using an excessive amount of oxygen is wasteful.

Rebreathing circuits generally use a high O_2 flow rate for induction and recovery, with large-volume delivery of gas. This perpetuates a speedy induction and assists in a quick recovery. Maintenance flows for rebreathing circuits are significantly less than the induction and recovery flow rates. Only enough oxygen to match the patient's tidal volume is needed because, in addition to the fresh gas being supplied, the patient is rebreathing some of the gases already in the system. Usually a buffer is added in calculating the flow to allow for large breaths that may be given to or taken by the patient (Box 3.4).

Nonrebreathing systems also use high O_2 flow rates (see Box 3.4), but the flows remain at a constant high flow whether the patient is undergoing induction, maintaining the desired depth of anesthesia, or recovering. Continuous high flow rates are necessary to provide adequate gases to the patient. Smaller patients cannot rebreathe any of the gases because of the difficulty in moving that much air with each respiration. Fresh gases need to be provided to these patients at all times.

BOX 3.4 Oxygen Flow Rate Values

Rebreathing System: Patients >7 kg*
Induction: 50 to 100 mL/kg/min with a maximum of 5 L/min
Maintenance: 20 to 40 mL/kg/min but not less than 500 mL/min
Recovery: 50 to 100 mL/kg/min with a maximum of 5 L/min
Nonrebreathing Systems: Patients <7 kg†
Induction: 200 mL/kg/min
Maintenance: 200 mL/kg/min
Recovery: 200 mL/kg/min

*Large-breed patients (<60 kg) may require higher induction and recovery flows (3–5 L/min).
†Formulas range with recommendations from 100 to 400 mL/kg/min; however, 200 mL/kg/min is typically used.

CONCLUSION

Anesthesia can be a stressful time for the veterinary technician. However, a thorough understanding of the components of the machine, the flow of gas through the machine, and the options available to deliver the anesthetic gases to the patient can reduce the stress level and can even make surgery a rewarding part of the technician's day.

KEY POINTS

1. Each component of the anesthesia machine has a specific purpose and must be in good working order for the machine to function.
2. The flowmeter reduces the oxygen pressure to the atmospheric pressure of 15 psi, which is well tolerated by the patient.
3. The use of the fast flush valve should be avoided whenever a patient is connected to the anesthetic machine.
4. Only the liquid anesthetic for which a vaporizer has been calibrated should be used in the vaporizer.
5. The pressure reading on the manometer should not exceed 20 cm H_2O when a patient is being ventilated.
6. The CO_2 absorber removes carbon dioxide from the exhaled breath of the patient.
7. Appropriate scavenging of waste anesthetic gas is essential for the safety of the staff.

REVIEW QUESTIONS

1. When reading a flowmeter with a ball float, read where the
   a. point sits.
   b. top of the ball sits.
   c. middle of the ball sits.
   d. bottom of the ball sits.
2. The oxygen flush valve of the anesthetic machine is used to
   a. prevent atelectasis in an anesthetized patient.
   b. increase flow of inhalant anesthetic to the patient.
   c. allow quick infusion of oxygen into the breathing circuit.
   d. improve oxygen flow in a nonrebreathing anesthesia circuit.
3. The function of the vaporizer is to
   a. change the liquid inhalant anesthetic to a gas form.
   b. change the gas inhalant anesthetic to a liquid form.
   c. carry the oxygen needed for respiration into the body.
   d. allows gas flow only one way within the anesthesia circuit.
4. What is the approximate tidal volume of a 40-lb dog?
   a. 180 mL
   b. 400 mL

   c. 900 mL
   d. 1,500 mL
5. Which valve is used for a vent to prevent excessive pressure in the anesthesia system?
   a. Negative-pressure relief valve
   b. Unidirectional expiratory valve
   c. Unidirectional inspiratory valve
   d. Adjustable pressure relief valve
6. The only time the pop-off valve should be closed when a patient is attached to a semi-closed rebreathing anesthesia circuit is when
   a. inducing the patient.
   b. using lower oxygen flow rates.
   c. using higher oxygen flow rates.
   d. the anesthetist is providing manual ventilation.
7. What part of the anesthesia machine measures the pressure in the system?
   a. Flowmeter
   b. Manometer

c. Tank pressure gauge

d. Negative-pressure relief valve

8. Which is the correct flow of oxygen in the anesthesia machine?

a. Oxygen source, pressure-reducing valve, flowmeter, vaporizer, unidirectional expiratory valve, breathing tube, patient

b. Oxygen source, flowmeter, pressure-reducing valve, vaporizer, unidirectional inspiratory valve, breathing tube, patient

c. Oxygen source, pressure-reducing valve, flowmeter, vaporizer, unidirectional inspiratory valve, breathing tube, patient

d. Oxygen source, vaporizer, flowmeter, pressure-reducing valve, unidirectional expiratory valve, breathing tube, patient

9. When should the CO_2 absorbent crystals of an anesthesia machine be changed?

a. Once per week

b. Every 14 days

c. After 6 to 8 hours of use

d. When ¾ of the crystals change color

10. Which part of the anesthesia machine regulates how much oxygen enters the anesthetic circuit?

a. Flowmeter

b. Manometer

c. Pop-off valve

d. Unidirectional inspiratory valve

11. When should a passive waste anesthetic gas canister be disposed of?

a. When the canister weighs 50 g

b. When the canister is ⅓ to ½ full

c. When ½ of the granules have changed color

d. When the canister weighs 50 g more than its initial weight

12. How often should an anesthesia machine be leak tested?

a. Daily

b. Before each use

c. Once per week

d. Once per month

13. When manual ventilation is being performed, the pop-off valve should be

a. opened and remain open after the manual ventilation breath is complete.

b. open and then closed after the manual ventilation breath is complete.

c. closed and remain closed after the manual ventilation breath is complete.

d. closed and then opened after the manual ventilation breath is complete.

14. Negative pressure exists in the anesthesia system when

a. using a closed system.

b. the oxygen source is depleted.

c. using chamber induction.

d. high-flow anesthesia is being used.

15. What rebreathing bag would you choose for a 32-lb dog?

a. 0.25 L

b. 0.5 L

c. 1 L

d. 2 L

16. What is the function of oxygen in the anesthesia circuit?

17. What are the three factors that affect vaporizer function?

BIBLIOGRAPHY

Bassert JM, McCurnin DM, editors: *McCurnin's clinical textbook for veterinary technicians*, ed 8, St Louis, 2014, Saunders.

Tear,M, Burcham S: *Practical math for veterinary technicians*, Minneapolis 2019, Bluedoor.

Thomas JA, Lerche P: *Anesthesia and analgesia for veterinary technicians*, ed 5, St Louis, 2017, Mosby.

4

Preoperative Patient Considerations

Megan Terry

LEARNING OBJECTIVES

After completion of this chapter, the reader will be able to:
- Understand the importance of and be able to perform a complete physical examination on the day of a scheduled surgery.
- Know the legal significance of a signed surgical consent form.
- Explain to clients the details in a surgical consent form.
- Collect and analyze preanesthetic diagnostic tests.
- Describe what is considered a minimum database for surgical patients.

- Bring the veterinarian's attention to any abnormal or invalid results.
- Understand the reasons for premedicating surgical patients.
- Explain the importance of preemptive analgesia.
- Describe the drug options available for preemptive analgesia.
- Explain the mechanisms of action of the different types of analgesics.

KEY TERMS

Agonists
Anticholinergic
Auscultation

Balanced anesthesia
Chief complaint
Nociception

Premedication
Prophylaxis
Signalment

HISTORY TAKING

The ability to collect a history that is both concise and chronologically accurate is a skill that takes practice. After the client (owner, guardian) and patient (animal) have been brought into the examination room and introductions have been made, a good starting point for collecting the history is to confirm the patient's signalment. Confirming the patient's age, gender, and reproductive status with the owner, then comparing this information with the patient's medical record, ensures the record's accuracy and clarifies any confusion should a discrepancy be found.

Once the patient's signalment has been established and verified, the client should be asked about the chief complaint (or reason for the visit). This is usually a brief but complete description of the current problem; for example, "HBC [hit by car] 2 days ago and fractured right femur." Once the chief complaint has been established or confirmed, ask the client to explain the sequence of events, starting from the beginning of the particular problem.

While collecting a history, the technician should avoid asking leading questions. Leading questions make the client feel compelled to answer a certain way; for example, "You don't feed your dog anything other than dog food, do you?" The owner feels compelled to answer in the negative because the question is leading toward or encouraging a specific answer. Asking the question in an open-ended format encourages the owner to answer the question truthfully, without prejudice. "What do you feed your dog?" is a nonleading, nonthreatening question that usually yields more useful information than the first example. Follow-up questions should be asked when appropriate. If there is a concern regarding the dog's nutritional status or body condition, it would be appropriate to ask how much and how often the dog is fed, in addition to what the dog is fed. A concluding question for the specific topic is often revealing as well. A final question about the dog's diet could be asked as follows: "Is there anything else your dog eats?" Again, this is a nonleading question and allows the owner to share information that may be helpful or significant.

During the history it is important to review what other treatments have been attempted to address the current problem, including any attempts by the owner to treat the problem at home. In addition, it is important to establish the nature of the treatment and the patient's response to each treatment. A review of the current medications and supplements that the animal may be given, including both over-the-counter (OTC) and prescription medications, and when they were last administered is an important part of the history. Certain medications and supplements may interact with diagnostic tests or pre medications and anesthetic drugs. The owner should also be asked if the patient has experienced any medication or anesthetic reactions and/or seizures in the past as anesthetic protocols may need to be altered due to these past occurrences.

Once the history of the current problem has been thoroughly investigated, a general question about any previous medical problems is appropriate. If a patient has had surgery or medical treatment in the past, additional follow-up questions may be in order. A good way to conclude the history-taking session is to ask the owner whether there is anything else that would be helpful to know but that was not addressed. Occasionally, this general question reminds clients about something else that is relevant to the situation or that they wanted to ask.

Allowing the animal to explore the examination room at will (e.g., letting the cat out of the carrier) during the history taking helps the technician determine the patient's general attitude and condition without even touching it. Most animals will take this opportunity to familiarize themselves with the scents and sounds of the hospital, and they may even relax if given a chance to explore the exam room on their own terms. An observant technician can establish a first impression of the patient's personality and degree of anxiety during the history.

After the history has been collected, the details need to be recorded in chronologic order in the medical record.

PHYSICAL EXAMINATION

The veterinary technician should be adept in the performance of the physical examination (PE), even though veterinarians may elect to perform the PE themselves. The veterinary medical team will consult the PE findings when determining the appropriate anesthetic and surgical protocols. The owner's presence during the PE allows for ongoing communication between the technician or veterinarian and the owner in regard to the findings and provides a historical perspective to unusual findings. This is especially true for any physical findings that might affect the surgical procedure or anesthetic protocols (e.g., retained testicles, pregnancy).

The complete PE should become a routine for the veterinary technician. This routine should be carried out in the same manner every time the PE is performed (e.g., head to tail or by body systems). This approach minimizes the possibility of forgetting to check a vital system and helps ensure patient safety. Being able to perform a complete PE is the first step in being the patient's advocate. The PE reveals the needs of the patient more than any other diagnostic procedure, and knowing their needs is the only way to advocate for patients.

Even if the animal was seen recently, it is imperative that a thorough PE is performed the day of the surgery, ideally with the owner present. The goal of this chapter is not to detail every aspect of a PE, but rather to give an abbreviated overview. Many wonderful textbooks have complete chapters dedicated to performing PEs.

General Body Condition and Mentation

The patient's general body condition (e.g., "strong and healthy" or "weak and emaciated") and mentation (e.g., "bright, alert, and responsive" [BAR] or "dull and depressed") should be observed and noted during the history taking. The patient's ability to see and hear is assessed during the history taking as well. If the patient is clearly distressed or aggressive, it is appropriate to request an assistant and to use a restraint device (e.g., muzzle) before the hands-on portion of the PE. If the patient is scared and timid, a slow, calm, and soft-spoken approach may sufficiently relax and calm the patient to allow for a thorough PE. Any gait abnormalities (lameness, ataxia), muscle atrophy, or asymmetry should be noted while observing the animal during the history taking and should be examined more closely during the hands-on examination.

The complete examination should include an evaluation of the temperature, pulse, and respiration (TPR).

Thoracic Auscultation

Thoracic auscultation requires using a stethoscope to listen to the chest for both heart and lung sounds (Fig. 4.1). The heart and lungs are heard best with the animal standing still on all four legs. A talented veterinary technician will quickly learn how to keep a cooperative animal standing or lying quietly while auscultating the thorax without an assistant (Fig. 4.2). Occasionally it is necessary to prevent a dog from panting or a cat from purring. To stop a dog from panting, use the hand with the wristwatch to extend the neck by gently lifting up on the dog's mandible using the top surface of the hand, while the other hand holds the stethoscope to the patient's chest (Fig. 4.3). Clamping the mouth shut to try to prevent a dog from panting should be avoided as it often results in excessive movement as the dog tries to wriggle out of the technician's grip and creates undo stress for the animal. Most dogs tolerate a gentle lift of the mandible with the top of the hand better and stand quietly long enough to count a heart rate. To stop a cat from purring, it may be necessary to restrain the cat firmly near a sink and turn on the water to a slow stream or hold a cotton ball soaked in 70% isopropyl alcohol near the cat's nose.

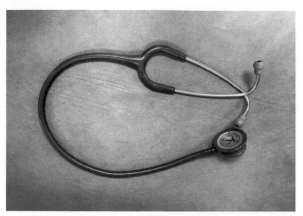

Fig. 4.1 Typical stethoscope, with both diaphragm and bell in chest piece. Swiveling the chest piece determines whether the diaphragm or bell is used for auscultation. Note the curvature in the stems of the earpieces. The stems should be placed in the examiner's ear canals and point toward the nose.

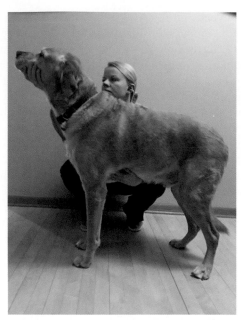

Fig. 4.3 Preventing a dog from panting by using a hand on the mandible to gently extend the head, while auscultating the thorax, helps the examiner hear heart sounds over breath sounds.

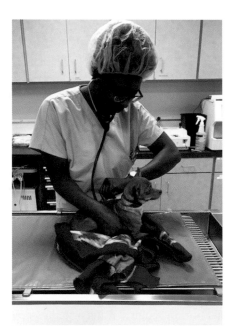

Fig. 4.2 If the patient is cooperative, one technician can easily restrain the patient in sternal recumbency while auscultating the thorax.

Begin auscultating the heart by placing the diaphragm of the stethoscope's chest piece just caudal to the point where the dog's left elbow meets the chest. For cats, a more ventral placement of the chest piece may be necessary to hear the heart best. One heartbeat normally has two sounds; that is, the "lub-dub." Both sounds are audible but signify only one complete heartbeat. Once the distinctive lub-dub heart sounds have been identified, time 15 seconds on a watch and count the number of heartbeats heard. To determine the heart rate, multiply the number of beats heard in 15 seconds by 4; this number is the heart rate in beats per minute. Systolic murmurs are usually heard as a swishing sound between the lub-dub ("lub-shh-dub"). Moving the stethoscope one rib space cranially or caudally may amplify the sound of the murmur. The rib space where the murmur is heard the loudest is the point of maximum intensity (PMI). The rib

space can be identified by counting backward, as the technician moves cranially, from the last (13th) rib. Keep in mind that some murmurs are heard loudest on the right side of the chest. The presence of a murmur and the PMI of the murmur should be noted in the medical record.

The lungs should fill up the pleural space when fully expanded during maximum inhalation. Normal lung sounds should be distinct but soft and free of any wheezing, crackling, and popping sounds. Normal lung sounds should be heard equally well on the left and the right sides of the thorax. Be sure to listen to both sides (cranial and caudal, dorsal and ventral) for lung sounds. One breath is a two-part movement: inhalation and exhalation. To determine the respiratory rate (number of breaths per minute), count the number of breaths in 15 seconds and multiply that number by 4. Any increased effort by the animal to breathe (dyspnea) and any increase or absence of lung sounds must be noted in the medical record and addressed. Usually, addressing respiratory abnormalities includes giving the patient supplemental oxygen. The lungs should be assessed not only for respiratory rate but also for crackles, wheezes, and any other abnormalities. Any abnormalities or noteworthy findings in the PE need to be recorded in the medical record and brought to the attention of the attending veterinarian.

Taking the Temperature

Ideally the temperature is taken rectally with a well-lubricated thermometer. Some patients strongly resist this part of the PE, and therefore taking the temperature should be saved for the end of the examination so that the patient may be more cooperative for most of the PE. Most digital thermometers emit a series of audible beeps within 60 seconds to indicate that the final temperature has been recorded (Fig. 4.4). It is important

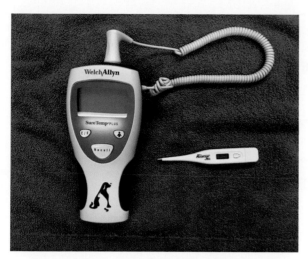

Fig. 4.4 Digital thermometers.

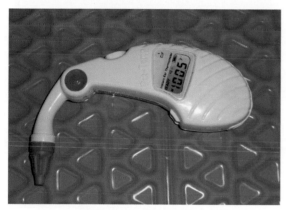

Fig. 4.5 Ear thermometer.

to use a thermometer that registers a wide range of temperatures for accurate diagnosis of hypothermia and hyperthermia cases.

If it is not possible to take the temperature rectally, an aural temperature measurement can be taken. There are several styles of ear thermometers on the market. Ear thermometers read the temperature of the tympanic membrane using infrared technology. The probe sits several millimeters off the eardrum as it records the temperature. This space and the shape of the animal's ear canal can lead to inaccurate readings (Fig. 4.5).

CONSENT FORM

A consent form is a piece of paper that identifies the patient (name, signalment, and descriptors such as hair coat color and body weight), the specific procedures to be performed along with the potential risks to the patient associated with the surgery and anesthesia, and the veterinarian(s) who will perform the procedures. The owner's information (name, address and phone number) may be contained on this form as well. The consent form requires the signature of the owner consenting to the procedures. Many clinics offer an estimate of costs with a low-end and high-end range directly on the consent form. Because the consent form contains such important information, a

veterinary technician familiar with the surgical procedure should review the form in detail, typically line by line, with the owner at completion of the PE. This gives the owner the opportunity to ask any last-minute questions about the procedure before the animal is admitted to the hospital. Open and clear communication is essential to avoid any confusion and to prevent miscommunication that could lead to legal complaints later. Many legal complaints originate with poor or rushed attempts at client communication.

Descriptions of the procedures should be written out and should be all inclusive; that is, everything that will be done to the animal needs to be listed. This form also should document whether or not the patient was fasted appropriately, include a notation that the owner received an estimate for the procedures to be performed, and provide a way of contacting the owner during the time the procedures will be performed. It is extremely important that the owner can be contacted during the procedure, should the need arise (Fig. 4.6). One such consent form suggested the owner provide a phone number where he or she could be reached within 2 minutes in case of emergency.

PREANESTHETIC DIAGNOSTIC TESTS

With the ever-increasing standards of care in veterinary medicine and the owner's expectations for the surgical patient's optimum health care, the minimum preanesthetic diagnostic database, or minimum database (MDB), is continually growing in scope. Information collected in the history and PE help determine which diagnostic tests should be performed before the patient is anesthetized. What is considered the MDB for an elective surgical procedure on a young, healthy animal is different than the MDB for a procedure on a geriatric patient with preexisting health problems. The MDB results may suggest that additional diagnostics are indicated or that the original anesthetic protocol may have to be amended.

Minimum Database

A minimum database for a young, healthy surgical candidate should include a packed cell volume (PCV), total solids (TS), blood glucose (BG), blood urea nitrogen (BUN), and alanine aminotransferase (ALT). These tests should be considered a starting point, and other diagnostic tests should be performed if any of these four basic parameters cause any concern. These tests are generally easy to run, can usually be performed as point-of-care or in-house tests, and require only a small amount of blood. With minimal time and effort, much useful information can be gained from these tests. Several laboratories and in-house analyzer companies sell packaged preanesthetic test panels, making the process even easier.

Packed Cell Volume (Hematocrit)

The packed cell volume (PCV), or hematocrit (HCT), is the percentage of whole blood that is made up of red blood cells (RBCs). Low PCVs are found in cases of decreased RBC production (as in chronic renal failure), decreased RBC life span (as with some autoimmune diseases and parasite infections), and blood loss (secondary to trauma, blood-clotting disorders,

DATE_____ CASE NUMBER_____

COMPANION ANIMAL CLIENT/PATIENT INFORMATION FORM

Please provide the following information for our records: **PLEASE PRINT!**

OWNER INFORMATION

OWNER'S NAME	SOCIAL SECURITY NUMBER

STREET ADDRESS

CITY STATE	ZIP CODE	PARISH OR COUNTY

TELEPHONE NUMBER(S) (Area Code, if long distance) ➔	HOME	BUSINESS

DRIVER'S LICENSE NUMBER	PLACE OF EMPLOYMENT	HOW LONG?

ANIMAL INFORMATION

ANIMAL SPECIES (Dog, Cat, Other)	BREED

ANIMAL'S NAME	SEX	HAS ANIMAL BEEN SEXUALLY ALTERED? ☐ Yes ☐ No

COLOR	BIRTHDATE (Month/year, or approximate)	The undersigned owner or agent certifies that the herein described animal has a maximum value of approximately **$**

REFERRAL INFORMATION

WERE YOU REFERRED BY A VETERINARIAN? ☐ Yes ☐ No	IF YOU WERE REFERRED BY A VETERINARIAN, PLEASE COMPLETE THE FOLLOWING:

VETERINARIAN'S NAME	PHONE

STREET ADDRESS

CITY/STATE	ZIP CODE

You will be advised of estimated cost and anticipated procedures. Please feel free to discuss the proposed treatment and its cost with the veterinarian. A minimum deposit of 50% of the initial estimated charges will be required for hospitalization of an animal patient.

STATEMENT OF OWNERSHIP AND CONSENT: I am the owner of the above described animal, or have authorization from the owner to consent to its treatment.

I hereby authorize the performance of professionally accepted diagnostic, therapeutic, anesthetic, and surgical procedures necessary for its treatment.

I accept financial responsibility for these services.

I have read the above consent and understand why the above procedures may be necessary. I also have been told of the possible complications and alternatives to the listed procedures.

PAYMENT CHOICE: ☐ Cash ☐ Check ☐ Bank Card

SIGNATURE (Owner/Agent)	DATE

Fig. 4.6 Companion animal client and patient information form. (From Bassert JM, Thomas JA, editors: *McCurnin's clinical textbook for veterinary technicians*, ed 8, St Louis, 2014, Saunders.)

or gastric ulcers). Increased PCV may indicate dehydration (common) or absolute polycythemia (rare). Any values outside the normal ranges need to be brought to the attending clinician's attention.

Checking a PCV requires microhematocrit tubes, a tube sealant (e.g., Critoseal), a centrifuge, and a hematocrit card reader (Fig. 4.7). If whole blood is collected in a syringe without an anticoagulant, heparinized microhematocrit tubes should be used for this test. If blood is collected into a heparinized syringe or placed in a Vacutainer tube with anticoagulant (ethylenediaminetetraacetic acid [EDTA]) in it, a plain microhematocrit tube should be used. Glass microhematocrit tubes are generally easier to work with than the plastic variety.

After spinning the microhematocrit tube for the appropriate time in the centrifuge (Fig. 4.8), the tube is placed on the card reader. Line up the top of the clay sealant with the 0% line on the card reader. Roll the tube across the card until the top of the plasma lines up with the 100% line on the card. Read the percentage line that crosses the point where the packed RBCs are separated from the plasma, at the buffy coat; this percentage is the PCV (Fig. 4.9). The buffy coat usually appears as a small

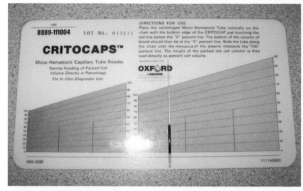

Fig. 4.9 To read packed cell volume (PCV) on a card, line the top of the clay sealant on the 0% line and the top of the plasma on the 100% line. PCV is read on the line where plasma and packed red blood cells meet. On this sample, PCV is approximately 40%.

column of white between the packed RBCs below it and the clear plasma above it. The buffy coat contains white blood cells (WBCs), nucleated red blood cells (nRBCs), and platelets. The area just above the buffy coat can be examined under a microscope to perform a heartworm screening for live microfilaria. The packed cell volume is also routinely performed while running a complete blood cell count (CBC) with an automated hematology analyzer.

Normal Range of Packed Cell Volume
• Canine: 37% to 55%
• Feline: 30% to 45%

Plasma is the liquid (noncellular) component of blood that separates out from the packed RBCs after whole blood is placed in a microhematocrit tube, sealed with the clay, and spun in a centrifuge. Normally, plasma is clear and colorless. If the plasma has any color, the color should be noted next to where the PCV percentage is recorded in the medical record and brought to the attention of the veterinarian.

Total Solids or Proteins

Total solids (TS) or total proteins (TP) provide information on the animal's plasma protein levels. There are three major plasma proteins: albumin, globulin, and fibrinogen. These levels have a direct effect on serum oncotic pressure. The lower the TP value, the lower the serum oncotic pressure. Changes in serum oncotic pressure directly affect changes in the patient's fluid shifts between the interstitium and the vasculature. With a low serum oncotic pressure, fluid tends to accumulate in the interstitium, resulting in edema. On the other hand, with a high serum oncotic pressure, fluid shifts out of the interstitium and back into the vasculature (blood vessels).

Elevated plasma protein values are associated with dehydration, malignancies (e.g., lymphosarcoma), and infections. Decreased plasma protein values are associated with inadequate production (albumin is made in the liver), inadequate intake (starvation), increased loss (renal disease, blood loss, parasites), and inadequate absorption from the gastrointestinal tract (pancreatic disease, inflammatory bowel disease).

In addition, plasma protein levels are important because some anesthetics (e.g., some barbiturates) are highly bound to

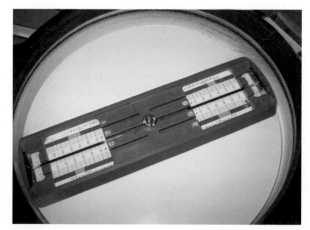

Fig. 4.7 Heparinized (red) and plain (blue) microhematocrit tubes (top), packed cell volume (PCV) card reader (bottom left), and clay to seal blood in microhematocrit tube (bottom right).

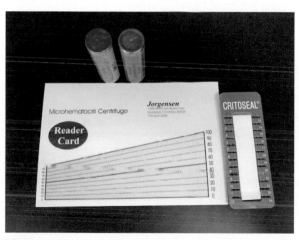

Fig. 4.8 Place microhematocrit tube in centrifuge with clay plug toward the outside.

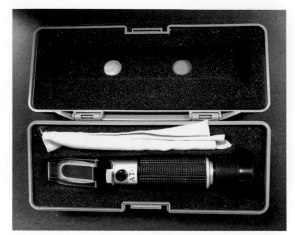

Fig. 4.10 A refractometer is needed to determine the total solids in plasma.

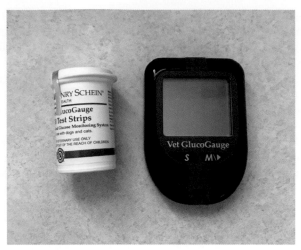

Fig. 4.11 A small glucose meter can be purchased from most veterinary distributors; shown is Vet GlucoGauge (Henry Schein Animal Health, Dublin, OH).

proteins. If a patient is hypoproteinemic, more free drug (not bound to plasma proteins) will be available to function as an anesthetic, effectively increasing the dose. Therefore, the animal's protein levels should be noted when deciding which anesthetics to use because the anesthetic dose may need to be adjusted accordingly.

Supplies needed to check plasma proteins include a refractometer (Fig. 4.10) and microhematocrit tubes. After the PCV level is checked, snap the glass microhematocrit tube in the area of the plasma column. Take care not to touch or scratch the prism cover glass of the refractometer with the sharp edges of the microhematocrit tube. Allow the plasma to drip onto the refractometer out of the microhematocrit tube. The TP level is read on the scale seen in the refractometer. It is important to read the appropriate scale within the refractometer as many refractometers are used to read urine specific gravity as well. Total protein can also be analyzed using commercial blood chemistry analyzers as well.

Normal Range of Total Protein
- Canine: 5.4 to 7.5 g/dL
- Feline: 5.7 to 7.6 g/dL

Blood Glucose

Blood glucose (BG) levels indicate carbohydrate metabolism and measure the endocrine function of the pancreas. Eating raises BG levels, and fasting lowers them. Stress will elevate BG levels in cats. In juvenile patients and diabetic patients, BG values may need to be checked preoperatively, intraoperatively, and postoperatively if the procedure is especially long.

Glucometers are available at most pharmacies and are easy to use (Fig. 4.11). Usually, only a drop of fresh whole blood is required. Some glucometers (e.g., Vet GlucoGauge, Covetrus Animal Health, Dublin, OH) can determine BG levels using whole blood collected in EDTA or heparin, two types of anticoagulants, but they will not accurately measure BG in serum. It is important to use recently collected blood because glucose values are affected by how long the blood sits before it is analyzed. Likewise, it is important to follow the manufacturer's guidelines and directions. Any invalid results should be addressed (e.g., repeat with another sample), and any abnormal

results should be brought to the attending veterinarian's attention and addressed. Blood glucose can also be evaluated using a commercial blood chemistry analyzer.

Normal Range of Blood Glucose
- Canine: 76 to 120 mg/dL
- Feline: 58 to 120 mg/dL

For both canine and feline patients, less than 40 mg/dL indicates hypoglycemia.

Blood Urea Nitrogen

Urea is a nitrogenous compound that is a product of amino acid breakdown in the liver. BUN levels are used to evaluate the kidney's ability to remove nitrogenous wastes (urea) from the blood. If the kidneys are not working properly or if the patient is dehydrated, an insufficient amount of urea is removed from the plasma, resulting in increased BUN levels.

An estimate of the patient's BUN value can be assessed quickly using a reagent strip (e.g., Azostix, Siemens Healthcare Diagnostics, Washington, DC; Fig. 4.12). Blood mixed with the anticoagulants EDTA or heparin (not containing an ammonium salt) will not affect the estimated BUN of an Azostix; however, neither serum nor plasma should be used for this test. Supplies needed to check BUN on a reagent strip include the reagent strip, a fresh blood sample, a watch with a second hand, and a strong stream of water to rinse the strip. The color change on the reagent strip is compared with the color scale on the bottle for the strips. The corresponding color match between the reagent strip and the bottle indicates the estimated BUN (Fig. 4.13). Because this method tends to be less accurate, it should only be used as a quick screening test. Photometric tests for the measurement of BUN have an acceptable level of accuracy and precision.

Some anesthetics are primarily metabolized by the kidneys; if there is any question regarding the patient's renal function, choosing a drug that is not primarily metabolized by the kidneys ought to be considered. Further diagnostic tests assessing kidney function (e.g., urinalysis, blood creatinine level) should be considered as well.

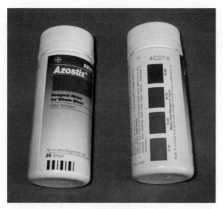

Fig. 4.12 Bottle of reagent strips (Azostix, Siemens Healthcare Diagnostics, Washington, DC) used to estimate blood urea nitrogen (BUN); color scale is used to estimate BUN value.

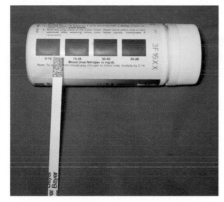

Fig. 4.13 Comparing sample reagent strip with color scale on bottle provides estimated blood urea nitrogen (BUN) level.

Normal Range of Blood Urea Nitrogen
- Canine: 9 to 27 mg/dL
- Feline: 18 to 34 mg/dL

Alanine Aminotransferase

Alanine aminotransferase (ALT) is an enzyme found in high concentration in the liver cells of dogs, cats, and primates. Damage to hepatocytes can elevate blood ALT levels. Certain drugs, such as anticonvulsants and corticosteroids, can also raise blood levels. ALT, although not indicative of specific liver disease, can be used as a general hepatic screen. The patient's ALT level can be assessed using a commercial blood chemistry analyzer.

Normal Range of Alanine Aminotransferase
- Canine: 8.2 to 109 U/L
- Feline: 25 to 97 U/L

Additional Tests

Other diagnostic tests specific to the patient's history and PE findings should be performed before any surgery. Generally, preanesthetic diagnostics are noninvasive and may eliminate ("rule out") the need for more invasive procedures. However, these diagnostic tests may support the need for additional, more invasive diagnostics or procedures. For example, the logical progression of diagnostic testing for a puppy with vomiting

and diarrhea would start with an intestinal parasite test ("fecal") and a parvovirus ("parvo") test, followed by abdominal radiographs, then an abdominal ultrasound, and finally an abdominal exploratory procedure. In addition, the puppy with vomiting and diarrhea should receive a CBC, serum chemistry panel, and electrolyte panel to aid in determining what type of intravenous fluid or additional support (e.g., antibiotics, parenteral nutrition, plasma transfusion) is indicated.

It is important to note that preanesthetic diagnostic tests will not be the same for every patient and that not all preanesthetic diagnostics are limited to blood tests (e.g., CBC; serum chemistry, electrolyte, thyroid, and clotting panels; heartworm, feline immunodeficiency virus, and feline leukemia virus tests; blood cultures). For example, intestinal parasite tests, radiographs, diagnostic ultrasounds, urinalyses, and electrocardiograms may need to be performed before surgery on certain patients, depending on the history and PE findings.

PREOPERATIVE MEDICATIONS

Once all the preanesthetic diagnostic tests have been performed and analyzed, if the results still indicate that surgery is necessary and is the appropriate next step, the patient is premedicated for anesthesia.

Surgical patients are routinely premedicated with a combination of agents, including analgesics and sedatives. The purpose of administering these agents before induction is threefold. First, the patient is more relaxed, allowing a less stressful transition to anesthesia. Second, pain management is provided at the optimum time, before surgical tissue trauma occurs. Third, appropriate premedications ("premeds") ease the transition out of anesthesia, facilitating a smooth recovery.

Balanced Anesthesia

Premedication is an important part of balanced anesthesia. The objective of balanced anesthesia is to combine several agents, in smaller dosages, to maximize the positive effects, such as analgesia and muscle relaxation, while minimizing the negative effects, such as cardiac and respiratory depression. The goal is to calm the patient, minimize pain, and reduce the adverse effects of the agents used (Box 4.1).

Principles of Pain Management

The basic principles of current pain management involve (1) preemptive (preventive) analgesia, (2) multimodal analgesia (using different classes of drugs simultaneously to interrupt the pain pathway at various points), and (3) appropriate follow-up analgesia. Using this strategy, veterinarians design an analgesic

BOX 4.1   **Components of Balanced Anesthesia**
Premedication
Induction
Maintenance
Recovery—pain medication

plan for each patient that maximizes pain control, keeps patients on an analgesic plane, and reduces unwanted side effects.

These simple principles have evolved from our current understanding of the pain pathway, or **nociception**. Pain signaling occurs in a distinct pathway that begins at the onset of a noxious stimulus. The stimulus may be tissue trauma, surgical incision, or even heat. When tissue is traumatized, the first phase of the nociceptive pathway is triggered, and the event is converted to a signal that can be sent to the central nervous system (CNS) for processing. This phase is called *transduction*. The second phase, *transmission*, is the propagation of the impulses up toward the spinal cord. Once in the spinal cord, pain signals may undergo a number of different effects. Some signals are handled locally by the release of endogenous opioids, whereas others are sent to the brain for further processing. This sorting process is called *modulation*, the third phase; pain signals are said to be "modulated" in the spinal cord. The fourth and final phase of nociception, *perception*, occurs only in the conscious patient. Perception is "knowing" that pain is present and usually results in such reactions as withdrawal, vocalization, and, in some cases, aggression. Anesthesia interrupts the perception phase only. It is important to remember that interfering with perception alone does not address transduction, transmission, or modulation. Patients who undergo surgery only with anesthesia have essentially no pain management; the spinal cord is continually bombarded by pain signals, which will become evident as soon as the animal wakes.

The four distinct phases of the pain pathway allow pain to be interrupted at more than one juncture. Pain management specialists believe that interrupting nociception or pain perception can be achieved most effectively by targeting multiple points along the pathway. The analgesic drugs currently available target one or more of the nociceptive phases, although each class of agents exerts a major effect on one of the four phases (Fig. 4.14). This is the rationale for combining different analgesics as premedications for surgery, a process called *multimodal analgesia*.

Analgesics

Optimum premedication for surgery is likely to include several agents, as just discussed. Four classes of drugs can be effectively used to deliver preemptive analgesia: opioids (e.g., butorphanol, buprenorphine, morphine, fentanyl), nonsteroidal antiinflammatory drugs (NSAIDs; e.g., carprofen, meloxicam, deracoxib, robenacoxib for use in cats and dogs), local anesthetic agents

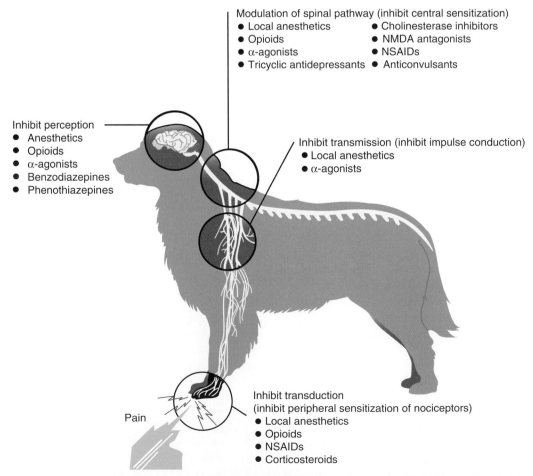

Fig. 4.14 Analgesic drugs work at one or more of the phases of nociception. *NMDA,* N-methyl-d-aspartate; *NSAIDs,* nonsteroidal antiinflammatory drugs. (From Tranquilli WJ, Grimm KA, Lamont LA: *Pain management for the small animal practitioner,* Jackson, WY, 2000, Teton New Media.)

(e.g., bupivacaine, lidocaine), and α_2-adrenergic agonists (e.g., medetomidine, xylazine). The most effective time to administer analgesia is before tissue trauma or damage occurs. Preemptive analgesia, the anticipation of pain and its treatment in advance, is a critical pain management strategy. Most patients require less anesthesia and actually experience less pain on recovery with smaller doses of analgesics when effective preemptive analgesia is administered.

Table 4.1 summarizes the side effects of analgesics. Note that not all the agents described in this table are approved for use in veterinary patients. Some are approved for use in dogs but not cats, and some are approved for use as single agents rather than in combination with other drugs. However, although the U.S. Food and Drug Administration (FDA) has not approved all the previously cited analgesics for use in veterinary medicine, the Animal Medical Drug Use Clarification Act of 1994 (AMDUCA) permits veterinarians to use them on an "extralabel" basis.

Opioids

Opioids, the mainstay of acute pain management, provide analgesia by binding to specific opioid receptors in both the CNS and the peripheral nervous system (PNS). Opioids work at several locations along the pain pathway, affecting nociceptive signal transduction, modulating signals at the spinal level, and inhibiting perception of pain. In addition to providing analgesia, opioids help reduce anxiety and nonpainful distress.

Almost every patient expected to experience pain is a candidate for opioid analgesia. As a class, opioids produce minimal side effects in animals. The only cases in which opioids may be contraindicated are patients with head trauma, because even mild respiratory depression associated with opioids may worsen potential intracranial pressure. Opioids are most effective when administered before the onset of pain. Opioids can be administered through the conventional intravenous (IV), intramuscular (IM), and oral (PO) routes. Other, less common but effective routes of administration are transdermal (e.g., fentanyl), epidural, and intraarticular, as well as constant-rate infusion. Buccal administration has become a popular route for buprenorphine in the cat, whose unique oral pH allows for excellent absorption by this route.

How opioids work. Opioids bind to opioid receptors in the spinal cord. The mu (μ) and kappa (κ) opioid receptors are primarily responsible for producing analgesia, with the μ receptor producing the most profound analgesia. The κ receptors produce much milder analgesia. Both receptor types are also responsible for producing respiratory depression, euphoria, sedation, and miosis. An opioid can interact with one or more types of opioid receptor. Drugs that bind to a receptor and cause expression of activity are called **agonists**. Drugs that bind to receptors and block their action are called **antagonists**. There are further subclassifications into full (pure) agonists, partial agonists, and mixed agonist-antagonists. The opioid drugs are classified by these subdivisions, which describe their potential action and duration.

Pure agonists (e.g., morphine, hydromorphone) bind and stimulate all types of opioid receptors, causing maximum analgesia. They are extremely effective but of only moderate duration, typically about 4 hours. Full agonists are also the most likely to have side effects.

Partial agonists function much the same as full agonists, but the interaction occurs with less than full activity at the receptors. Buprenorphine is a μ partial agonist. Although buprenorphine only partially binds to the μ receptor, it does so with great affinity. Therefore, although it provides analgesia of less intensity than morphine, buprenorphine has a much longer duration of action, up to 8 to 12 hours. A newer formulation of buprenorphine injectable (Simbadol™), is FDA approved and offers 24 hours of postoperative pain control in cats. Sustained release formulations of buprenorphine, lasting 72 hours, are currently available from some compounding pharmacies. Buprenorphine may potentially antagonize some analgesic effects and may also reverse some of the sedative and respiratory depressant effects of pure agonists.

Agonist-antagonist opioids (e.g., butorphanol) bind to more than one type of opioid receptor, having an effect at one type but blocking effects at another receptor. Butorphanol binds and activates κ receptors to produce analgesia and sedation; it also binds with μ opioid receptors, blocking (antagonizing) the receptors. For this reason, butorphanol is considered a mild analgesic with extremely short duration, less than 1 hour in most cases. Butorphanol does produce profound sedation for up to 2 hours, outlasting the analgesia provided. Co-administration with butorphanol may result in reversal of the μ effects of full opioid agonists.

TABLE 4.1 Side Effects of Analgesics

Agent	Adverse Effects	Monitoring
Opioids	Sedation, low blood pressure, respiratory depression, vomiting	Mentation, blood pressure, respiratory rate and quality
Local anesthetics	Tissue irritation, allergic reaction With CRI: nausea, vomiting, neurologic signs, seizures	Monitor injection site for skin rash and/or hives. Observe regularly for muscle tremors and GI upset.
Nonsteroidal antiinflammatory drugs	GI disturbances, GI bleeding, renal disturbances	General observation, hydration status, stool quality, urine production
α_2-Agonists	Bradycardia, cardiac arrhythmias, hypertension, peripheral vasoconstriction	Palpate femoral pulse rate and quality, auscultate heart, monitor blood pressure

CRI, Constant-rate infusion; *GI*, gastrointestinal.

Antagonist opioids fully or partially reverse the effects of opioid agonists. Naloxone is a pure opioid antagonist that completely reverses the effects of all opioid agonists at all receptor sites. Butorphanol can be used as a partial reversing agent, reversing μ activity but not κ effects.

Side effects. Opioids have few clinically significant cardiovascular effects, other than bradycardia, in dogs and cats when administered at recommended doses. However, opioid-induced bradycardia is responsive to anticholinergics. Respiratory depression is a common side effect with opioids in humans but rarely is clinically significant in veterinary patients. Emesis (vomiting) is a common side effect of some opioids, particularly morphine and hydromorphone. Vomiting typically occurs when opioids are used as a premedication rather than when administered to an animal already in pain. Incidences of vomiting can be decreased with concurrent use of antiemetics such as ondansetron or maropitant citrate. Panting is a fairly common side effect of many opioids, especially at higher doses. This potential side effect may not be clinically important, but it can make patient monitoring difficult postoperatively because it is difficult to differentiate between panting as a sign of pain and panting as a reaction to an opioid.

Nonsteroidal Antiinflammatory Drugs

NSAIDs have been used in human and veterinary medicine for many decades to treat fever, inflammation, and pain. More recently, NSAIDs have been found to be quite efficacious for treating inflammation and pain associated with surgery, and several NSAIDs have been approved for preoperative use in dogs. Robenacoxib has been approved preoperative use in both dogs and cats. NSAIDs can be incorporated into premedication protocols to control mild to moderate pain associated with surgery. For maximum effect, NSAIDs should be administered preoperatively, up to 1 to 2 hours before tissue trauma. When they are used in this way, controlling inflammation before it begins, dramatic results can be observed in the postoperative period. Patients who receive preemptive NSAIDs tend to recover with significantly less pain and often require less postoperative analgesia than those who do not. This class of drugs can be safely combined with opioids to provide excellent multimodal analgesia. NSAIDs are available in several formulations, including oral tablets, chewable forms, liquids, and injectable solutions.

How nonsteroidal antiinflammatory drugs work. When cells are damaged as a result of trauma, surgery, or disease, fatty acids such as arachidonic acid (AA) are released from cell membranes. The release of AA triggers a cascade of biochemical activities that ultimately produce prostaglandins, which serve many functions in the body; some prostaglandins are essential for normal homeostasis, and some result in inflammation and pain. The enzyme cyclooxygenase (COX) metabolizes AA to prostaglandin and is the target of NSAIDs. To date, two forms of COX enzymes have been identified. These enzymes are closely related and are now known as COX-1 and COX-2. Each converts AA to prostaglandins, although the prostaglandins produced by each COX enzyme appear to serve very different functions. COX-1 is continuously present in most cells

and is important for normal body functions. In the stomach, COX-1 plays a key role in maintaining integrity of gastric mucosa. In platelets, COX-1 is essential for thromboxane A_2 production. In contrast, COX-2 is not readily present in the cells, but it is rapidly synthesized in response to various inflammatory stimuli. Once induced by tissue injury, COX-2 converts AA into prostaglandins that create inflammation and pain. Both COX-1 and COX-2 play a vital role in the kidney as important mediators of salt and water balance, rennin (chymosin) release, and vascular tone. NSAIDs exert their antiinflammatory effects by inhibiting activity of COX-1, COX-2, or both. This inhibitory activity varies between NSAID compounds and with animal species.

Side effects. As a class, NSAIDs are associated with specific types of potential side effects. Some of these are species specific and drug specific, as in the case of acetaminophen metabolism in cats. Possible side effects associated with NSAIDs include gastrointestinal tract damage, hepatopathy, renal toxicity, impaired platelet function, and cartilage destruction. Administration of NSAIDs should be restricted to well-hydrated, normotensive animals with normal hepatic and renal function, no hemostatic abnormalities, and no evidence of gastric ulceration.

Alpha₂-Adrenergic Agonists

Alpha₂-adrenergic agonists (α_2-agonists) are short-duration sedative-analgesic–muscle relaxants that can be rapidly reversed with α_2-antagonists. This characteristic makes these drugs suitable for procedures requiring short-term restraint and analgesia as well as premedication for longer surgical procedures. Use of α_2-antagonists as premedications may result in substantial reduction in both induction and inhalant anesthetic dosages. α_2-Agonists are nonnarcotic and nonscheduled agents. Medetomidine or dexmedetomidine and xylazine are the two α_2-agonists currently approved for use in dogs and cats in the United States. Medetomidine is a dose-dependent sedative-analgesic often used as a preanesthetic agent in healthy animals. Onset of effect is 5 to 15 minutes depending on route of administration, which can be IV or IM, and sedation can last up to 2 hours.

How α_2-agonists work. α_2-Agonists inhibit release of the excitatory neurotransmitter norepinephrine to produce analgesia and sedation. These agents interrupt the pain pathway by inhibiting nerve impulse transmission, modulating nociceptive signals in the spinal cord, and inhibiting perception within the brain. Because α_2-adrenoceptors are found in various sites throughout the body, α_2-agonists normally induce a number of physiologic changes in addition to sedation, analgesia, and muscle relaxation. Administration results in physiologically normal peripheral vasoconstriction, which creates a transient increase in blood pressure. Because the normal cardiovascular response to these events is a reflexive decrease in heart rate, patients are expected to become bradycardic. All cardiovascular parameters smoothly return to presedation levels on reversal of the agent with an α_2-antagonist (atipamezole or yohimbine).

Side effects. α_2-Agonists can have profound effects on the CNS and cardiovascular system, but using low dosages can minimize these adverse events. Bradycardia and vomiting are the most common side effects. All α_2-agonists have potential side effects, including initial hypertension followed by prolonged hypotension, bradycardia and heart block, respiratory depression, excessive CNS depression, vomiting, increased urine production, and peripheral vasoconstriction.

Candidates for α_2-agonist administration should be healthy, have sound cardiovascular systems, and be exercise tolerant. An α_2-agonist should never be administered to an animal with a compromised cardiovascular or respiratory system.

Local Anesthetics

Local anesthetics are inexpensive to use and quite effective in blocking the transmission of nociceptive signals at the source. Use of local anesthetics offers three major benefits. First, these agents produce true analgesia, that is, a complete absence of pain. Second, they are nonscheduled agents, requiring no cumbersome paperwork. Third, the techniques used to administer local anesthetics are relatively easy to perform. Most blocking techniques are well within the skill level of licensed veterinary technicians. Local anesthetics can and should be used in any surgical patient with an identifiable site for nerve blockade. For example, local anesthetics can be used effectively in patients undergoing thoracotomy, elbow surgery, maxillomandibular procedures, local excisions, feline declawing, and knee or cruciate repair. Anesthetic agents can be administered to create local and regional anesthesia and analgesia (Box 4.2).

In addition, local anesthetics are most often the drugs of choice for epidural anesthesia and analgesia. This technique is a good alternative to general anesthesia or as an adjunct to inhalant anesthesia, especially for patients at high risk during general anesthesia and those undergoing painful orthopedic surgeries of the hind limb. Finally, an IV constant-rate infusion of a local anesthetic can provide sustained pain control in a variety of patients undergoing extensive nerve trauma, such as limb amputation. Lidocaine and bupivacaine are the agents most often used for dogs and cats. Lidocaine is characterized by rapid onset (5–10 minutes) but short duration (45–90 minutes). In contrast, bupivacaine has a longer onset (15–20 minutes) but provides up to 6 hours of analgesia (Table 4.2).

TABLE 4.2 Comparison of Local Anesthetic Agents

Drug	Onset	Duration
Lidocaine	5–10 minutes	45–90 minutes
Bupivacaine	15–20 minutes	Up to 6 hours

How local anesthetics work. Local anesthetics act by inhibiting transduction and transmission of nerve impulses and by modifying the signals at the spinal cord. Local anesthetics inhibit generation and transmission of nerve impulses by blocking sodium channels in the neuron's cell membrane. This effect slows the rate of depolarization of the neuron cell membrane and prevents the threshold potential from being reached.

Side effects. When administered at an appropriate dose, local anesthetics have relatively few, if any, adverse side effects. The potential systemic side effects of local anesthetics involve the CNS and cardiovascular system. Other potential side effects include development of methemoglobinemia, nerve and skeletal muscle toxicities, and allergic reactions, including hypersensitivity and anaphylaxis.

Sedation and Tranquilization

Sedatives alone do not possess any analgesic properties but are an important adjunct to premedication protocols. Sedation should be incorporated into preoperative regimens to reduce stress, fear, and anxiety, all of which exacerbate pain and vice versa. However, sedatives alone should never be administered to an animal without analgesia when pain is anticipated. Sedation alone may decrease the animal's ability to express pain and give the false impression that the animal is pain free. Commonly used sedatives for premedication include the tranquilizing agents phenothiazines (acepromazine) and benzodiazepines (diazepam, midazolam).

ANTICHOLINERGICS

Historically, anticholinergic drugs such as atropine and glycopyrrolate were routinely added to premedication protocols that were expected to produce profound, sustained bradycardia. Anticholinergics were given to reduce episodes of bradycardia and to dry oral secretions. Anticholinergics can increase the incidence of cardiac arrhythmias and sinus tachycardia. Increasing the heart rate is not always beneficial to the patient because higher heart rates do not necessarily translate into better perfusion. The best approach is to avoid "routine" use of anticholinergics, and instead administer them on a case-by-case basis only to patients in need.

Atropine sulfate has a quick onset of action and rapid elimination and can be given subcutaneously (SC), IM, or IV to treat bradycardia and to dry oral secretions. Glycopyrrolate can be given SC, IV, or IM, although onset of action is substantially increased when given SC or IM. Glycopyrrolate also treats bradycardia and dries oral secretions. The effects of glycopyrrolate are much longer lasting than those of atropine.

BOX 4.2 Local and Regional Anesthesia and Analgesia

- Field block, such as an incisional line block, produces regional anesthesia.
- Infraorbital nerve block provides anesthesia and analgesia to the upper lip and nose, the dorsal aspect of the nasal cavity, and the skin ventral to the infraorbital foramen.
- Mandibular nerve block provides anesthesia of the teeth, skin, and mucosa of the lower lip and chin.
- Intercostal block provides analgesia after thoracotomy and for desensitizing the area around broken ribs.
- Intraarticular administration of a local anesthetic provides analgesia to a joint before and after a surgical procedure.
- Circumferential ring block provides anesthesia and analgesia around a given area, such as a foot or claw.

Whether or not an anticholinergic should be routinely administered in conjunction with α_2-agonists that lower heart rate has been the subject of considerable scientific debate. Initially, treatment of α_2-agonist–induced bradycardia with anticholinergics was thought to be beneficial. Currently, however, anticholinergic drugs are not generally recommended to prevent periods of expected transient bradycardia. α_2-Antagonist reversal agents, in full or partial doses, should be used, rather than anticholinergics, to reverse bradycardia if it occurs.

ANTIBIOTICS

An important consideration is whether or not the surgery patient needs intraoperative antibiotics and, if antibiotics are indicated, which type is appropriate. If the procedure is elective and a possible break in sterility intraoperatively is not a concern, antibiotics are generally unnecessary. However, if the surgical procedure is done specifically to treat contaminated or infected wounds, or if possible contamination during an elective procedure is a concern, intraoperative antibiotics may be indicated. When determining whether antibiotics are indicated, it is helpful to know what type of wound is present. See Chapter 11 for a discussion on wound classifications.

Prophylaxis refers to the measures taken in the prevention of disease. The administration of antibiotics just before and during surgery is known as *perioperative prophylaxis*. The purpose of this practice is to decrease the chances of postoperative infection of the surgical site. Few surgical cases or circumstances warrant prophylactic antibiotic treatment; one example is an orthopedic procedure involving the placement of implants.

The choice of antibiotic depends on the type of bacterial contamination expected. For example, staphylococci from the skin are of concern in orthopedic procedures. Gram-negative bacteria (e.g., *Escherichia coli*) are of concern in large-bowel procedures. The antibiotic's spectrum of activity should be narrow and limited to the predicted bacterial contaminant.

The antibiotic must be administered by injection (IV, IM, or SC) just before induction. The dose may be repeated during the surgical procedure to ensure adequate serum levels throughout the surgery. Antibiotic administration may be discontinued or may be altered to the oral route once the procedure is completed.

If an animal is taken to surgery with an infection that is already established, the clinician may have prescribed antibiotics for a period before the surgery. This situation is not considered prophylactic in nature. The antibiotics have been prescribed in response to an already established infection. In this case it is important to continue the administration perioperatively and postoperatively, during the recuperative period. The antibiotic may need to be administered by injection (SC, IM, or IV) immediately before the surgery. Oral antibiotic administration can be reinstituted as soon as the animal can tolerate food and water after the surgery.

KEY POINTS

1. Taking an accurate history and recording it in a concise, chronologic order create the foundation for the treatment plan for each surgical patient.
2. During the interview process of the history taking, the technician needs to confirm the patient's signalment (age, gender, breed) and chief complaint (reason for the visit to the surgical hospital).
3. While the client is being interviewed, the patient should be allowed to explore the examination room at will; this will allow the patient to acclimate itself to the surgical hospital and allow the technician to make a mental note of the patient's overall condition and mentation (mental status, attitude).
4. The physical examination needs to be thorough and systematic and performed the day of surgery with the owner present.
5. Any abnormalities found on the physical examination need to be brought to the attention of the attending veterinarian and recorded in the medical record.
6. The consent form should identify the patient, the procedures to be performed on the patient, the potential risks associated with those procedures and anesthesia, and the name(s) of the veterinarian(s) performing the procedures and include a place for the owner to sign indicating consent.
7. The consent form should provide confirmation that the patient was fasted appropriately before admission, that the owner was given an estimate for the costs of the procedures, and that the owner's phone number is readily available so he or she can be contacted during the procedure if necessary.
8. Selection of the preanesthetic diagnostic tests depends on the patient's age and health status, type of surgery to be performed, and results of initial diagnostic screening tests.
9. Preoperative medications should provide preemptive analgesia and tranquilization and allow for easier anesthetic induction and smoother anesthetic recovery.
10. To provide the most effective pain prevention and relief, different types of analgesics with different mechanisms of action (multimodal analgesia) need to be administered to surgical patients.

REVIEW QUESTIONS

1. The patient's signalment includes which information?
   a. Age, gender, breed
   b. Diet and clinical signs (history, screen
   c. Owner name and address
   d. Temperature, pulse, respiratory rate (PE)

2. A consent form should include
   a. blood test results for the patient.
   b. instructions for care of the patient at home.
   c. a thorough description of the surgical procedure.
   d. the physical exam results of the patient.

3. What is a method of interrupting a cat's purring during thoracic auscultation?
   a. Scratch the cat's ears.
   b. Lift the head with the top surface of the hand under the mandible.
   c. Hold the cat's mouth closed.
   d. Hold a cotton ball soaked in alcohol near the cat's nose.
4. Decreased plasma proteins on a preanesthetic bloodwork may be due to
   a. infections.
   b. dehydration.
   c. malignancies.
   d. inadequate albumin production in the liver.
5. What blood test is used to assess the patient's kidney function?
   a. Total solids
   b. Blood glucose
   c. Blood urea nitrogen
   d. Alanine aminotransferase
6. It is best to administer analgesics
   a. prior to the painful procedure.
   b. immediately after surgery ends.
   c. when the patient shows signs of pain.
   d. when the patient has recovered from anesthesia.
7. Combining different classes of analgesics to maximize the pain relief is called
   a. modulation.
   b. extralabel.
   c. multimodal analgesia.
   d. preemptive analgesia.
8. Where does the modulation portion of the nociceptive pathway occur?
   a. Tissues
   b. Spinal nerves
   c. Spinal cord
   d. Brain
9. Which drug class has the ability to provide complete absence of pain, at least temporarily?
   a. Alpha 2 adrenergic agonists
   b. NSAIDs
   c. Local anesthetics
   d. Opioids
10. Sedatives are used as part of a premedication anesthesia protocol because they
    a. reduce fear and stress.
    b. prevent bradycardia.
    c. increase perception of pain.
    d. block transmission of pain.
11. The goal of balanced anesthesia is to
    a. charge the client the least amount possible.
    b. use a single drug that is safe for all patients.
    c. minimize the positive effects of the drugs used.
    d. combine smaller doses of multiple medications to minimize side effects.
12. Thoracic auscultation is best performed with the patient in what position?
    a. Sitting
    b. Standing
    c. Lateral recumbency
    d. Sternal recumbency
13. The reason for a patient's visit is also called
    a. signalment.
    b. history.
    c. chief complaint.
    d. diagnosis.
14. Which description could be used to appropriately note a patient's mentation?
    a. Obese
    b. Weak
    c. Healthy
    d. Depressed
15. When microscopically examining a PCV tube to assess for heartworm microfilaria, where on the sample would you find the microfilaria?
    a. At the top of the plasma
    b. Just above the buffy coat
    c. Within the buffy coat
    d. In the packed red blood cells
16. Which drug class is an NSAID?
    a. Maropitant
    b. Robenacoxib
    c. Buprenorphine
    d. Dexmedetomidine
17. Which drug is a partial opioid agonist?
    a. Naloxone
    b. Butorphanol
    c. Buprenorphine
    d. Hydromorphone
18. A contraindication to using an opioid in a patient is
    a. anxiety.
    b. hypertension.
    c. head trauma.
    d. feline species.
19. Why is it important to review all medications and supplements that a patient is taking before beginning the surgery?
20. Why are leading questions inappropriate to ask during the history taking?

BIBLIOGRAPHY

Bassert JM, Thomas JA, editors: *McCurnin's clinical textbook for veterinary technicians*, ed 8, St Louis, 2014, Saunders.

Cunningham JG: *Textbook of veterinary physiology*, ed 4, St Louis, 2008, Saunders.

Fossum TW: *Small animal surgery*, ed 5, Philadelphia, 2019, Elsevier.

Plumb DC: *Plumb's veterinary drug handbook*, ed 8, Stockholm, WI, 2015, Pharma Vet Inc.

Romich JA: *An illustrated guide to veterinary medical terminology*, Stamford, CT, 2015, Cengage Learning.

Sirois, M: *Laboratory procedures for veterinary technicians*, ed 7, St Louis, 2020, Elsevier.

Stoeberl TA: Preparing the small animal patient for surgery, *AHT*, 4:271, 1983.

Thomas JA, Lerch P: *Anesthesia and analgesia for veterinary technicians*, ed 5, St Louis, 2017, Elsevier.

Patient Preparation

Marianne Tear

LEARNING OBJECTIVES

After completion of this chapter, the reader will be able to:

- Discuss the indications for placement of an intravenous (IV) catheter.
- Identify appropriate sites for placement of IV catheters.
- List the supplies required for IV catheter placement.
- Discuss the technique for IV catheterization of peripheral vessels.
- Identify the components of an endotracheal (ET) tube.
- Discuss factors considered for determining ET tube size.
- List supplies required for ET intubation.
- Discuss the differences between the one-person technique and the two-person technique for performing ET intubation.
- Discuss methods of assessing proper ET tube placement.
- Describe hair removal protocols for a variety of soft tissue, orthopedic, neurologic, and miscellaneous surgical cases.

- List antiseptic products available for use to prepare patients for surgery.
- Discuss different patterns used in applying materials for the surgical preparation.
- Discuss potential patient reactions from clipper or chemical irritation.
- Explain the process to secure the patient to the surgery table in a safe, accessible manner.
- Properly position the patient for various surgical procedures, providing access to the (1) surgical site, (2) IV catheter site, (3) ET tube, (4) other venous access sites, and (5) monitoring sites.
- Explain the steps to perform a sterile preparation of the surgical site.
- Describe the final preparation before surgery.
- Use appropriate techniques to conserve body heat.

KEY TERMS

Aseptic
Bactericidal
Butterfly catheter
Central venous pressure
Fungicidal

Fungistatic
Injection cap
Macrodrip set
Microdrop set
Over-the-needle catheter

Peripheral catheter
Urine scald
Viricidal

INTRAVENOUS CATHETERS

An intravenous (IV) catheter is placed after the patient has received the appropriate premedication. In addition to the analgesic benefits provided by these agents to the surgical patient, premedication makes for a more sedate and cooperative patient when the catheter is placed.

The placement of an IV catheter offers many benefits. When an IV catheter is in place, performing a venipuncture for every injection is unnecessary. This reduces stress for the patient who may need to receive multiple IV medications. Many drugs needed by a surgical patient are only able to be administered intravenously, and the IV catheter allows for easier administration of these drugs. For example, induction agents for general anesthesia, analgesics, antibiotics, and fluids may need to be given to the surgical patient at some point during its hospital stay. Having established access to the vascular system through an IV catheter aids in the efficiency of administering these medications. From a safety standpoint, having venous access also allows for immediate administration of emergency drugs if necessary. The type and placement site of the catheter greatly influence its capabilities. **Peripheral catheters** (a catheter placed in a peripheral vessel such as the saphenous or cephalic vein) are completely adequate for anesthesia induction and medication and fluid administration.

Peripheral Catheters

Peripheral catheters are most often placed in the following sites:
  Canine: cephalic and lateral saphenous veins
  Feline: cephalic and medial saphenous veins

Almost any palpable vessel can be used to place a catheter. The vessel should be examined for overall integrity and ability to withstand catheterization. Vessels that have been catheterized multiple times may not be suitable. If a vessel has scar tissue as a result of multiple injections or catheters, placement of a smaller gauge catheter may be required.

Supplies

Regardless of the site, the basic supplies needed to place the catheter remain the same (Fig. 5.1).

Catheter. Many styles of catheter are available for use. The choice of catheter style is primarily determined by the site of placement and the intended use. The three most common styles are the **over-the-needle catheter** (a catheter in which the catheter is mounted over the needle), the through-the-needle catheter, and the **butterfly catheter** (a small-gauge catheter with a plastic set of wings below the hub that allows for ease of griping and more stability) (Fig. 5.2). The over-the-needle type is typically used for short-term and surgical catheters. It is placed in a peripheral vein (e.g., cephalic vein). The butterfly catheter is useful when vascular access is required for medications that need to be administered once (as in outpatient treatments) and slowly (i.e., over 1–3 minutes). Butterfly catheters are sharp and rigid and are not intended to remain in a patient that is not being directly monitored (i.e., with hands-on monitoring). Through-the-needle catheters are often placed in the jugular veins of patients that will need intensive nursing care postoperatively (Fig. 5.3).

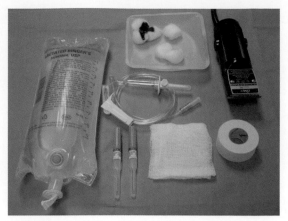

Fig. 5.1 Supplies required for placement of intravenous (IV) catheter and administration of IV fluids. *From left:* IV fluid bag (1 L bag of lactated Ringer's solution shown), cotton balls and scrub product, IV fluid administration set, IV catheters, gauze squares, tape, and clippers.

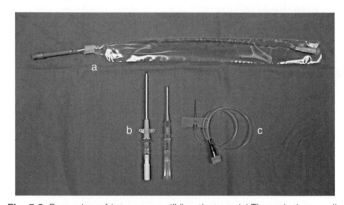

Fig. 5.2 Examples of intravenous (IV) catheters. (a) Through-the-needle catheter. (b) Over-the-needle catheters. (c) Butterfly catheter.

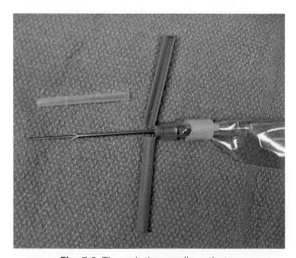

Fig. 5.3 Through-the-needle catheter.

The choice of catheter size is primarily influenced by five factors: (1) site of placement, (2) length of time the catheter will be needed, (3) reason for placement, (4) diameter of the vessel, and (5) length of the vessel working area. The gauge (diameter) of the catheter should be chosen after evaluation of the vessel's size and the reason for placement. The length of the catheter

TABLE 5.1 Intravenous Catheter Selection Guidelines

Patient Size (LB)	Vein	Type of Catheter	Catheter Diameter (Gauge)	Catheter Length (Inches)
CANINE				
0–5	Saphenous/cephalic	Over the needle	24	¾
5–25	Saphenous/cephalic	Over the needle	22	1–1¼
25–80	Saphenous/cephalic	Over the needle	20	1–2
80 and up	Saphenous/cephalic	Over the needle	18	1–2
0–5	Jugular	Through the needle	21	1–1½
5–25	Jugular	Through the needle	18	1–1½
25–80	Jugular	Through the needle	16–18	1–1½
80 and up	Jugular	Through the needle	16	1–1½
0–5	Saphenous/cephalic	Butterfly	24–23	¾–1
5–25	Saphenous/cephalic	Butterfly	22	¾–1
25–80	Saphenous/cephalic	Butterfly	20	¾–1
80 and up	Saphenous/cephalic	Butterfly	18	¾–1
FELINE				
0–4	Femoral/cephalic	Over the needle	24	¾
4 and up	Femoral/cephalic	Over the needle	22	1
0–4	Jugular	Through the needle	21	1–1½
4 and up	Jugular	Through the needle	18	1–1½
0–4	Cephalic	Butterfly	24	¾
4 and up	Cephalic	Butterfly	22	¾

needs to be considered after the vessel has been chosen so that the length of the working area is known. For example, a 2-inch catheter placed in the cephalic vein of a dachshund is inappropriate, because once completely seated, the catheter would be proximal to the patient's elbow and would be more likely to kink every time the leg was bent. Table 5.1 provides guidance in making appropriate catheter selections based on the factors listed.

Injection caps, T-ports, and fluid administration sets. Injection caps may be placed on the catheter if occasional injections are anticipated (Fig. 5.4). An **injection cap** (a rubber diaphragm under a plastic cap that permits a needle insertion) allows for repeated punctures without resulting in damage or leaking. Needleless styles of injection caps are available and are a good option because they reduce accidental needle punctures of workers.

T-ports (or T-sets) serve the same purpose as an injection cap and also allow easier access to the catheter (see Fig. 5.4). The short tubing incorporated into the design of the device allows sample collection or medication administration to be done more easily. A fluid administration set of the appropriate size should be used if continuous infusion of fluids or IV medication is anticipated, and the set can be connected to the T-port.

Usually an administration set called a **macrodrip set** (an IV fluid line that delivers fluids, usually 10 or 15 drops per milliliter; this allows for a high volume to be delivered in a short time) is used for patients weighing more than 7 kg. A **microdrop set** (an IV fluid line that delivers fluids at a rate of 60 drops per milliliter; this allows for greater precision) is used for patients

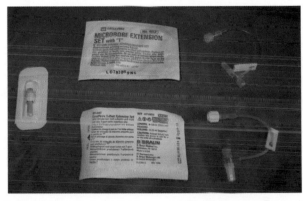

Fig. 5.4 Injection cap *(left)* and two examples of T-ports or T-sets *(right)*.

weighing less than 7 kg. For extremely small patients, a Buretrol solution administration set (Baxter, Deerfield, IL) can be employed for the most accurate measurement of fluids administered, and it is especially useful if an electric fluid infusion pump is not available (Fig. 5.5).

Extension sets. An extension set may be used in conjunction with an administration set to add length to the line and allow for better animal mobility in the cage postoperatively. The administration sets are often not long enough to be practical, so the addition of an extension set may be used to allow the patient more freedom. Care must be taken that the patient does not become entangled in the line.

Tape. The tape is one of the most important components of the catheter. Without proper anchoring, even the best placed

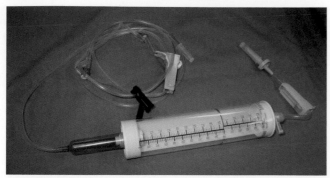

Fig. 5.5 Buretrol administration set can be attached to a bag of intravenous (IV) fluid and the chamber filled with the amount of fluid to be administered. These sets are generally used on small (e.g., pediatric) patients when an electric infusion pump is not available.

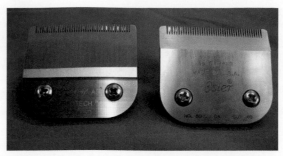

Fig. 5.6 Two types of clipper blades, a No. 50 (left) and a No. 40 (right), that can be used to clip hair in preparation for surgery or placement of an intravenous (IV) catheter.

catheter is useless. The technique for taping can vary from technician to technician, the only constant being that the catheter must be secure without being too tight. A loose tape job would allow the catheter to lose patency, but applying the tape too tightly could occlude blood flow. Typically, 1-inch and ½-inch tape are used in varying orders to secure the catheter. The first piece of tape should be long enough to encircle the patient's limb or neck, depending on where the catheter is placed. Two additional pieces of tape, the same length as the first, will be needed to secure the catheter further in place.

Catheter "prep" materials. Clippers with a number 40 (No. 40) blade are required for hair removal from the catheter site (Fig. 5.6). The amount of hair to remove depends on the catheter site and the patient's size. In general, for peripheral veins, a margin of 1½ to 2 inches on all sides of the proposed puncture site is appropriate. Clipping an area of this size often requires clipping the entire circumference of the patient's limb. For catheters placed in the jugular vein, a larger area should be clipped. This larger area is necessary to assist with the sterile placement and maintenance of the jugular catheter.

Preparation materials include cotton balls saturated with either diluted (50:50) povidone-iodine scrub or chlorhexidine scrub for the cleansing step. Cotton balls saturated with 70% isopropyl alcohol or saline should be used for the rinsing step. Jugular catheter sites may be prepared with saturated gauze sponges instead of cotton balls.

Fluids or saline flush. Either continuous infusion of IV fluids or regular flushing of the catheter is necessary to maintain patency of the catheter once it is placed. Frequent inspection of the catheter site is important. Any changes to the vessel, the catheter, or the patient should be immediately evaluated by the veterinary technician and the veterinarian. If fluids are used, the choice is usually an isotonic crystalloid (e.g., Lactated Ringer's solution or 0.9% sodium chloride).

Bandage materials. Bandage materials are needed if the catheter is to remain in place after the surgical procedure is completed. Elastic gauze and elastic tape (or Vetrap, 3M, St Paul, MN) are the materials of choice. Usually, 1-inch widths of all materials work best, given the area that will be bandaged on most dogs and cats, but personal preference eventually becomes the determining factor. Tegaderm (3M) is a sterile, transparent,

breathable adherent dressing used to cover the insertion site of the catheter. This dressing is impervious to liquids and bacteria and therefore is effective in maintaining a catheter. Other sterile wound dressings may be used, depending on the indication for and placement site of the catheter.

Daily evaluation of the catheter and insertion site helps prevent phlebitis and detects any problems early. The date, time, and initials of the technician placing the catheter can be placed on the outer bandage and the inner tape and should be noted in the patient's chart. This information ensures that the catheter is replaced in the appropriate time frame.

Placement Technique
Box 5.1 details the placement of IV catheters in a peripheral vein.

Jugular Catheters
Some surgical patients require intense postoperative critical care. If part of this care requires **central venous pressure** (CVP; a measure of blood volume and venous return used to monitor fluid volume status) measurements or long-term fluid therapy, a jugular catheter (central line) should be placed.

Supplies
The supplies required for placement of a jugular catheter are similar to those used for a peripheral vein catheter. Jugular catheters are longer, 8 to 12 inches, and can be single lumen or double lumen. The extra length is needed to ensure placement of the catheter close to the right atrium of the heart, which is required to measure CVP. Because they are long-term catheters, jugular catheters should always be secured with a sterile bandage in addition to the tape. Antimicrobial ointment, elastic gauze, and elastic tape can be used for the bandage.

Placement
With the animal in lateral recumbency, a large area is clipped over the ventrolateral neck to reveal the jugular vein. The site is **aseptically** prepared as done for a peripheral catheter. Because these catheters are generally left in place for a longer time, a final preparation of antiseptic is applied after the last rinse. The person placing the catheter should wear sterile gloves, and a sterile drape should cover the prepared area. Different catheters need to be inserted with different techniques, so it is best to consult and follow the manufacturer's recommendation for the catheter used.

BOX 5.1   Technique for Placement of a Peripheral Intravenous Catheter

1. Before beginning the placement of the catheter, be sure all supplies are available and readily accessible.
2. Clip an ample amount from the area where the catheter is to be placed. Bear in mind that no component of the catheter and no accessories (e.g., injection cap, end of fluid line) should be resting in hair once the catheter has been placed. When in doubt, clip more than would seem necessary.
3. After clipping, remove all loose hair from the tabletop and dispose of it in the waste can.
4. To begin, the restrainer should occlude the vessel to be catheterized. Proper restraint must be used to prevent contamination of the prepped catheter site (Fig. 5.7).
5. Cleanse the area using a surgical scrub product and rinsing agent combination, either povidone-iodine/70% isopropyl alcohol or chlorhexidine/70% isopropyl alcohol (Fig. 5.8). Cotton balls are best used to help prevent depositing excessive amounts of fluid on the area. The target pattern should be used when preparing the area. Begin at the proposed puncture site and move in a circle progressively toward the hair margins. Cotton balls that have left the center of the area must never return to the center. A rinsing agent should be used in the same manner to remove the scrub from the skin. A minimum of three "cycles" of scrub/rinse should be performed. If, however, after the third rinse the skin is still dirty, continue cleansing until the skin is clean. No final prep solution is necessary unless the catheter will be left in place after the surgery is completed. In this case apply the solution using the target pattern as previously described.

6. Open the catheter using aseptic technique. Remove both the injection plug at the end of the catheter and the cover on the catheter. If the cap at the end of the catheter has a paper filter, the cap may be left in place as the catheter is placed. The filter will allow the blood to "flash back" while preventing excessive bleeding. Take care to avoid touching the exposed catheter.
7. Place the thumb of the nondominant hand parallel to, but not touching, the prepared vessel. The same hand should be holding the leg in extension as well.
8. Hold the catheter at the junction of the catheter and stylet with the thumb and index finger of the dominant hand (Fig. 5.9).
9. Ensure that the bevel of the stylet is facing up.
10. Using a 10- to 20-degree angle, quickly penetrate the skin with the catheter and then insert it into the vessel.
11. Check the stylet for blood flow (Fig. 5.10). If flow is present, advance both the catheter and the stylet 1 to 2 mm, and check the stylet again. If blood flow is still present, grasp the stylet with the hand that is holding the leg. Using the other hand, advance only the catheter into the vessel (Fig. 5.11). *(It is possible to use one hand to hold the stylet and advance the catheter; grasp the stylet with the middle and ring fingers while using the index finger to advance the catheter.)* Be sure to advance the catheter all the way to the hub. If blood flow is not present, redirect the catheter until blood flow is established.

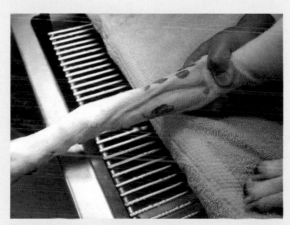

Fig. 5.7 Scrubbing clipped area before catheter placement.

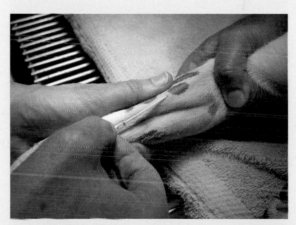

Fig. 5.9 Proper holding of catheter and appropriate approach to vessel.

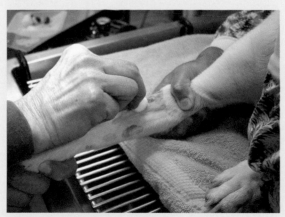

Fig. 5.8 Aseptically prepared and properly restrained catheter site.

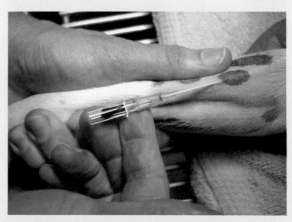

Fig. 5.10 "Flash" of blood in stylet of catheter ensures proper placement in vessel.

Continued

BOX 5.1   Technique for Placement of a Peripheral Intravenous Catheter—cont'd

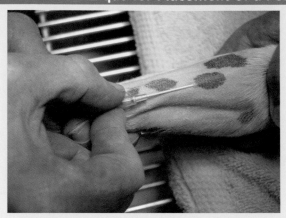

Fig. 5.11 Advancing catheter into vessel.

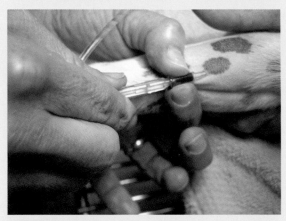

Fig. 5.12 Attachment of injection port, T-port, or fluid administration set to catheter hub. Note hand placement to stabilize hub.

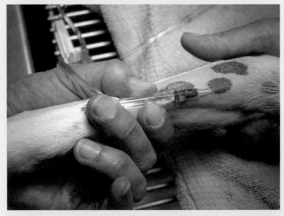

Fig. 5.13 Attached fluid line.

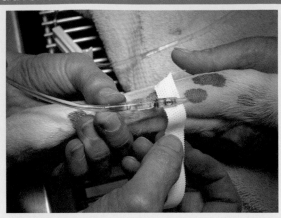

Fig. 5.14 Placement of ½-inch piece of tape, sticky side up, under hub of catheter.

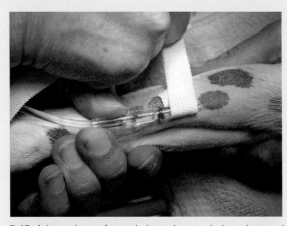

Fig. 5.15 A long piece of tape is brought over hub and around leg.

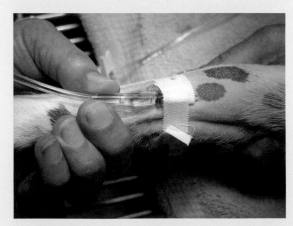

Fig. 5.16 Anchor piece of tape properly placed.

12. Using the other hand, quickly remove the stylet and connect either an injection cap, a T-port, or a fluid administration set to the catheter hub (Figs. 5.12 and 5.13).
13. If using a fluid administration set, be sure to turn on the fluids to maintain a patent line. If using an injection cap or a T-port, flush the catheter with 2 mL of heparinized saline. *(It may be easier to insert an injection cap, secure the catheter with the first piece of tape, and then hook up the fluid line. The weight of the fluid line may otherwise pull the catheter out.)*

14. Use a dry gauze sponge to remove any blood on the clipped area or hair near the catheter.
15. Begin securing the catheter by using a ½-inch-wide piece of tape long enough to encircle the limb at least once. Place the tape, sticky side up (Fig. 5.14), under the hub of the catheter all the way up to the puncture site. Bring the long side of the tape over the hub (Fig. 5.15) and tape all the way around the leg, leaving a tab of tape folded over (Fig. 5.16) to aid in removal of the tape when the catheter is removed later. This piece

BOX 5.1 Technique for Placement of a Peripheral Intravenous Catheter—cont'd

should be snug, but not occlusive, because it is the "anchor" for keeping the catheter in place.

16. Place a 1-inch-wide piece of tape, sticky side down, under the catheter all the way up to the first piece of tape (Fig. 5.17). Bring the long side of the tape over the catheter hub and around the leg, securing the hub of the catheter. Be sure the connection of the fluid line and the catheter is not covered.

17. The final step in securing the catheter is to use the piece of tape to secure the fluid line with a stress loop (Fig. 5.18). When making the stress loop, be sure not to kink the line to impair or obstruct the flow of fluid. Tape the loop to one of the other pieces of tape to ensure that it is secure.

18. Ensure that the catheter is still patent by checking the limb for any swelling or "blebs." Generally, the fluid will not run if the catheter is not in the vessel. The drip chamber of the fluid administration set can also be observed to see that the fluid is flowing. Another trick to check catheter placement is to place the bag of fluid lower than the patient's heart and see whether blood flows back into the catheter.

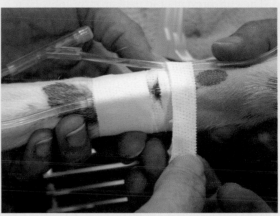

Fig. 5.18 A stress loop is made by carefully folding a length of the intravenous (IV) fluid line and taping it securely to patient's leg. The stress loop relieves direct pressure at the connection between catheter (or T-port) and fluid administration set should patient exert tension on administration set, making it less likely that patient will pull the catheter out while shifting positions and moving about the cage.

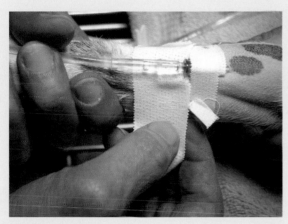

Fig. 5.17 A 1-inch piece of tape, sticky side down, is placed under catheter.

After the catheter has been placed and is secured, it is essential to maintain the patency of the line. The administration of fluids will aid in ensuring line patency. If fluids are not being administered, saline should be used to flush the line at regular intervals (e.g., every 6 hours). The catheter site should also be checked daily for any problems that may necessitate the removal of the catheter.

Central Venous Pressure

CVP monitoring is done to assess how well blood is returning to the heart as well as how effectively blood is pumped from the heart. This procedure is helpful in monitoring a patient with right-sided heart failure because blood backs up into the vena cava in such a patient. CVP monitoring also helps to assess overhydration with fluids because as blood volume increases, CVP rises. A water manometer is connected to the catheter to determine the measurement. A normal reading for cats and dogs is less than 8 cm H_2O.

ENDOTRACHEAL INTUBATION

Endotracheal (ET) tubes are an important piece of anesthetic equipment. They are used for three main reasons: administration of oxygen and inhalation anesthetics, protection of the airway, and assistance with resuscitative needs.

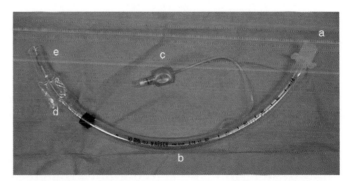

Fig. 5.19 Endotracheal tube. (A) Hose connector. (B) Body. (C) Cuff indicator. (D) Cuff. (E) Murphy eye.

Components of Tube

All ET tubes have several components (Fig. 5.19). It is important to know each of these components in order to use the tubes properly and evaluate the integrity of each tube before use.

- The hose connector is found at one end of the ET tube. It connects the tube to the Y piece, nonrebreathing system, or Ambu bag.
- The body is the major portion of the ET tube. Several numbers may be found on the tube body. The length measurements are in 2-mm increments and identify the length of the

tube. The manufacturer's name may also be seen on the body. The large bold number is the size of the internal diameter in millimeters. The most common tubes are available in sizes ranging from 3.0 to 12.0 mm in 0.5-mm increments.

- The cuff indicator is used to determine the pressure of the cuff on the trachea once air has been infused into the cuff.
- The cuff is present to permit the creation of a leak-proof system. Air is infused into the cuff, via the cuff indicator, to ensure a seal between the ET tube and the lumen of the trachea. The cuff prevents the patient from inhaling room air, which would dilute the gas delivered to the patient during anesthesia. The cuff also prevents the patient from exhaling anesthetic gas into the operating room and from aspirating any vomitus while intubated.
- The Murphy eye is found at the tip of the ET tube. It allows airflow in the event that the end of the tube becomes occluded with respiratory secretions (mucous plugs).

Selection of Proper Tube Size

The largest size ET tube possible, without being traumatic, should be used. Generally, tube size is based on a patient's weight, although palpation of the trachea and experience will aid in this decision. Table 5.2 is provided as a reference. Because of the variability in patient size, multiple tubes should be set aside for possible use. An acceptable practice is to choose the size thought to be needed, in addition to a tube 0.5 mm smaller and a tube 0.5 mm larger. Each tube chosen should be checked for leaks. Box 5.2 explains how to check an ET tube for leaks before using it in a patient.

Supplies

Using the proper supplies in the proper manner will significantly increase the success rate of intubation (Fig. 5.20).

Endotracheal Tube

Both clear and colored ET tubes are available. Although the two types work equally well, the clear tubes have two distinct advantages. First, any type of occlusion in the tube (e.g., blood, mucus) is more easily identified in a clear tube than in a colored or

BOX 5.2 How to "Leak Check" an Endotracheal Tube

The endotracheal (ET) tube must be checked for leaks each time it is used, as follows:

1. Completely submerse the tube in a pan of clean water.
2. Attach a syringe to the cuff indicator.
3. Fully inflate the cuff and observe for any bubbles. Bubbles in the water, seen coming from any spot on the tube, indicate a leak in the tube.

The ET tube may be thrown away, or it may be kept and identified as a leaky tube if that type of equipment would be needed (e.g., as a tracheostomy tube).

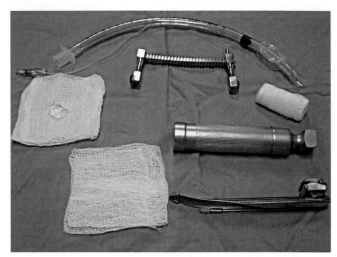

Fig. 5.20 Supplies needed for endotracheal intubation.

nonclear tube. Second, clear tubes allow visualization of the fog that moves along the lumen of the ET tube as the patient breathes. This is another useful means of quickly confirming that the patient is breathing.

Securing the Tube

A method of securing the tube in place is necessary. Rolled gauze is most commonly used to secure the ET tube to the patient once proper placement has been established. Any width can be used, although 2-inch gauze is most often employed. The gauze should be a nonstretch type, like muzzle gauze. Kling gauze can stretch, leading to tube slippage. The gauze is placed on the tube to indicate the depth of placement of the ET tube in the patient. Another method of securing the tube is using pieces of IV lines or plastic ties. The plastic can be cleaned and used with many different patients; it can also be less messy for performing dental procedures. The plastic or tubing is placed in a similar fashion to the gauze. Proper depth of insertion is determined by measuring the tube before placement. Box 5.3 describes the procedure for measuring the tube for proper placement in the patient.

Lubricant

A water-soluble lubricant is needed to lubricate the tip and cuff of the ET tube to permit easier passage of the tube through the

TABLE 5.2 Approximate Sizes for Endotracheal Tubes Based on Body Weight

Body Weight (KG)	Internal Diameter (MM)
CANINE	
2	3–4
5	5–6
10–12	7–8
14–16	8–9
18–20	9–10
>20	11 and up
FELINE	
2	3.0–3.5
4–5	3.5–4.0
>5	4.0–4.5

BOX 5.3 Measuring an Endotracheal Tube for Proper Placement in Patient

1. Position the patient in sternal recumbency if possible.
2. Identify the thoracic inlet and the larynx. The ramus of the mandible may be used as a landmark for the larynx.
3. Without touching the tube to the patient's hair coat, place the tip of the endotracheal (ET) tube halfway between the larynx and the thoracic inlet.
4. Identify the part of the tube that is just caudal to the canine tooth.
5. Place the gauze tie on the tube at the point on the tube that is just caudal to the canine tooth.
6. Ideally, the connector end of the tube should be at the incisors. If too much tube extends beyond the incisors, the ET tube may need to be cut to decrease the "dead space."

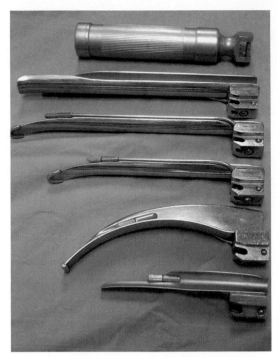

Fig 5.21 Laryngoscope handle and various blades.

larynx. The lubricant should be placed on a clean gauze sponge or clean paper towel and then applied to the tube. Water can also be used to lubricate the tube.

Cuff Syringe

The cuff syringe, or "puffer cuffer," is needed to inflate the cuff of the ET tube. A 6- or 12-mL syringe is used. It should be readily available throughout the procedure. Securing a syringe case to an accessible area of the anesthesia machine provides reliable storage for constant availability.

Laryngoscope or Light Source

The use of some type of light source significantly enhances the process of intubation. Easy visualization of the larynx permits greater success of first attempts to intubate. Laryngoscopes are composed of two major parts: the blade and the handle (Fig. 5.21). The blade houses the light bulb and can be curved or straight. Curved blades are commonly identified as Macintosh blades, and straight blades are often called Miller blades. The numbers included in the identification process refer to the length of the blade. The higher the number, the longer the blade. Often, "0" blades work well with cats, No. 1 blades for small dogs, No. 2 blades for medium-sized dogs, and No. 3 blades for large dogs. The handle houses the batteries that power the laryngoscope. Alternative light sources include floor lamps and overhead lights.

Tube Placement
Patient Anatomy

Proper knowledge of the laryngopharynx is critical to placement of the ET tube. Recognition of structures assists in the detection of abnormalities and helps ensure proper placement of the tube. Fig. 5.22 displays the region involved. When one is viewing this area, the following structures can be seen: vocal folds, epiglottis, and glottis. The epiglottis is a triangular flap of tissue that covers (or protects) the glottis when in the up or most dorsal position. The epiglottis must be lying down for intubation to be accomplished. The vocal folds are located on the lateral edges of the glottis. The glottis is the most ventral opening in the throat. The esophagus runs along the dorsal surface of the trachea, just left of center.

One-Person Technique

Box 5.4 describes the technique for performing single-person ET intubation.

Two-Person Technique

Box 5.5 describes the technique for performing two-person ET intubation.

Laryngospasms

Certain species, most often cats and rabbits, experience laryngospasm during ET intubation. If excessively stimulated, the muscles of the larynx spasm, and the vocal folds clamp shut. Application of 0.05 mL of 2% lidocaine to each vocal fold (dripping the lidocaine out of a tuberculin syringe onto the vocal folds with the needle removed) just before attempting intubation will significantly decrease the occurrence of laryngospasm. Care must be taken with this step because laryngeal paralysis can occur. A safer tactic to avoid laryngospasm is good technique. Repeated stimulation of the area may cause the muscles to spasm, so avoiding unnecessary touching of the area until the tube is actually passed is beneficial. The best technique is to try to pass the ET tube on inspiration when the vocal folds are open.

Confirmation of Proper Tube Placement

The following methods are used to confirm proper placement of the ET tube:

Cough: Many animals cough as the tube is passed into the trachea. Although fairly accurate, this method can be deceiving because as the animal coughs, the ET tube may move off the glottis and into the esophagus as it is advanced.

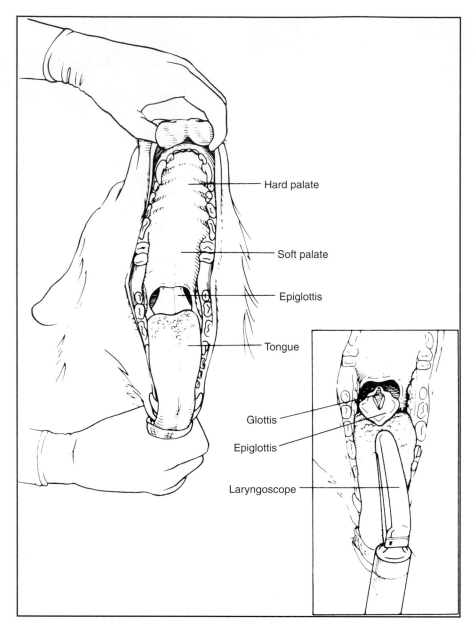

Fig. 5.22 Anatomy of the throat. (From McKelvey D, Hollingshead KW: *Veterinary anesthesia and analgesia,* ed 3, St Louis, 2003, Mosby.)

BOX 5.4 Single-Person Endotracheal Intubation

1. Place the animal in sternal recumbency.
2. Place the mouth speculum in the mouth.
3. Position a floor lamp or overhead light if being used.
4. Holding the mandible with the nondominant hand, fully extend the tongue and hold it in place with the thumb. The thumb should be caudal to the canine tooth, and the rest of the hand should be on the ventral surface of the mandible.
5. Visualize the glottis. If the epiglottis is lying dorsally, it will need to be pulled down with the endotracheal (ET) tube to ensure visualization of the glottis.
6. Pass the lubricated tube through the glottis to the predetermined length, as indicated by the gauze tie placed on the tube.
7. Secure the tube to the patient.
   a. For dogs, tie the gauze in a bow on the muzzle, just caudal to the canine teeth.
   b. For cats or brachycephalic dogs, tie the gauze in a bow behind the ears at the base of the skull.
8. Leave the mouth speculum in place until the patient has reached a surgical plane of anesthesia to avoid accidental biting of the tube.

Alternatively, a blind technique can be used, as follows:

1. Place patient in lateral or dorsal recumbency.
2. Place the mouth speculum in the mouth.
3. Insert the nondominant hand into the mouth and feel for the epiglottis with the index finger.
4. With the dominant hand, pass the lubricated ET tube through the glottis /using the index finger of the nondominant hand as a guide.
5. Follow steps 7 and 8 from above.

BOX 5.5 Two-Person Endotracheal Intubation

1. The restrainer holds the patient in sternal recumbency.
2. The restrainer opens the mouth by holding the maxilla in one hand and the mandible in the other hand.
   a. In a dog, the maxilla should be held caudal to the canine teeth.
   b. In a cat, the maxilla should be held just caudal to the ear pinna so that the skull is in the palm of the restrainer's hand.
3. The hand holding the mandible grasps the tongue and fully extends it over the mandibular incisors (Fig. 5.23).
4. The restrainer lifts the head and extends the neck to aid the intubator's visualization.
5. Using the laryngoscope, the intubator illuminates the larynx for proper visualization (Fig. 5.24).

6. The intubator visualizes the glottis and passes the tube between the vocal folds into the glottis (Fig. 5.25).
7. The intubator advances the tube to the predetermined depth as indicated by the preplaced gauze tie.
8. The intubator secures the tube to the patient.
   a. For a dog, tie the gauze in a bow on the muzzle (Fig. 5.26). The gauze should be snug but should not constrict circulation.
   b. For a cat or brachycephalic dog, tie the gauze in a bow caudal to the ears at the base of the skull.

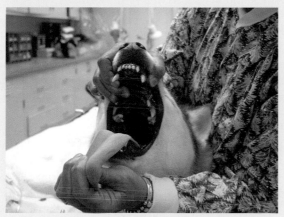

Fig. 5.23 Proper positioning for endotracheal intubation.

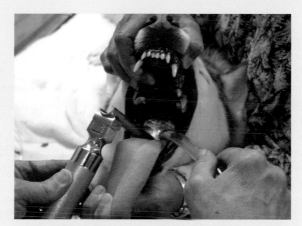

Fig. 5.25 Passing endotracheal tube.

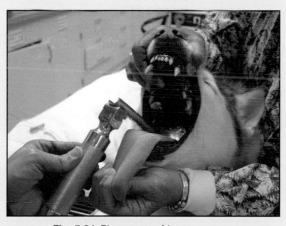

Fig. 5.24 Placement of laryngoscope.

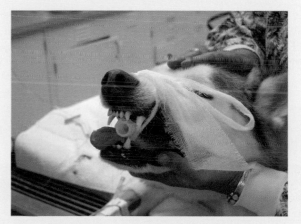

Fig. 5.26 Endotracheal tube tied in place.

Fogging in the tube: When an ET tube has been properly placed in the trachea, there should be fogging of the lumen of the tube with each expiration. This method can be employed only if a clear tube is used.

Blowing of gauze or hair: A few strands of gauze or hair placed at the connector end of the ET tube blow away with each expiration if the tube is correctly placed. A disadvantage is that the hair may move from the tube because of excessive movement of room air rather than expiration.

Air movement: If the ET tube is in the trachea, forced air should be felt at the connector end of the tube with each expiration. Bilateral chest compressions can be used with this method to ensure placement. Care must be taken to avoid compressing the abdomen, because an incorrectly placed tube may provide a false-positive assessment.

Palpation: Palpation of the ventral neck should result in the identification of one "tube." If the ET tube is in the trachea, only one firm, tube-like structure should be felt. If the ET tube is in the esophagus, however, two firm, tube-like structures are palpated.

Whatever method is used to ascertain correct tube placement, it should be performed before the patient is connected to the anesthesia machine. Once the patient is connected to the machine, a double check of placement can be done. Movement of the flutter valves and the rebreathing bag with each inspiration and expiration confirm proper placement. A stethoscope can also be used to auscultate bilateral lung sounds, the presence of which ensures that the tube has not migrated too far down in the trachea. It is a good idea to recheck cuff inflation at this point.

Once the patient is successfully intubated, the intended surgical site can be prepared.

PATIENT PREPARATION

Proper preparation ("prepping") of the surgical patient is a critical part of the surgical process. The veterinary technician should be the primary staff member responsible for this task. Proper prepping should include the following steps:

- Double-check (with the neck identification [ID] band, cage card, and medical record) and triple-check (with the surgeon) the patient's correct identity and exact procedure. Cross-check that the consent form has been signed by the client for the correct procedures. If the procedure is an amputation, double-check (with the record and consent form) and triple-check (with the surgeon) that the correct limb is being prepared. Any radiographs taken before anesthesia should be in the surgery room and hung on the view boxes.
- Extremely dirty patients may require a bath before surgery. The bath decreases overall body soil and aids in reducing the risk of postoperative complications from iatrogenic contamination. However, the patient's hair coat must be completely dry before general anesthesia is induced. Wet animals are at an increased risk of hypothermia while under anesthesia.
- Ensure that the anesthesia form has been started.

Anesthesia Form

The anesthesia form "tells the story" of the anesthesia event from beginning to end. It is an important piece of the patient's medical record and serves as a legal document. It can help guide the choice of anesthetic protocols to follow in the future. The anesthesia form documents vital signs and their trends intraoperatively. For example, a graph of the patient's blood pressure may be a line that goes down over time, with an occasional spike as the procedure proceeds, indicating that the trend for the overall blood pressure is dropping, which is a cause for concern.

The anesthesia form should be filled out completely and accurately, starting the minute the patient is given any premedication. The following paragraphs demonstrate the information typically found in each section of the form.

Demographics

The demographics section records the owner's name and the patient's signalment, with date of birth (DOB). The technician should fill in the blanks using the information from the medical record.

Preanesthetic Values and Disposition

The preanesthetic values and disposition section of the anesthesia form records the date and patient's weight, identifies the clinician, and lists the surgical procedures to be performed, as follows:

Weight: Be sure to enter both pounds (lb) and kilograms (kg).

Procedures: List the procedures in the order they will be performed. More than one procedure may be done.

Preanesthetic values: May include temperature (Temp), heart rate (HR), respiratory rate (RR), mucous membrane color and capillary refill time (MM/CRT), packed cell volume (PCV), total protein (TP), renal function, and hydration status. This information should be recorded before premedication is given.

ASA status: The American Society of Anesthesiologists (ASA) rating system is used to assess a particular patient's risk for an anesthetic procedure, helping to define the patient's anesthetic risk category (Table 5.3).

TABLE 5.3 American Society of Anesthesiologists (ASA) Rating System for Anesthetic Risk (ASA Status)*

Category	Physical Condition	Examples of Possible Situations
Class I: Minimal risk	Normal healthy patient with no underlying disease	Ovariohysterectomy; castration; declawing procedure; hip dysplasia radiographs
Class II: Slight risk	Patient with slight to mild systemic disturbances; patient able to compensate; no clinical signs of disease	Neonatal or geriatric patients; obese patients; fracture without shock; mild diabetes; compensated heart or kidney disease; full-blown estrus
Class III: Moderate risk	Patient with moderate systemic disease or mild clinical signs	Anemia; anorexia; moderate dehydration; low-grade kidney disease; low-grade heart disturbances, heart murmur, or cardiac disease; moderate fever
Class IV: High risk	Patient with preexisting systemic disease or severe disturbances	Severe dehydration; shock; anemia; uremia or toxemia; high fever; uncompensated heart disease; diabetes; pulmonary disease
Class V: Grave risk	Surgery often performed in desperation on patients with life-threatening systemic disease or disturbances not correctable by surgery; includes all moribund patients not expected to survive 24 hours	Advanced cases of heart, kidney, liver, lung, or endocrine disease; profound shock; major head injury; severe trauma; pulmonary embolus

*ASA recommends that every patient with ASA status of III, IV, or V have a responsible person solely dedicated to managing the patient during the anesthetic period. However, more veterinarians are finding it advantageous to have an anesthetist assigned to all patients under anesthesia.

Preanesthetic disposition: Circle the descriptive term that best describes how the patient appears before any premedication is given.

Preanesthetic Drugs

Preanesthetic drugs are usually given via an intramuscular (IM) or subcutaneous (SC) route to relax and sedate the patient. This relaxed state generally allows for a more willing patient when it is time to place the IV catheter and induce anesthesia. The following information should be entered in the preanesthetic drug section:

Drug: Write out full name of drug.

Dose: Write in a weight unit, such as milligrams (mg). It is important here to avoid units of volume, such as milliliters (mL), because one drug may be available in different concentrations. Depending on which concentration of the drug is used, the amount of milligrams in 1 mL of the same drug varies. The important amount to know is how many milligrams of the drug the patient received, not how many milliliters, which depends on the concentration.

Route: IM, IV, or SC.

Time: Note the time when the drugs are administered.

Premedication Results

Sedation: Record results after administration of premedication. How well did the patient seem to be sedated?

Resistance: How much did the patient resist manipulation, such as catheter placement?

Anesthetic Induction

Anesthetic induction drugs are generally given through an IV line and have a rapid onset and short duration. Anesthesia induction should be a rapid and smooth event that brings the patient to a level of anesthesia that allows the patient to be quickly and safely intubated with an ET tube. The following information about anesthetic induction should be noted on the anesthesia form:

Drug: Full name of drug.

Dose: Use a weight unit (e.g., mg) only. Remember that this information cannot be filled in before the drug is given. IV induction agents are given to effect. The desired effect is sufficient muscle relaxation of the jaw and diminished gag reflex such that the patient can be intubated. For example, the calculated IV dose may be 2 mL, but the patient may require only 1 mL for sufficient relaxation to be intubated. The amount of milligrams of induction drug in the 1 mL administered is what needs to be recorded here. This underscores the importance of filling out the dose box after the induction drug is administered. Induction agents given by the IM or oral (PO) route are based on the calculated dosage rate.

Route: This is the route of administration of the induction drug (IV, IM, mask).

Time: Note the time the drug was administered. In the case of gas induction, note the time the anesthetic gas was first turned on.

Breathing System

Breathing system: Check that appropriate breathing system is used (rebreathing or nonrebreathing system).

Size of tube: Record the size of the ET tube used. The size is stamped on the side of the ET tube. If a patient's medical history includes recent general anesthesia, the anesthesia form for that procedure may help in tube selection for this procedure.

Recumbency: Enter the position in which the patient is placed for the procedure. For example, "LL" may be entered here for left lateral recumbency (patient's left side is in contact with surgery table). Recumbency is important to note, especially if a complication occurs (e.g., nerve paralysis in a limb, burn from heating pads). If more than one procedure is performed, the patient may be in more than one position during this anesthetic period.

Intraoperative Updates

It is important to keep the anesthesia form as current as possible throughout the surgical procedure. Record all information every 5 to 10 minutes (heart and respiratory rates, level of anesthetic, oxygen flow rate, patient's depth of anesthesia). If any additional medications are given intraoperatively or if the fluid rate is altered, that should also be recorded.

Fig. 5.27 describes the graph component of the anesthesia form.

Postoperative Values

Measure and record the postoperative values after extubation, as follows:
1. Temperature.
2. Pulse.
3. Respiration.
4. Total fluids: Total volume administered and type of fluids given.

Hair Removal

Once the patient has been stabilized under anesthesia, the process of clipping may begin. It is ideal to have the patient positioned for the preparation in the same way as for the procedure (Fig. 5.28). Although this may be easily accomplished (for an exploratory laparotomy) or may be more of a challenge (perineal surgery), it is an important step to ensure an appropriate prep of the surgical area can be accomplished. Except in an emergency, it is recommended that the anesthetist be comfortable with the patient's level of anesthesia before any manipulation begins. Emergency procedures are more critical, and time is of the essence; therefore the anesthetist may not have the patient at the ideal anesthetic depth before the prep begins. While waiting for the nonemergency patient to stabilize at the appropriate anesthetic level, the surgery technician can complete some of the prep tasks.

The area of hair clipped needs to be neat, tidy, and symmetric (Fig. 5.29). The appearance of the clipped area may influence the client's impression of the enter clinic and staff. Clipping should be done only with a surgical clipper blade (No. 40). This design has close-set teeth to achieve the closest possible

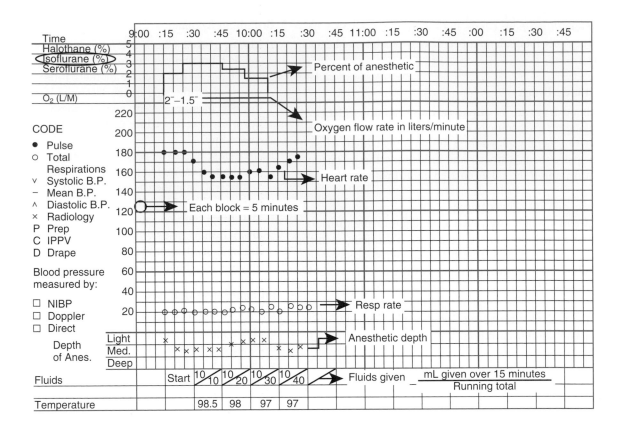

Fig. 5.27 Graph component of the anesthesia form.

Time: Each block (or small square) represents 5 minutes. If "start anesthesia" time is 9:15, start recording all the parameters at the 15-minute mark (see graph).

Percentage of anesthetic: A record of the percentage of anesthetic gas being delivered to the patient. It corresponds to the settings on the vaporizer (%).

Oxygen flow rate: A record of the flow of oxygen throughout the procedure. This corresponds to the rate of flow at which the flowmeter is set on the anesthesia machine.

Heart and respiratory rates: Record every 5 minutes. See *Code* at far left.

Anesthetic depth: Subjective assessment of the patient's depth of anesthesia graphed over time reveals whether the patient may be "getting light" or "getting too deep" for the specific procedure. Assessment is affected by trends in heart and respiratory rate, pupil position, and presence or absence of reflexes.

Fluids given: A record of how many milliliters (mL) of fluid the patient received throughout the procedure. *Top number* is the number of mL given over 15 minutes (mL/hour divided by 4). *Bottom number* is a running total of how much the patient has received at that particular point in the procedure, again in 15-minute blocks. First box is usually written as "start," but "0/0" is also acceptable.

Temperature: Measured every 15 minutes; however, you may not be able to obtain a body temperature measurement once the procedure has started and the patient has been draped.

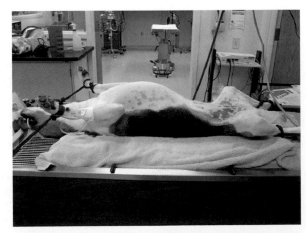

Fig. 5.28 Patient positioned for ovariohysterectomy (OHE, "spay").

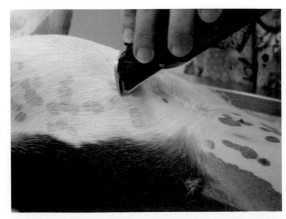

Fig. 5.29 Holding clipper at 90-degree angle to skin creates an even, neat margin for clipped area.

shave. When clipping, the person performing the clip needs to hold the clippers in a pencil grip (Fig. 5.30). This grip permits the greatest amount of control and maneuverability. Other grips will prove to be cumbersome and may strain the wrist and arm. The clipper should be held flat against the patient's skin for the closest clip. The hand not holding the clipper can tense the skin to encourage as easy a movement as possible for the clipper (Fig. 5.31).

The amount of hair to be removed depends on the surgery being performed. For general soft tissue surgery, a good rule of thumb is to clip two clipper-blade widths in every direction from the proposed incision site. Depending on the size of the animal, its length of hair, and the procedure being done, the clip may be altered. For example, a gastrotomy will require a very different clip than a prostatic biopsy. The technician should be sure to check with the surgeon for any special circumstances or anticipated additional procedures. Preoperative clipping and prepping need to include preparations for any ancillary procedures that may be done (e.g., chest tube placement, drain placement, feeding tube placement). Table 5.4 provides clipping guidelines for specific procedures.

Orthopedic preps use the rule of thumb of clipping the limb from the joint distal to and the joint proximal to the surgical incision. The limb needs to be clipped circumferentially to allow complete limb draping and manipulation. As with soft tissue

procedures, the rule for clipping may need to be adjusted according to the patient's size, the surgeon's preference, and additional procedures to be performed (e.g., bone graft harvest, drain placement). Tables 5.5 (forelimb) and 5.6 (hind limb) provide clipping guidelines for most orthopedic procedures.

Neurologic surgical patients are usually quite easy to clip, especially when the surgical site is a caudal thoracic or lumbar vertebral space. Clipping two vertebral spaces cranial and two vertebral spaces caudal to the affected site is usually adequate. As with other surgical procedures, communication with the surgeon is critical to ensure adequate prepping of the neurologic surgical patient. Particularly in the event of a cervical vertebral procedure, the technician should be sure to ascertain whether the surgeon will make a ventral or dorsal incision. If multiple intervertebral spaces are affected, clipping should extend from the most cranial to the most caudal space affected. Table 5.7 provides clipping guidelines for neurologic surgical procedures.

Some procedures may fall into either the soft tissue category or the orthopedic category, depending on the reason for surgery. For example, aural surgeries are generally considered soft

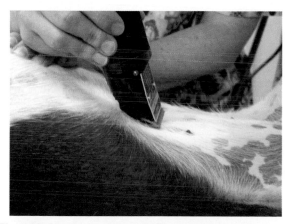

Fig. 5.30 Clipper should be held like a pencil for best control.

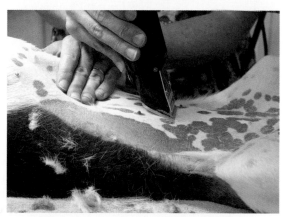

Fig. 5.31 Proper hand position for clipping.

TABLE 5.4 Clipping Guidelines for Selected Soft Tissue Surgical Procedures

Soft Tissue Procedure/Area	Guidelines
Exploratory laparotomy	Midsternum to pubis; laterally to edge of ribs
Gastric, liver, splenic	Midsternum to pubis; laterally to edge of ribs
Urinary bladder	Umbilicus to caudal pelvis; laterally to edge of ribs
Kidney	Midsternum to pubis; laterally to edge of ribs
Prostate	Umbilicus to caudal pelvis, including prepuce; laterally to edge of ribs
Uterine, ovarian	Xiphoid to pubis; laterally to edge of ribs
Ventral neck	Cranially to midmandible; caudally to thoracic inlet; laterally to commissure of lips

TABLE 5.5 Clipping Guidelines for Selected Forelimb Orthopedic Procedures

Forelimb Area	Guidelines
Digit	Nails to midhumerus; use towel clamp through nail to suspend limb
Metacarpal	Nails to midhumerus; use towel clamp through nail to suspend limb
Carpus	Second metacarpal to midhumerus
Radius, ulna	Midmetacarpals to shoulder; ventrally to midline; cranially to thoracic inlet; caudally to seventh rib
Elbow	Carpus to dorsal midline; ventrally to ventral midline; cranially to thoracic inlet; caudally to seventh rib
Humerus	Carpus to dorsal midline; ventrally to ventral midline; cranially to base of neck; caudally to seventh rib
Scapula	Midradius to two clipper-widths past dorsal midline; cranially to base of neck; caudally to tenth rib

TABLE 5.6 Clipping Guidelines for Selected Hind Limb Orthopedic Procedures

Hind Limb Area	Guidelines
Digit	Nails to midfemur; use towel clamp through nail to suspend limb
Metatarsal	Nails to midfemur; use towel clamp through nail to suspend limb
Tarsus	Second metatarsus to midfemur
Tibia, fibula	Midmetatarsals to hip; ventrally to midline; cranially to last rib
Stifle	Tarsus to hip; cranially to last rib; caudally to tuber ischii
Femur	Tarsus to dorsal midline; cranially to last rib; caudally to tuber ischii
Hip	Tarsus to two clipper-widths past dorsal midline; cranially to last rib; caudally to tail head
Pelvis	Depends on area of pelvis to have surgery (ilium vs. pubis vs. ischium); consult surgeon

TABLE 5.7 Clipping Guidelines for Selected Neurologic Procedures

Vertebrae	Guidelines
Cervical: ventral approach	Midventral mandible to midsternum; laterally to halfway between dorsal and ventral midline
Cervical: dorsal approach	Midskull to two vertebral spaces caudal to affected space; laterally to halfway between dorsal and ventral midline
Thoracic	Two vertebral spaces cranial and caudal to affected space; laterally to edge of transverse process
Lumbar	Two vertebral spaces cranial and caudal to affected space; laterally to edge of transverse process

TABLE 5.8 Clipping Guidelines for Miscellaneous Surgical Procedures

Procedure/Area	Guidelines
Aural	Lateral canthus of eye; dorsal midline on head and neck; ventrally to ventral midline
Ophthalmic: intraocular	Trimming of eyelashes; limited skin clip because of potential irritation
Ophthalmic: extraocular	Entropion, ectropion: one clipper-width past lateral canthus, lower lid, and medial canthus. Enucleation: midline of muzzle to cranial edge of ear pinna; dorsally to midline; ventrally to commissure of lip
Facial	Procedures vary widely among nasal, maxillary, and mandibular; best to consult surgeon
Perineal	Dorsally to tail head; laterally to tuber ischii (bilaterally); ventrally to midthigh (caudal aspect)

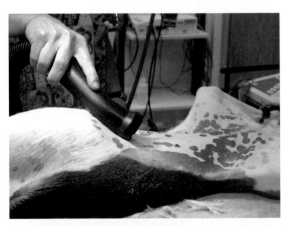

Fig. 5.32 The area should be thoroughly vacuumed after clipping.

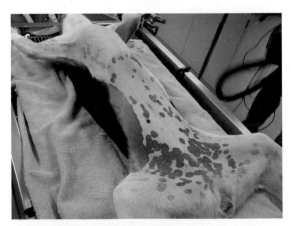

Fig. 5.33 Clipped abdomen ready to be prepared.

tissue, but if a bulla osteotomy is done, it is more of an orthopedic procedure. Likewise, facial surgery is soft tissue surgery if it is a tumor removal or nasal procedure, but if there is maxillary or mandibular involvement, the procedure is considered orthopedic. Table 5.8 provides guidelines for clipping for these types of surgical procedures.

After clipping, the patient and the area must be thoroughly vacuumed (Fig. 5.32). The hair removed from the animal must be cleared from the surgical site as well as from the work area. Loose hair can be a source of contamination in the surgery room, so it is important to avoid transporting any hair into the surgical suite. Brushing away loose hair from the clipped site with a hand is not as effective as vacuuming (Fig. 5.33).

Urination

The urinary bladder should be emptied independently by the animal or manually by the technician before the surgical prep. Caution should be used if the abdomen has been traumatized or if the procedure will involve the urinary bladder. Expression of the bladder may be contraindicated and may do more damage to the bladder in these situations. The technician should discuss with the surgeon whether to attempt manual expression

or to state in the patient's record that the bladder was not expressed. The patient undergoing nonabdominal surgery must also undergo bladder emptying if possible. Otherwise, the patient may urinate during the surgical procedure, soaking the table linens as well as the patient's hair coat and skin. Lying in urine for any period exposes the patient to the risk of **urine scald** (the moist, irritating effect of urine in contact with the skin). Even if the animal does not urinate during the surgery, it will probably do so during recovery. The patient soaked in urine is at increased risk not only of urine scald but also of contamination of the surgical wound with urine. For patients that will require critical care nursing postoperatively, a urinary catheter may be placed to prevent these problems.

The bladder can be expressed with the patient either in dorsal or in lateral recumbency. Some type of receptacle should be used to collect the expressed urine to avoid saturating the fur with urine or having the urine pool under the animal. During expression of the bladder, care is taken to use gentle, constant pressure rather than a pulsating action.

SURGICAL SITE PREPARATION

The skin of a patient cannot be sterilized, in the true definition of the word, but reducing the contaminants on the skin can greatly reduce the risk of wound infection. Multiple options exist for the products used to prep the patient as well as for the applicators used to apply these products. The use of the particular antiseptic products, in a particular fashion and in a particular order, is done to render the skin as clean as possible by eliminating or decreasing as many of the skin flora as possible.

Antiseptics

The first product used in the preparation of the patient is a scrub product. A scrub has a soap or detergent base and therefore creates a sudsy appearance when used. Some properties of the scrub product are desired for maximum effect. Although no available scrub product has all the desired qualities to achieve maximum effect, the choice of product should contain as many of these qualities as possible.

One product available for use as a patient scrub is povidone-iodine. This scrub is an iodine-based product that has a detergent and a wide spectrum of antimicrobial activity. Povidone-iodine is bactericidal (kills bacteria), viricidal (kills viruses), fungistatic (inhibits growth), and fungicidal (kills fungus). Its toxicity to tissues is relatively low, and it is inexpensive and readily available. Because of the iodine base, it does stain clothing and discolor the white hair of animals. Povidone-iodine has a better residual activity level than hexachlorophene but is not as effective as chlorhexidine. The povidone-iodine scrub is generally diluted 50:50 with tap water when used.

Chlorhexidine gluconate is another scrub product available. Its residual effect is the best of any available product. Chlorhexidine has shown bactericidal action against 30 bacterial genera, including *Escherichia coli* and *Pseudomonas* species. It also has demonstrated viricidal and fungicidal properties. Chlorhexidine scrub has relatively low tissue toxicity, except for mucous membranes. It also has the advantage of not staining clothing or skin. Chlorhexidine is generally used in a 60:40 dilution with tap water.

Rinsing Agents

After the application of a scrub product, a rinsing agent is needed to remove the detergent. A common rinsing product is 70% isopropyl alcohol, which is effective against most gram-negative bacteria. Alcohol coagulates protein, contraindicating its use on open wounds and mucous membranes. Isopropyl alcohol is generally well tolerated by patients, and it is inexpensive and readily available. Alcohol can be used with either povidone-iodine or chlorhexidine scrub. Residual properties of the chlorhexidine seem to be enhanced when it is used with 70% isopropyl alcohol, whereas povidone-iodine does not show any increase in residual activity.

Alcohol's tendency to evaporate rapidly is both an advantage and a disadvantage. The advantage of rapid evaporation is the ability to move quickly through the prepping process without diluting subsequent products. The extreme cooling effect that results from rapid evaporation is a disadvantage. Use of excessive amounts of alcohol to prepare the patient can significantly contribute to the hypothermia experienced by the anesthetized patient. Alcohol that is allowed to pool under an animal or saturate the fur can contribute to the risk of thermal burn if electrocautery is used. Therefore, alcohol should not be used as a rinsing agent if electrocautery will be used intraoperatively.

Another rinsing agent available is bottled sterile water or sterile saline. Sterile water or saline is effective at removing the detergent product, although it has no antimicrobial properties itself. For prepping of open wounds, compound fractures, or mucous membranes, this is the rinsing agent used. Because 70% isopropyl alcohol is not appropriate in certain situations, sterile water or sterile saline is a practical and reasonable alternative.

Applicators

Regardless of the prepping products used, applicators used can vary widely depending on the site being prepared. The most common applicator used is a gauze sponge. Sponges can be used individually as needed and saturated with the product by squirting the liquid from a bottle onto a dry sponge, or sponges can be mass produced and stored in jars or plastic containers. If mass produced, the prep sponges and the containers need to be discarded and cleaned weekly to inhibit the growth of contaminants. It is best to place the sponges needed in a separate, smaller container (e.g., "weigh boat") to avoid reaching into the large storage container with dirty hands.

As applicators, cotton balls usually are practical only when prepping small areas, so their use is limited. Cotton balls are indicated for IV catheter sites and perhaps ophthalmic procedures.

Similarly, a cotton-tipped applicator is usually chosen only for intraocular procedures. The limited amount of preparation needed for the eye can be best accomplished with the delicate control provided by a cotton-tipped applicator.

A spray bottle is an appropriate applicator only for application of the final paint solution (e.g., povidone-iodine solution). This is an efficient method of application but can be messy. The mist from the spray bottle can easily be deposited on the patient's skin as well as other areas. Monitoring devices, table linens, and even the rest of the animal may be covered with a mist of paint solution.

Special Male Dog Preparation

In preparation of the abdomen of a male dog, one task must be done before the surgical site prep is started. After all the hair has been removed from the prepuce, the sheath must be flushed to remove potential contaminants, as follows:

1. Combine 1 mL of povidone-iodine solution with 9 mL of tap water.
2. Insert the syringe tip into the prepuce and inject 5 mL of solution (Fig. 5.34). Pinch the prepuce around the syringe tip before removing the syringe.
3. While still pinching the prepuce closed, gently massage the solution in the prepuce.
4. Place a towel over the end of the prepuce to absorb the solution.
5. Release the pinch hold on the prepuce.
6. Repeat the process with the remaining 5 mL of solution. This step is required only for intraabdominal procedures when the prepuce will be in the draped surgical field.

Patterns for Scrubbing

Depending on the area of the body that is undergoing surgery, one of three patterns of action should be used to prepare the site: target, orthopedic, or perineal.

Target Pattern

The most common pattern is the target pattern, which resembles a target or bull's-eye. This pattern is used to prepare surgical sites for abdominal, thoracic, and neurologic procedures. The prep begins after the hair has been removed by the clipper and vacuumed from the area. The first step is to take one of the rinsing sponges and wipe around the periphery of the clipped margin. This action moistens the hair and flattens it down, helping to keep the hair from flying onto the clipped area once the prep begins.

To begin preparation of the surgical site, pick up one scrub sponge and fold it in half and then in half again, or bring all four corners to the center and hold the sponge by the corners. Either method produces a smaller contact surface that will be easier to control. Always start at the proposed incision site (Fig. 5.35), and then move the sponge progressively outward in a circle until the hair is reached (Fig. 5.36). Excessive pressure is not encouraged because it may abrade the skin; the wound may be more prone to healing complications if the dermal layer is compromised. Once the hair or any other dirty or contaminated area has been touched with the sponge, the sponge must never return to the incision site.

The surgical site should be rinsed with 70% isopropyl alcohol. The same target pattern should be used with the alcohol rinsing sponges as with the scrub sponges (Fig. 5.37). The process of scrubbing and then rinsing should be performed a minimum of three times. If dirt is still present with the last rinse, repeat the process until the last rinse gauze is clean.

Orthopedic Pattern

The second prep pattern is used with orthopedic procedures. After the hair has been removed from the surgical site (Fig. 5.38), any hair remaining on the foot must be covered. An inverted

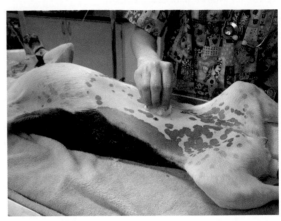

Fig. 5.35 Target pattern for preparing surgical site begins at proposed incision site.

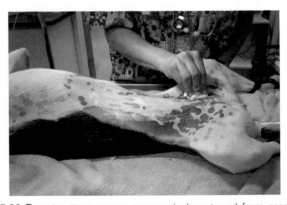

Fig. 5.36 Target pattern moves progressively outward from proposed incision site.

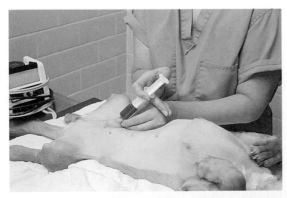

Fig. 5.34 Prepuce of a male dog should be flushed before surgical site is prepared for abdominal procedure.(From Fossum TW, Hedlund CS, Hulse DA, et al: *Small animal surgery*, ed 3, St Louis, 2007, Mosby.)

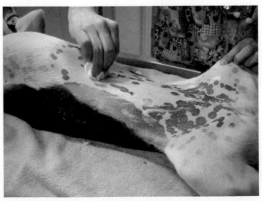

Fig. 5.37 Rinsing agent is applied with the same target pattern.

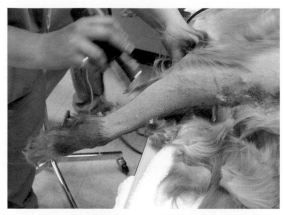

Fig. 5.38 Clipping of a forelimb.

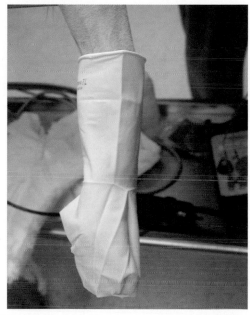

Fig. 5.39 Inverted glove placed over an unshaven foot.

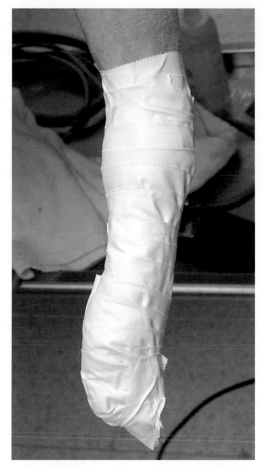

Fig. 5.40 Tape covering an examination glove.

examination glove is placed over the foot (Fig. 5.39) and secured with tape (Fig. 5.40). To avoid a tourniquet effect, be sure the tape is not applied too tightly. Cover with tape (or Vetrap), again not too tightly. Also, make a stirrup to allow suspension of the limb for preparing and draping; take a long piece of white tape (2–3 feet), leaving 2 to 3 inches at either end, then fold the remainder of the tape on itself to make it ½-inch wide. Place the ends of the stirrup on either the medial and lateral or the anterior and posterior sides of the gloved foot. Secure the stirrup to the foot with tape (Fig. 5.41). The limb should be suspended for the preparation to allow access to all surfaces of the limb. Place the stirrup over the hook of an IV pole and then fully extend the pole to elevate the limb (Fig. 5.42). In the event of a fracture, it is imperative that the limb and bones be supported as the pole is extended. With fractures, the extension of the limb may actually provide some distraction and traction to fatigue the muscles, which will aid in reduction of the fracture. Once the limb is suspended, clipping can be completed (Fig. 5.43), and the scrub prep can begin.

With a scrub sponge in hand, begin the prep at the tape edge of the suspended limb. Scrub the limb from distal to proximal, moving circumferentially around the limb. As the sponge dries out, discard it and continue with a new sponge. As with the target pattern, the wrist must be kept moving to provide the scrubbing action. Repeat the scrub a minimum of three times before rinsing to achieve the best antimicrobial efficacy. The rinsing agent is applied in the same pattern, starting at the taped foot and moving proximally to the dorsal midline (Fig. 5.44). Generally, a final solution is not applied because another prep will be done once the patient is positioned on the surgery table.

After the final rinse, place a clean towel over the medial surface of the down limb. This provides a clean surface on which the prepped limb can lie. The final prep is performed in the surgery room, so the towel only needs to be clean, not sterile. Carefully lower the limb, supporting any broken bones, to the towel (Fig. 5.45). The patient is now ready to be transported to the surgical suite.

Perineal Pattern

The third pattern that can be used is that for perineal surgery. It is important that a purse-string suture be placed in the anus before the preparation is begun. This suture prevents the evacuation of fecal material onto the surgical site during the procedure. The purse-string suture needs to be placed carefully to

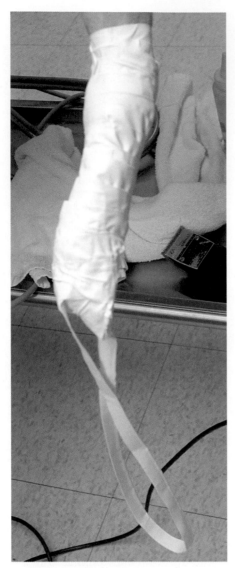

Fig. 5.41 Stirrup is secured to the foot.

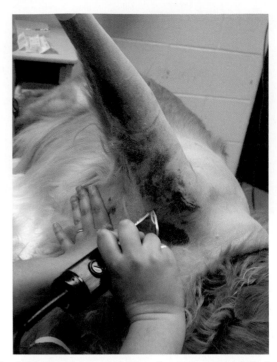

Fig. 5.43 Completion of clipping after suspension of the limb.

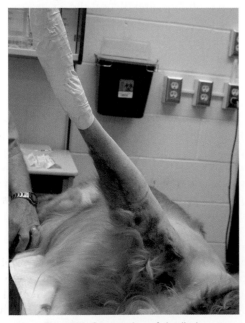

Fig. 5.42 Suspension of the limb.

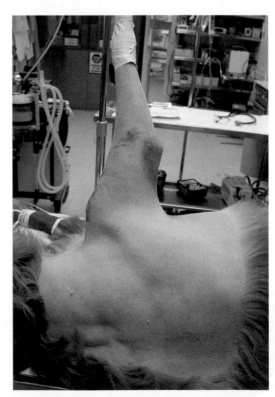

Fig. 5.44 Completed orthopedic preparation.

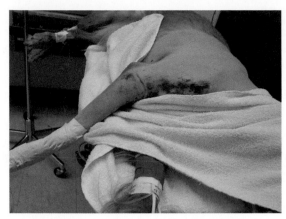

Fig. 5.45 Patient ready to be transported to surgery room.

avoid puncturing the anal glands. It is the technician's responsibility to ensure that the suture is removed after the procedure; a reminder note on the anesthetic monitoring sheet helps the technician remember this task.

The perineal pattern is basically three separate target patterns performed in a particular sequence. The first step is to do a target pattern on the clipped area to the right of the anus. The second step is to perform another to the left of the anus, and the third pattern is done on the anus itself. The "dirty" area should always be prepared last to minimize contamination. As with other patterns, the scrub is followed by a rinsing agent.

Potential Reactions

Clipper-Related Reactions

If dull clipper blades are used or the technique is harsh, clipper burn can occur. Clipper blades should be checked before use for chipped or missing teeth, rust, and other inhibitors of performance. Such inhibitors will pull on the skin and can cause clipper burn. Using excessive pressure with the clippers can also cause clipper burn. Irritation of the skin can inhibit wound healing if the irritation is over the proposed incision site. Irritation can also promote bacterial growth, which could cause an infection. Clipper burns on the peri-incisional skin can be an irritation to the patient, promoting excessive licking, which can also compromise the healing process.

Chemical-Related Reactions

Reactions to prepping products generally manifest as plaques or wheals. Certain breeds (Labrador, Shar Pei) seem more prone to these reactions, although any breed may be affected. Povidone-iodine tends to cause more reactions than chlorhexidine. If a patient has a chemical-related reaction, a notation should be made in the medical record so that an alternative product can be used the next time.

SITE PREPARATION AND POSITIONING

Securing Patient in Position on Surgery Table

Properly securing the animal to the table aids in the aseptic preparation of the surgical site and ensures that the surgeon has an immobile subject with adequate room for working. The techniques used are dictated by the surgical procedure. The patient's limbs may be tied to the table. The body may be braced in position by a V-trough or sandbags. The head, neck, or abdomen may need to be elevated through the use of a foam rubber tube or rolled towels. The patient's legs should not be forced to bend or extend beyond their natural anatomic limitations. Bony prominences should be cushioned to protect against excessive compression.

The use of a sturdy, flexible cord is common practice for securing the animal's limbs in position to the table. Most surgery tables are fitted with four stays (supports) located near the corners of the table. Some tables have adjustable stays that can slide and thus accommodate patients of various sizes. The end of the cord can be wrapped in a figure-eight fashion around the stay with a half-hitch loop to secure the cord in place. It is important to tie the cord to the table with a quick-release method because the patient may need to be untied quickly. The cord should be wrapped around the stays only two or three times and then locked with a half-hitch loop at the end (Fig. 5.46). If the surgery table does not have stays to secure the cords, they can be tied to each other under the tabletop. The knot used should be a quick-release knot such as a bow tie (Fig. 5.47).

It is best to spread out the distribution of pressure around the limb by placing two half-hitch loops, one proximal to and

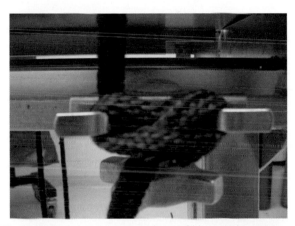

Fig. 5.46 Figure-eight wrap with a half-hitch as the last loop.

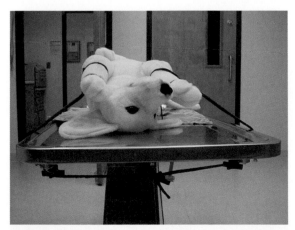

Fig. 5.47 Two half-hitch loops are placed on each foreleg; then the end of each rope is extended underneath the tabletop and tied with a bow tie.

the other distal to the elbow, carpus, or hock (Fig. 5.48). If the patient has a catheter in its leg, both loops should be placed distal to the catheter. The tie may prevent the administration of fluid to the animal during the procedure if the cord loop is placed proximal to the catheter. The paws should be checked throughout the surgical procedure. If the paw becomes swollen or the toes feel unusually cold compared with the opposite paw, the ties are too tight and are cutting off circulation to the paw. In this situation the cord needs to be loosened and repositioned.

Positioning for Specific Procedures
Abdominal Surgery
For abdominal procedures, the patient is placed in dorsal recumbency and secured by all four limbs to the table. Patients with deep-chested conformation can be challenging when it comes to keeping them in perfect dorsal recumbency. Deep-chested dogs need to be placed in a V-trough or braced by sandbags (Figs. 5.49 and 5.50). Some surgery tables are designed with built-in adjustability to form a V-trough (Fig. 5.51). Another technique to keep the patient balanced on the table involves tying the forelimbs crossed over the chest (Fig. 5.52).

Castration
For canine castration, the veterinary surgeon may prefer dorsal recumbency or a modified version of this position. For modified dorsal recumbency, the hind limbs are secured to the table. The forelimbs are not tied, and the cranial half of the dog rolls toward the side on which the surgeon stands (Fig. 5.53).

For feline castration, the cat is placed in dorsal recumbency with the hind legs pulled toward the head. The legs may be taped into position, held by the assistant, or tied to the surgery table (Fig. 5.54).

Orthopedic and Extremity Surgery
The patient is placed in lateral recumbency for procedures involving the extremities. If the left limb is the focus, the patient is positioned in right lateral recumbency. If the right limb is the surgical site, the patient is placed in left lateral recumbency. The paw may be wrapped in gauze and tape. The limb is suspended from above by tying the tape around the paw and tying the tape to an IV pole. The limb is clipped and scrubbed in this position. All sides of the limb are prepared (Fig. 5.55).

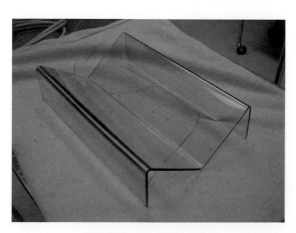

Fig. 5.48 Two half-hitch loops are tied around the limb. This technique distributes the pressure on the limb evenly between the two hitches. Care is taken to keep all the joints of the leg in anatomic alignment; that is, the limb is not forced into an unnatural position that may strain or torque the joints.

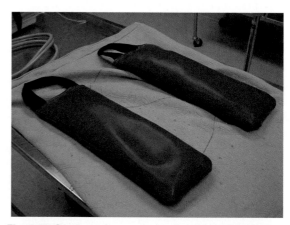

Fig. 5.50 Sandbags for supporting the sides of the patient.

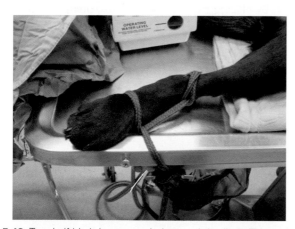

Fig. 5.49 Plastic V-trough.

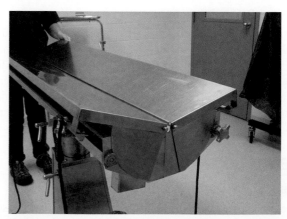

Fig. 5.51 Surgery table capable of forming a V-surface to help stabilize the patient in position.

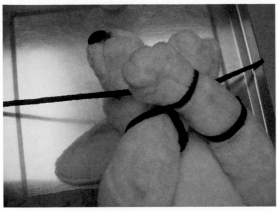

Fig. 5.52 Tying the legs in a crossed position across the chest helps stabilize the patient in dorsal recumbency. Care must be taken when this technique is used to avoid restricting chest excursions as the patient breathes.

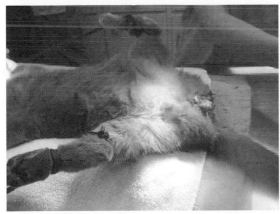

Fig. 5.53 Canine patient in position for castration procedure.

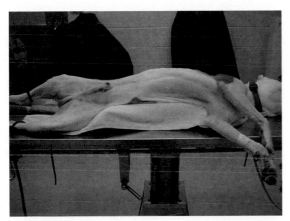

Fig. 5.54 Feline patient in position and surgically prepared for castration. The legs are secured to the table with two half-hitches on each leg and then carefully pulled in the cranial direction.

Tail and Perianal Surgery

The patient is placed in ventral recumbency for procedures involving the tail or perianal area. The forelegs are secured to the table, with the hind limbs hanging over the edge at the end of the table. A rolled towel is placed under the caudal abdomen for extra padding. A piece of adhesive tape is placed in a spiral on

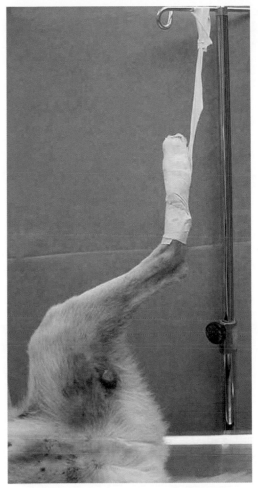

Fig. 5.55 Patient's leg is suspended by a piece of tape secured to an intravenous (IV) stand. This patient has a skin mass on the medial aspect of the thigh, so suspending the leg from the IV pole facilitates the preparation process.

the tail, with a long extension of the tape attached above to an IV pole or another object (Fig. 5.56).

Back Surgery

The patient having back surgery is placed in ventral recumbency. Positioning in a V-trough or placing sandbags on both sides helps brace the patient and prevents listing to one side. The forelimbs are extended cranially. The hind limbs are bent in a natural sitting or squatting position. A strip of adhesive tape may provide additional stabilization across the shoulders (Fig. 5.57).

Thoracic Surgery

The patient undergoing thoracic surgery is placed in lateral or dorsal recumbency, depending on the surgeon's intended approach. The forelimbs are extended cranially as much as possible and secured to the table.

Final (Sterile) Surgical Site Preparation

Once the patient has been transported and appropriately positioned on and secured to the surgery table, the final surgical prep is performed in the surgical room. The area is scrubbed

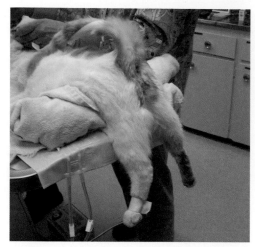

Fig. 5.56 Positioning patient for surgery of the tail or perineal area. Note the rolled towel placed under the abdomen for extra cushioning.

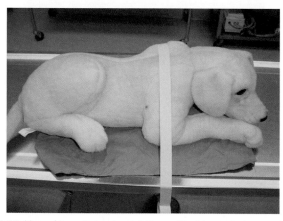

Fig. 5.57 Use of tape helps to stabilize patient in ventral recumbency.

and rinsed as described early in the chapter. In some university or specialty clinic settings, the doctor may wish the final prep to be performed sterilely (i.e., applied by the sterile surgical assistant); however, in most small animal settings this is not the case. Box 5.6 outlines the procedure for a sterile final prep.

Solutions (Paint)

The final step in the surgical site preparation is the application of the solution product, or paint. Povidone-iodine solution is in the same chemical family as the scrub, but the paint does not contain a detergent. The solution also has a stronger concentration of iodine, therefore increasing its potential for staining. It is corrosive when it contacts metal. The full-strength solution is applied to the patient and remains on the surgical site. It has much better efficacy when allowed to dry on the patient's skin before the drapes are applied or the incision is made.

A second current option for a final solution is chlorhexidine gluconate. As with povidone-iodine, chlorhexidine as a solution contains no detergent. This product is diluted to a 0.2% solution (30 mL/gallon of distilled water) when used as a final paint. Chlorhexidine also has better efficacy when allowed to dry on the patient's skin before the incision is made.

It is important to remember that only povidone-iodine scrub should be followed by povidone-iodine solution. Likewise, only chlorhexidine scrub should be followed by chlorhexidine solution. Using a povidone-iodine scrub with a chlorhexidine solution, or vice versa, is counterproductive and strongly discouraged.

Regardless of which product is used, the same method of application is utilized. The first squirt from the spray bottle should be directed into the kick bucket. This removes any debris and bacteria from the nozzle. Then, using a swiping motion, the technician applies a light mist from the spray bottle to the center of the proposed surgical site and allows it to dry.

BOX 5.6 Sterile Final Prep

1. Open the sterilized surgical bowl containing gauze sponges.
2. Pour off a small amount of surgical scrub solution into a trash can to cleanse the lip of the container, then pour the soap on the gauze sponges.
3. Open the container of sterile water and pour off a small amount into trash can to cleanse the lip of the container, then dilute the scrub soap in the bowl with sterile water.
4. Open a second sterile bowl containing sterile gauze.
5. After pouring a small amount of "rinse" (70% rubbing alcohol or sterile water) into the trash can, carefully pour the rinse on the sterile sponges until they appear soaked.
6. Aseptically perform the open-gloving technique (see Chapter 8).
7. Once you have put on surgical gloves, grasp a gauze sponge filled with scrub using your designated "clean hand," then squeeze out the excess liquid.
8. Transfer this sponge to your other hand, designated your "dirty hand," and start scrubbing. Use the same (clean) hand to retrieve each new sponge, and then transfer it to the other (dirty) hand to do the scrubbing; thus the phrase *clean hand, dirty hand technique*. Only the clean hand goes into the sterile bowl, and only the dirty hand touches the patient. (Rather than clean and dirty, both hands are actually sterile because they are covered with sterile gloves.)

9. The surgical site is scrubbed for the appropriate length of time recommended by the manufacturer of the scrub product, usually about 5 minutes. Scrubbing is done in a target pattern starting from the intended incision site and working outward to the edge of the shaved area. The time can be adjusted according to the duration of the initial surgical scrub performed in the surgery prep area.
10. Begin at the center of the clipped area over the proposed surgical incision.
11. Without touching the hairline, scrub the length of the incision with long, straight strokes. Scrub outward toward the periphery while slightly overlapping the previously scrubbed line in a circular fashion.
12. Never go back to the center of the area with the same gauze sponge.
13. After scrubbing the skin at the margin of the clipped area, discard the used gauze sponges and start again.
14. The skin should be cleansed thoroughly but gently. Excessive friction can result in hyperemia and bleeding of the skin and subcutaneous tissues.
15. The surgical scrub must have an overall contact time as recommended by the manufacturer. After the appropriate duration has elapsed, wipe the scrub away by using the "rinse"-soaked gauze.

TECHNIQUES FOR MAINTAINING BODY TEMPERATURE

Ideally, if the surgical suite has been thoroughly prepared for the day's procedures, any devices available to help maintain the surgical patient's body temperature will have been turned on and allowed to warm up before the patient is moved into the surgery room. It is preferable to place a patient on a warming device rather than arrange a warming element underneath a patient already positioned on the surgery table.

Several factors contribute to hypothermia in the surgical patient (see Chapter 4). The following devices and techniques should be used as available and appropriate to prevent hypothermia:

- A pad with circulating warm water is placed under the patient as soon as the animal is under anesthesia. Electric heating pads can become too hot and can burn the patient's skin and therefore should not be used. The circulating warm-water pad avoids the risk inherent with electric heating pads because the water is constantly circulating between the pad under the patient and the warming unit (Figs. 5.58 and 5.59).

Water bottles do not provide a constantly renewable source of heat and carry the risk of leaking. A wet patient can quickly become a cold patient.

- Warm-air convection blankets consist of an electrical unit that warms air and pumps it through a tube to a pad. The pad has a series of holes that allow the warm air to escape slowly. The pad is laid on top of the patient, or the patient rests on top of the pad; this creates a warm microenvironment. When used for the surgical patient, the unit is not activated until the surgeon has completed draping the patient (Fig. 5.60).
- Some stainless steel surgery tables are fitted with heating coils that warm the entire surface of the table to approximate body temperature. The need for warm-water blankets and bottles is eliminated while the patient is on the heated surgery table.
- The SnuggleSafe Microwave Heat Pad (SnuggleSafe, Lenric C21 Ltd., Littlehampton, West Sussex, UK) is a flat plastic disc that is placed in a microwave oven for a set number of minutes. This disc retains heat much longer than warm water bottles (Fig. 5.61).

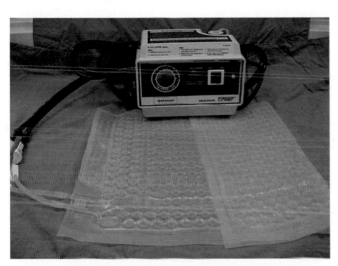

Fig. 5.58 Circulating warm-water blanket.

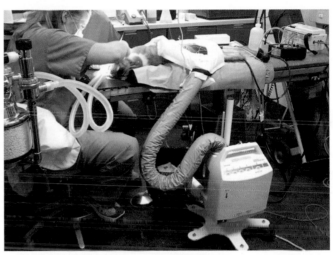

Fig. 5.60 Convection-current patient warming system (Gaymar Industries, Inc., Orchard Park, NY). The disposable blanket is lying on top of the patient. Air is warmed and pumped into the blanket, through which the warmed air slowly diffuses around the patient.

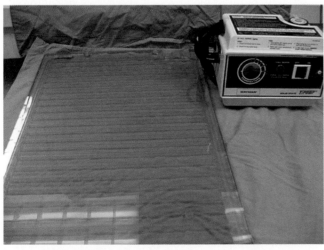

Fig. 5.59 Hard pad for circulating warm water.

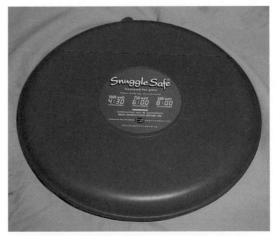

Fig. 5.61 SnuggleSafe Microwave Heat Pad (SnuggleSafe, Lenric C21 Ltd., Littlehampton, West Sussex, UK).

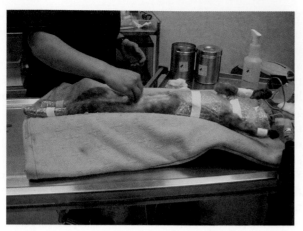

Fig. 5.62 Plastic bubble wrap around the extremities, head, and thorax helps to maintain the body heat as this cat is being prepared for a spay procedure.

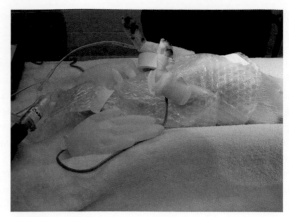

Fig. 5.63 Plastic bubble wrap and latex gloves filled with warm water laid across the pinnas help retain the body heat in the upper portion of this Chihuahua undergoing a spay procedure.

- A plastic bottle (e.g., soda bottle) can be filled with dry, uncooked rice and heated in a microwave oven. The bottle with rice holds heat longer than a water bottle and eliminates the risk of leaking water on the patient.
- The bag of IV fluids can be warmed in a microwave oven to approximately the same temperature as body temperature. The line for the IV administration set can run through a bowl of warm water to make the fluid warmer before going into the patient.
- Plastic bubble wrap can be wrapped around the patient's extremities, including the head. The plastic wrap is light but provides warmth by retaining the body heat that would be lost through the extremities (Figs. 5.62 and 5.63).

KEY POINTS

1. The benefits of placing an IV catheter for every anesthetic procedure outweigh any risks.
2. The five factors that should be considered in the choice of a catheter are site of placement, length of time the catheter will be needed, reason for placement, diameter of vessel, and length of vessel.
3. Catheter sites must be aseptically prepared to avoid complications.
4. Having all supplies readily available will aid in the success of the placement procedure.
5. Some surgical patients may require intensive care after surgery and may be better served by placement of a jugular catheter.
6. Successful ET tube placement depends on using the appropriate equipment and minimizing irritation to the patient.
7. Most patients can be intubated using the one-person technique, although the two-person technique is generally the more common practice.
8. Multiple options are available for checking the ET tube for proper placement in the trachea.
9. Clean, neat, symmetric clipping is an important skill to master for the patient's well-being as well as good client relations.
10. Appropriate hair removal helps to prevent contamination of the surgical site.
11. Contact time is the important consideration when one is using skin preparation materials.
12. When preparing a surgical site, the technician should always move the applicator from clean to dirty surfaces to avoid introducing contaminants to the proposed incision site.
13. Position the animal on the surgery table in the most natural position possible that does not put excess stress on joints, severely compress blood vessels and nerves, or compromise the well-being of the patient in any way.
14. Quick-release knots are tied in the cords securing the patient to the table so that the patient can be easily and efficiently untied.
15. The cords securing the animal to the table can cause problems if wrapped around the legs too tightly. Check the paws repeatedly throughout the procedure.

REVIEW QUESTIONS

1. A central catheter is placed in which vein?
   a. Jugular
   b. Cephalic
   c. Medial saphenous
   d. Lateral saphenous

2. What is a correct use of a butterfly catheter?
   a. Aid in monitoring central venous pressure
   b. Placement in the jugular vein for long-term critical care
   c. Short-term placement in peripheral vein for IV fluids during a surgical procedure

    d. One-time venous access for administration of medication over a 1- to 3-minute period

3. A macrodrip IV set should be reserved for patients that are:
   a. <7 kg
   b. >7 kg
   c. <7 lb
   d. >7 lb

4. Which central venous pressure would indicate a patient is overhydrated?
   a. 0 cm H_2O
   b. 6 cm H_2O
   c. 8 cm H_2O
   d. 12 cm H_2O

5. Which part of the endotracheal tube allows airflow if the end of the tube become occluded?
   a. Body
   b. Cuff
   c. Murphy eye
   d. Hose connector

6. Which laryngoscope blade is commonly used for cats?
   a. No. 0
   b. No. 1
   c. No. 2
   d. No. 3

7. What method is used to check that the endotracheal tube has not migrated too far down the trachea?
   a. Palpation of neck
   b. Check for fogging of tube
   c. Watch for movement of flutter valves
   d. Auscult the thorax for bilateral lung sounds

8. Intraoperative values should be recorded every:
   a. 1–5 minutes
   b. 5–10 minutes
   c. 10–15 minutes
   d. 15–30 minutes

9. Postoperative values recorded in an anesthesia log include:
   a. Pulse, RR, level of anesthesia.
   b. RR, temperature, total volume of fluids administered.
   c. Pulse, RR, intraoperative medications administered.
   d. Pulse, temperature, oxygen flow rate.

10. What is the appropriate area to clip for a spinal surgery?
    a. One vertebral space cranial and one vertebral space caudal to the affected site
    b. Two vertebral spaces cranial and two vertebral spaces caudal to the affected site
    c. Three vertebral spaces cranial and three vertebral spaces caudal to the affected site
    d. Four vertebral spaces cranial and four vertebral spaces caudal to the affected site

11. When is expressing the bladder of a patient prior to surgery contraindicated or not indicated?
    a. Orchiectomy in an adult patient
    b. Thoracotomy in a geriatric patient
    c. Abdominal exploratory in a hit-by-car patient
    d. Routine ovariohysterectomy in a pediatric patient

12. During the final scrub, what can be used as a rinse agent?
    a. Sterile water
    b. Chlorhexidine scrub
    c. Chlorhexidine solution
    d. Povidone-iodine solution

13. The use of alcohol as a rinse agent is contraindicated when prepping for:
    a. Feline oral surgery.
    b. Canine orchiectomy.
    c. Feline spinal surgery.
    d. Canine tibial plateau leveling osteotomy.

14. During the final scrub, what can be used as a rinse agent?
    a. Sterile water
    b. Chlorhexidine scrub
    c. Povidone-iodine solution
    d. Chlorhexidine solution

15. A patient would be placed in ventral recumbency for which procedure?
    a. Castration
    b. Thoracotomy
    c. Fracture repair of radius
    d. Perianal adenoma removal

16. What device is contraindicated for maintaining patient body temperature during surgical procedures?
    a. Plastic bubble wrap
    b. Thermal heating pad
    c. Warm-air convection blanket
    d. Circulating warm-water blanket

17. What is the disadvantage of bathing a patient prior to surgery?

18. List three ways to determine if the endotracheal tube is properly placed.

19. When recording the information about the anesthetic induction agent, dose should be recorded in what type of unit?

20. List four things that should be included on the anesthesia form in regards to the pre-anesthetic agent.

BIBLIOGRAPHY

Bassert J, Beal A, Samples O, editors: *Clinical textbook for veterinary technicians*, ed 9, St Louis, 2018, Elsevier.

Cunningham JG: *Textbook of veterinary physiology*, ed 4, St Louis, 2008, Saunders.

Fossum TW, Hedlund CS, Hulse DA, et al: *Small animal surgery*, ed 3, St Louis, 2007, Mosby.

Romich JA: *An illustrated guide to veterinary medical terminology*, Albany, NY, 2000, Delmar.

Thomas JA, Lerche P: *Anesthesia and analgesia for veterinary technicians*, ed 5, St Louis, 2017, Elsevier.

Patient Monitoring

Marianne Tear

LEARNING OBJECTIVES

After completion of this chapter, the reader should be able to:
- Perform complete monitoring of the patient under anesthesia, assessing cardiovascular, respiratory, and neurologic parameters.
- Discuss the special anesthetic considerations regarding monitoring of various surgical procedures and patient positions.
- List examples of anesthesia monitoring devices.
- Describe the functions of anesthesia monitoring devices.
- Discuss the cause and effect of various physiologic changes that may occur during anesthesia.

KEY TERMS

Adrenergic
Agonal breathing
Agonist
Anticholinergic
Assisted ventilation
Atelectasis

Capnography
Cyanosis
Dissociative anesthetic
Hypercarbia
Hypocarbia
Hypotension

Pulse deficit
Pulse oximetry
Pulse strength
Shock
Sphygmomanometer

ROLE OF THE VETERINARY TECHNICIAN ANESTHETIST

While under anesthesia, patients are completely vulnerable. They need to be carefully monitored to ensure that the procedure does not have a negative outcome. There is a fine line between safe, surgical anesthesia and inadvertent euthanasia. For this reason, anesthetic monitoring is one of the greatest responsibilities that a technician can undertake.

Ideally, every surgical procedure would have a dedicated technician anesthetist, whose only responsibility would be monitoring the patient, and a circulating assistant to help transport the patient from the surgery prep area to the surgical suite. This team approach allows the surgeon and surgical assistant to be scrubbing while the anesthetist and circulating assistant arrange the patient, anesthesia machine, and monitoring devices in the surgery room. When the circulating assistant takes responsibility for positioning the patient on the surgery table, attaching the monitoring devices to the patient, and performing the final skin prep and paint in the surgery room, the anesthetist is able to focus on the most important task, monitoring the patient. Without the help of a circulating assistant, the anesthetist would need to perform all these tasks alone in rapid succession. If the technician is working alone, the primary task is careful, constant monitoring of the surgical patient. This may mean delaying the final surgical scrub (or other, less critical tasks) until the patient is stable.

MONITORING

The patient that is monitored closely is the patient that is safely anesthetized. Close, constant monitoring allows the anesthetist to detect dangerous trends and to make appropriate adjustments. Monitor comes from the Latin *monere*, to warn. If the patient is showing signs of waking up, the anesthetist can increase the concentration of anesthetic. If the patient is showing signs of becoming too deeply anesthetized, the anesthetist can decrease the concentration of gas delivered. Table 6.1 summarizes the stages of anesthesia.

The patient should be monitored every 5 to 10 minutes with all findings recorded on the anesthesia form. More frequent monitoring may be required if the patient is compromised or if the inhalation agent used has a low solubility/parturition coefficient (allowing for quick changes in anesthetic depth). The observant surgeon and surgical technician can supplement intermittent, frequent monitoring by nonsterile personnel.

Patient parameters that should be monitored include heart rate and rhythm, respiratory rate and rhythm, capillary refill time, color of mucous membranes, eye position, muscle tone, and reflexes. The patient's temperature should be monitored at least every 15 minutes if possible. Several anesthetic and treatment parameters should be tabulated including volume of fluid administered, oxygen flow rate, anesthetic gas concentration, and any other medications administered.

The best monitoring device is the trained veterinary technician who knows the normal for their specific patient, what to expect from the anesthetic procedure, and how to troubleshoot the anesthetic and monitoring equipment. Hands-on, direct monitoring can give real-time empirical data on several important parameters. The technician can listen for the heart rate and respiratory rate through the stethoscope or esophageal stethoscope. The pulse can be palpated to obtain a general impression of pulse strength (Figs. 6.1 to 6.5). The reservoir bag can be observed for frequency and extent of movement. The color of the mucous membranes can be visually assessed, and the capillary refill time is directly measured. The technician's sense of smell can detect possible anesthetic leakage problems.

Heart Rate and Rhythm

Monitoring the cardiovascular system during anesthesia is very important. Most anesthetic agents depress the cardiovascular

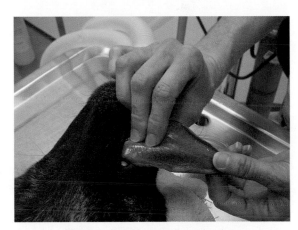

Fig. 6.1 Checking the lingual pulse.

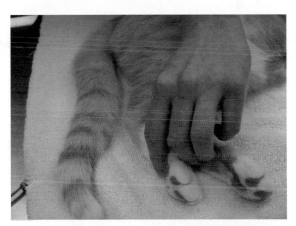

Fig. 6.2 Checking the digital pulse.

TABLE 6.1	**Expected Responses of Selected Monitoring Parameters**		
Stage of Anesthesia	**Behavior**	**Respiration**	**Cardiovascular Function**
I	Disorientation, struggling, fear	Respiratory rate increased; dogs may pant	Heart rate increased
II Excitement stage	Excitement: reflex struggling, vocalization, paddling, chewing	Irregular; may hold breath or hyperventilate	Heart rate often increased
III/Light stage III anesthesia	Unconscious; possible movement in response to surgical stimulation	Regular; rate—high, normal, or low	Heart rate often high normal; pulse strong
III/Surgical anesthesia	Unconscious; immobile	Regular and shallow; rate—often normal or mildly decreased	Heart rate often normal or mildly decreased, capillary refill time (CRT) normal; pulse strength decreased
III/Deep stage III anesthesia	Unconscious; immobile	Shallow; rate—often below normal; may see abdominal breathing	Heart rate low normal to well below normal; pale mucous membranes; CRT high normal or prolonged; pulse strength significantly decreased
IV	Unconscious; immobile	Apnea	Cardiovascular collapse

From Thomas J, Lerche P: *Anesthesia and analgesia for veterinary technicians*, ed 5, St Louis, 2017, Elsevier.

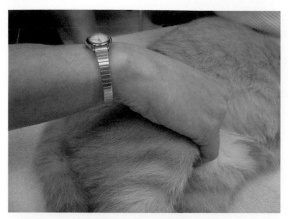

Fig. 6.3 Checking the femoral pulse.

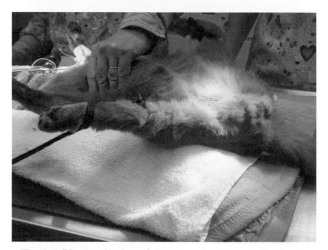

Fig. 6.4 Direct palpation of the heart through the chest wall.

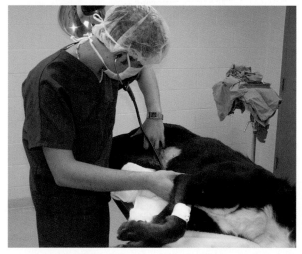

Fig. 6.5 Auscultating the heart and monitoring the femoral pulse simultaneously.

system, so the heart rate of an anesthetized patient is expected to be slower than the rate when awake. Hypothermia can also cause a decreased heart rate. When the heart rate falls below an acceptable limit, the surgeon should be notified, and interventions should be taken. Suggested guidelines for acceptable lower limits are 70 beats per minute (beats/min) for a large

dog, 80 beats/min for a small dog, and 100 beats/min for a cat. Rates lower than these warrant notifying the surgeon immediately.

The heart rate can be monitored through direct palpation of the thoracic wall or by listening through a stethoscope. The stethoscope can be the conventional type that is placed on the thoracic wall. However, the location of the surgical site may prevent the use of a conventional stethoscope. An esophageal stethoscope is a more convenient and less intrusive means of monitoring heart rate intraoperatively.

In positioning the esophageal stethoscope, special sensory plastic tubing is placed in the esophagus next to the heart. The tubing is passed through the mouth into the esophagus. The endotracheal (ET) tube prevents the esophageal stethoscope tubing from entering the trachea. The heart sounds can be heard through earpieces, or an amplifier can be attached to broadcast the sound (Figs. 6.6 and 6.7). If the end of the tubing is adjacent to the lung fields, breath sounds will be heard.

Anticholinergic drugs such as atropine sulfate and glycopyrrolate are administered to help maintain the heart rate above the acceptable lower limits (see Chapter 4). Dissociative anesthetics such as ketamine and tiletamine can also elevate the

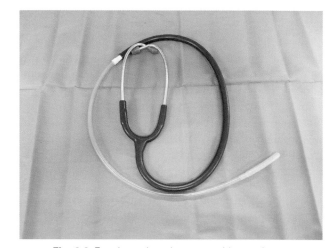

Fig. 6.6 Esophageal stethoscope with ear pieces.

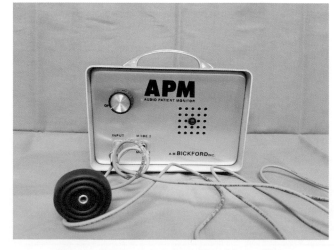

Fig. 6.7 Esophageal stethoscope with amplifier.

heart rate. When an animal is in shock or pain, the heart rate is usually rapid. Regardless of the reason, once the heart rate exceeds the acceptable limits, the surgeon should be notified. Suggested guidelines for acceptable upper limits are 180 beats/min for a large dog, 200 beats/min for a small dog, and 220 beats/min for a cat.

An irregular heart rhythm may be detected through auscultation of the thorax or on an electrocardiogram (ECG). Some anesthetic agents sensitize the heart muscle to arrhythmias. When the heart beats arrhythmically, the heart is inefficient at pumping the blood through the body. This inefficiency leads to poor tissue perfusion, acidosis, poor oxygen delivery to the tissues, and buildup of waste products in the body tissues. These irregular beats may spontaneously disappear. If the arrhythmic beats are frequent or continuous, the veterinarian should be alerted.

Detection of a pulse deficit is cause for concern. A pulse deficit occurs when the heart contracts (beats) but does not generate enough push to produce a palpable peripheral pulse. Pulse deficits are detected when the heartbeat is arrhythmic; tissue perfusion is poor, and the patient may quickly go into shock. The veterinarian should be alerted immediately. Skipped beats are detected when one is listening to the heartbeat with a stethoscope but is unable to palpate that individual beat simultaneously as a peripheral pulse. In this case the single skipped beat is a result of a single premature depolarization of the heart muscle.

Respiratory Rate and Rhythm

A patient's oxygenation and ventilation need to be closely evaluated. A dog or cat in the surgical plane of anesthesia has a rate of 8 to 20 breaths/min. A respiratory rate of less than 8 breaths/min is cause for concern and most likely indicates an excessive anesthetic depth. As anesthetic depth becomes dangerously deep, respiration ceases before the heart stops beating.

The respiratory rate can be determined by watching the patient's chest movement. The reservoir bag on the anesthesia machine can also be observed. The reservoir bag collapses and fills synchronously with the patient's breathing. The anesthetist can listen for breath sounds through the stethoscope or esophageal stethoscope and should note their character and intensity. An increase in intensity, crackles, or wheezing indicates pulmonary airway narrowing through constriction or the presence of fluid.

The depth and rhythm of the respirations should also be assessed. The inspiratory phase is about half as long as the expiratory phase. A short pause occurs before the next inspiration. If the animal feels pain during the surgery, the respiratory rate will increase. Dissociative anesthetic agents will cause the animal to inhale, hold its breath, and then exhale. As anesthetic depth increases, respiratory rate usually decreases. Gasping or labored breathing is of particular concern. An obstruction of the trachea or the endotracheal (ET) tube or a lack of fresh gas flow can cause exaggerated respiratory effort. Check the patency of the ET tube, check for the appropriate oxygen flow rate on the anesthesia machine, and confirm that the pressure in the reservoir bag is not too high. If the ET tube is not patent, it may need to be suctioned, or the patient may need to be reintubated.

If the desired setting on the oxygen flowmeter is not being maintained, the oxygen tank supplying the anesthesia machine may need to be changed. If the reservoir bag is overinflated and has a high pressure, assuming the pop-off valve is open, the anesthetist can try decreasing the oxygen flow rate on the anesthesia machine.

The animal that spasmodically contracts its diaphragm may be exhibiting agonal ("death agony") breathing. Agonal breathing, or agonal gasping, is not real breathing, that is, no physiologic exchange of gases is occurring in the lungs. Agonal gasps can be mistaken for deep breaths if the respiratory rate has not been sufficiently monitored. Agonal gasps typically occur after a long period of apnea and are often detected as rapid movement in the patient's diaphragm, jaw, or larynx. Agonal gasps occur after cardiac arrest, and the veterinarian must be alerted immediately of their presence.

The practice of manually ventilating the patient every 2 to 5 minutes during the anesthetic period is recommended. Assisted ventilation, bagging, opens up collapsed alveoli, preventing atelectasis. Anesthetized patients tend to breathe more shallowly; combined with the weight of other internal organs on the lungs, the shallow breathing contributes to atelectasis (lung collapse) (Box 6.1).

While administering a ventilating breath, the anesthetist should listen at the patient's mouth for any sound of air rushing past the ET tube. Some anesthetic agents, such as isoflurane, have a pungent odor, which indicates leakage if detected. If a sound is heard or the odor of gas detected, the cuff seal is incomplete. The cuff on the ET tube should be further inflated or the patient reintubated with a larger ET tube.

Tissue Perfusion

To maintain healthy and functioning tissues and organs, adequate tissue perfusion must be maintained. If not, adverse long-term effects may be sustained. The kidneys are particularly sensitive to states of low perfusion. During inadequate perfusion states, waste products from cellular metabolism are not removed, and nutrients such as oxygen and glucose are not delivered to the cells.

Mucous Membranes

The color of the mucous membranes is a general indicator of tissue perfusion. The pink color of the mucous membranes results from the color of the blood in the capillaries seen through the nonpigmented areas. Mucous membrane color may be evaluated by looking at the gums, conjunctiva, and mucosal surface of the vulva or prepuce.

BOX 6.1 Technique for Administration of a Ventilating Breath

1. The pressure relief valve is closed.
2. The reservoir bag is squeezed while the technician ensures that the manometer does not exceed 20 cm H_2O or that the chest does not exceed a normal excursion.
3. The pressure relief valve is opened.

Pale mucous membranes may indicate a state of poor tissue perfusion or anemia (Fig. 6.8). Preanesthetic diagnostic blood tests, such as complete blood cell count (CBC) and measurements of hematocrit and hemoglobin, will identify the anemic patient. Preferably, the severely anemic patient will not go to surgery before receiving appropriate blood component therapy. Pale mucous membrane color can also be an indicator of shock. Efforts must be made before the anesthetic episode to identify and begin correction of the poor color.

Dark-red mucous membranes may be seen if an animal is septic, meaning that the patient has a severe blood infection. Bacteria may be cultured from the blood. The immune system is reacting to the infection by releasing vasoactive chemicals that cause postcapillary venous dilation and increased permeability in the vessel walls. This can lead to congestion in the capillary beds and thus the brick-red color of the mucous membranes.

A bluish color to the mucous membranes (cyanosis) suggests that the red blood cells are not carrying adequate oxygen. The red cells may not have exchanged oxygen in the lungs, suggesting a respiratory problem such as obstruction of oxygen flow to the lungs or lack of breathing. The ET tube should be evaluated immediately for a kink or obstruction. A bluish color in the buccal mucosa may also result if a tie on the ET tube is too tight around the cheeks, causing stagnant blood flow. The buccal mucosa should be compared with the conjunctival mucosa to determine whether a tight tie could be the cause of the bluish color and needs to be loosened.

Capillary Refill Time

The capillary refill time (CRT) normally should be less than 2 seconds. The same areas used to assess the color of mucous membranes may be used to assess CRT. When CRT is longer than 2 seconds, perfusion in these tissues is poor. This condition may be caused by low arterial blood pressure or peripheral vasoconstriction. Release of epinephrine can cause peripheral vasoconstriction, and slow CRT is often seen in nervous and frightened animals. α_2-Adrenergic agonist drugs such as medetomidine cause significant peripheral vasoconstriction, thus slowing the CRT. A normal CRT can be detected shortly after some animals are deceased, reinforcing the importance of constant monitoring of several vital signs, not just one.

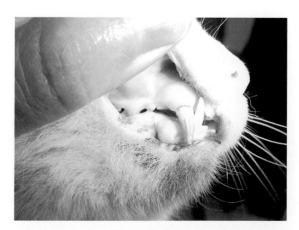

Fig. 6.8 Cat with pale mucous membranes.

PULSE AND BLOOD PRESSURE

Pulse strength can be defined as the ease or difficulty of palpating the blood flowing through the artery. Pulse strength is a general indicator of the blood pressure. If the patient's pulse becomes more difficult to palpate, the blood pressure has fallen. If the patient's pulse becomes more easily palpable or bounding, the blood pressure has increased. Pulses can be monitored at the following arteries: lingual, femoral, carotid, dorsal metatarsal, and digital (see Figs. 6.1 to 6.3). The heart may be palpated directly through the chest wall. In cats the examiner's thumb and fingers are placed on either side of the chest, and light pressure is applied to feel the beating heart (see Fig. 6.4). Obese patients and larger patients, such as medium- to large-sized dogs, are more difficult to palpate.

An ultrasonic Doppler or oscillometric device is needed to assess arterial blood pressure accurately. Normal mean arterial pressure (MAP) ranges in awake animals are from 85 to 120 mm Hg. MAP should be maintained above 70 mm Hg while the patient is under anesthesia and never allowed to drop below 60 mm Hg.

Hypotension

Hypotension (low blood pressure) in an anesthetized patient may be caused by the following factors:

Hypovolemia: Excessive blood loss or dehydration reduces the volume of the vascular space. With little blood to pump through the vessels, the blood pressure will be low.

Cardiac insufficiency: Patients with preexisting heart disease may have a weak myocardium or leaking heart valves, which can lead to inefficient pumping action.

Excessive vasodilation: Many preanesthetic and anesthetic drugs cause vasodilation to varying degrees. The effects can be additive and significant. When the blood vessels dilate, the blood pools, venous return to the heart is decreased, and blood pressure drops.

Anesthetic depth: In general, as the patient goes deeper under anesthesia, the blood pressure drops. The correlation between blood pressure and anesthetic depth is quite accurate.

Body Temperature

Body temperature is monitored before and during the anesthetic period. Monitoring every 15 minutes is common practice, although unless an esophageal thermometer probe or a rectal probe is used, this schedule may prove challenging.

In rare instances, hyperthermia may develop when inhalation anesthetics are used. Dangerously high body temperatures spontaneously manifest in patients that develop malignant hyperthermia. If the high temperature goes unnoticed, life-threatening cerebral edema can develop. Genetic predisposition may play a role in the phenomenon of malignant hyperthermia, which has been documented in humans, pigs, and dogs. If an abnormally high body temperature is detected, or if a temperature significantly higher than the preanesthetic body temperature is recorded, the anesthetic procedure should be terminated as soon as possible.

The development of hypothermia is common and a constant concern in patients undergoing general anesthesia. The following factors contribute to the decrease in body temperature:

- Anesthetic drugs relax muscles, significantly diminish the shivering response, and decrease the overall metabolic rate. Production of body heat decreases.
- The surgical site is shaved, washed with soap and water, and then rinsed with alcohol. Evaporation from the skin surface has a cooling effect on the body.
- Room-temperature fluids are administered.
- Cold gases are inspired.
- A body cavity may be opened, and internal organs are exposed to ambient temperatures.
- Measures to prevent body heat loss should be taken, as discussed earlier.

Neurologic Parameters
Reflexes

As anesthetic depth increases, reflex activity diminishes and eventually disappears. A reflex is an automatic reaction to a stimulus made by the patient without conscious awareness of the reaction. These reflex actions protect the patient from harm. For example, the swallowing reflex is triggered by the presence of saliva or other matter in the pharynx. The patient swallows the material into the gastrointestinal system rather than aspirating it into the respiratory system. Most reflexes monitored during anesthesia are located around the face, eyes, and throat. The return of the reflex or increasing strength of the reflex response indicates that the level of anesthesia is becoming lighter. The technician anesthetist may monitor the following reflexes:

- Auricular (ear flick) reflex: The fully conscious patient flicks its ear when the pinna is lightly touched or tickled. The intensity of the reaction varies among individuals. If the reflex is tested in rapid succession, the reaction to the stimulus may diminish quickly. Although this reflex can persist well into a moderate level of anesthesia, its variable nature renders it somewhat unreliable. It is best to monitor all available reflexes.
- Pedal (withdrawal, or toe pinch) reflex: When pressure is applied to a toe, the limb is withdrawn. The pressure applied should be significant. The withdrawal reflex is useful when the patient is being masked. The mask interferes with the ability to monitor other reflexes around the face. Once the pedal reflex disappears, the patient may be sufficiently anesthetized to attempt intubation.
- Palpebral (blink) reflex: The blink reflex protects the globe from injury by the eyelids quickly closing. The reflex can be elicited by lightly touching the medial canthus of the eye. The reflex disappears or is significantly diminished as the patient enters the surgical plane of anesthesia. The palpebral reflex usually returns just before the laryngeal reflex as the patient is recovering.
- Laryngeal (swallow) reflex: When saliva, food, or water is in the pharynx, the epiglottis and arytenoid cartilage close the entrance to the trachea, and the patient swallows. The laryngeal reflex can also be initiated by rubbing the ventral throat. The swallow reflex must be lost in order for intubation to proceed easily.
- Corneal reflex: The patient blinks or retracts the globe when the cornea is touched. This reflex persists well into the deep levels of anesthesia. The corneal reflex is seldom used in monitoring anesthesia; it is used more often to help assess the point of death during euthanasia.

Cats tend to retain the laryngeal reflex longer than dogs, so they need to be more deeply under anesthesia before intubation can be accomplished. If intubation is attempted too soon, the larynx may go into a spasm and remain closed. Cats also are more likely to develop laryngeal spasm than dogs during the intubation process. See Chapter 5 for a list of methods to avoid or reduce the likelihood of these spasms.

Muscle Tone

Muscles usually relax as the patient goes deeper under anesthesia. Dissociative anesthetics cause muscle rigidity; however, some muscle relaxants, such as benzodiazepines (e.g., diazepam, zolazepam), are usually added when these anesthetics are used. The most important muscles to relax are those that control the opening of the mouth. Once the mouth can be easily opened, intubation can be performed more easily.

It is important to monitor the intensity of the jaw tone during anesthesia. When jaw tone increases, the patient's depth of anesthesia is becoming lighter. The anesthetist can test the resistance to opening the mouth by carefully prying apart the upper and lower teeth with just two fingers (Fig. 6.9).

Depending on the procedure being performed, jaw tone may not be available for monitoring by the anesthetist. If the patient is undergoing a dental procedure or oral surgery, a mouth speculum may be placed in the mouth to keep it open. In such cases the anal opening may be inspected because it can indicate the degree of muscle relaxation the patient is experiencing. In the conscious patient, the anal opening is closed. In general, as the patient goes deeper under anesthesia, the anal tone becomes more relaxed and the anus opens more.

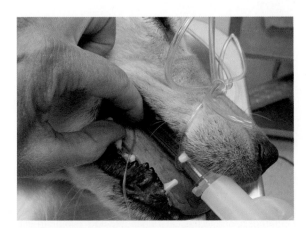

Fig. 6.9 Method for testing jaw tone involves prying the mouth open with just two of the examiner's fingers barely inserted into the mouth.

Eyes

The position of the eye in the socket, the pupil size, and the eye's responsiveness to light can be used to assess anesthesia depth. Although the responses may vary with the individual patient and the drugs given, the following general observations can be useful in assessing anesthetic depth:

- The eye rotates ventrally when the patient is in a moderate or surgical level of anesthesia (Fig. 6.10).
- At light and deep levels of anesthesia, the eye is in a central position.
- When dissociative anesthetics are given, the eye position may never change (Fig. 6.11).
- As the anesthetic depth increases, the pupil constricts more slowly in response to a light shined at it (pupillary light response [PLR]).
- Deeper stages of anesthesia and anticholinergic drugs cause pupillary dilation (mydriasis). The use of these drugs in the preanesthetic protocol interferes with the reliability of this reflex.

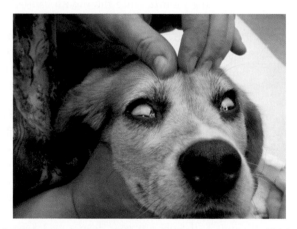

Fig. 6.10 The eyes have rotated ventrally. This dog is in stage III (plane 2) of anesthesia.

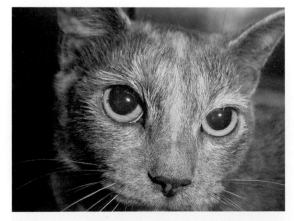

Fig. 6.11 Glycopyrrolate and Telazol (tiletamine/zolazepam) were administered intramuscularly to this cat 15 minutes ago. Eye ointment should be applied as soon as possible to protect the eyes from drying out. Tear production and the blink reflex are diminished. Note the widely dilated pupils.

It should be noted here as well that when a patient undergoes cardiac and respiratory arrest and expires, the pupils are fully dilated.

SPECIAL SURGICAL CASE CONSIDERATIONS

Although parameters to monitor for surgical patients are similar for all cases, certain anesthetic complications, reactions, and considerations must be given in special situations. Young, healthy patients that are undergoing an elective procedure are still at risk for anesthetic complications, although the risk is significantly lower. Patients experiencing a trauma or a disease process pose more of a challenge. A patient that is experiencing dystocia and now requires a cesarean section is compromised differently than a patient that has been hit by a car and now requires surgery to repair a fractured tibia.

Cranial Procedures

In most surgical procedures, the eyes are available for palpebral reflex evaluation, the jaw is available for muscle tone assessment, and the eye position is evaluated throughout the procedure. Mucous membrane color and capillary refill time are monitored by means of the gingiva for appropriate monitoring. Procedures that require the surgeon to be working on or near the head present unique monitoring challenges. When surgical procedures necessitate the removal of these options, technicians must redefine the options for monitoring. Ophthalmic, aural, or mouth procedures require the anesthetist to "rethink" the approach to anesthesia monitoring—using the vulva or prepuce to monitor mucous membrane color, for example. Attaching a reflectance probe to the underside of the base of the tail instead of on the tongue is another option. Using the femoral artery for pulse assessment instead of the lingual artery is another method to continue to effectively monitor the patient despite obstacles to the traditional methods used.

Respiratory Compromise

Patients that are experiencing dyspnea, for whatever reason, create a challenge for the technician anesthetist. For the patient in which thoracic trauma is the source of dyspnea, the use of a ventilator may be extremely beneficial. Once the chest cavity is opened, ventilator support needs to be provided anyway, so employing it earlier will do no harm. Patients in which abdominal issues are the cause of the respiratory compromise also benefit from ventilator support. Pressure on the aorta, for whatever reason (e.g., gastric dilation, gravid uterus, hemoabdomen), compromises return of venous supply as well as respiratory issues.

Patient Positioning Factors

Depending on the surgery being performed, certain necessary patient positions can create challenges for the anesthetist. Neurologic procedures that require the patient to be in ventral recumbency risk the development of respiratory problems. Patients lying on their abdomen and chest are not able to breathe as easily and effectively as if they were positioned in a different way. A patient in dorsal recumbency, with the neck in full extension or hyperextension (e.g., for thyroidectomy, ventral slot), will have respiratory issues as a result of the decreased ability to expand its chest. Animals undergoing perineal surgery (e.g., perineal urethrostomy) also present a respiratory challenge. With their hind legs draped over the end of the surgery table, much pressure is on their abdominal organs and diaphragm, inhibiting normal respiratory function.

ANESTHESIA MONITORING DEVICES

The monitoring of a patient that is under the effects of anesthetic drugs is an important responsibility of the veterinary technician. The veterinary technician must be prepared to anticipate and troubleshoot potential problems to ensure safety for the patient. Although there is no ideal monitoring device, multiple devices used together can provide useful information on the patient's status.

An educated, alert technician is the best device. The technician's sense of sight can watch for changes in mucous membrane color or patient movement or changes in respirations; the sense of sound is applied to listen to heart rate and rhythm; the sense of smell can detect the presence of anesthetic gas; and the sense of touch can feel for changes in peripheral pulses indicating changes in blood pressure.

Even the best technician has limitations, however, so the use of auxiliary monitoring devices is extremely helpful. Many types of monitors are available with varying capabilities and limitations. Some monitoring devices combine multiple capabilities into one unit for convenience and optimal anesthetic evaluation.

Table 6.2 lists normal values for anesthetic monitoring of dogs and cats.

Pulse Oximeter

Pulse oximetry, the estimate of saturated hemoglobin (SO2), has become a common piece of monitoring equipment in veterinary practices. The devices are noninvasive, relatively inexpensive, and in most cases portable. Most units also monitor the patient's pulse.

The pulse oximeter measures how much (or the percentage) of the available hemoglobin is saturated with oxygen. This measurement is achieved using two different wavelengths of light transmitted through tissue. The sensors (or probes) emit wavelengths of both red light and infrared light. The infrared light determines oxygen saturation, and the red light determines the pulse rate. The light is transmitted through the tissue, and the photodetector (located opposite the transmitter) senses the light. The software within the unit compares the absorption ratio of the two different wavelengths. Oxygen-rich blood (arterial) absorbs less light, so more of the light wavelength is sensed by the detector; therefore, a higher arterial oxygen saturation (Sao_2) reading is displayed.

Models

Units can be small handheld versions, whereas other versions are larger and more cumbersome (Fig. 6.12). Most models allow the user to set alarms for high and low limits of acceptable readings. These alarms emit an audio tone when the high or low limits of Sao_2 or pulse are reached. Other models are capable of monitoring multiple parameters, including Sao_2, heart rate, respiratory rate, and end-tidal CO_2 ($ETCO_2$).

Sensors

The choice of sensor depends on the placement site and species of patient being monitored (Fig. 6.13). One of the most common sensors is the lingual sensor, which resembles a clothespin in design and is available in large and small versions. Other common sensors are the reflectance probe and universal C clamp. The lingual sensor, as the name implies, is commonly used on the tongue but can be used on the ear pinna, toe webbing, external genitalia (vulva or prepuce), or any region with no hair. Using this probe on sites other than the tongue does cause increased pressure on the probe spring and can result in premature degradation of the probe. The reflectance probe can be used with a protective sleeve and placed in the rectum or used alone on the underside of the tail, at the base of the tail. The universal C clamp sensor can be used on feet, hocks, and other areas. Regardless of what sensor is used, certain factors can affect the efficacy of the unit and the reliability of the information. The site needs to be warm, motionless, nonpigmented, and hairless (or nearly hairless) in order to ensure accurate readings. If at any time the information being displayed by the unit appears unreasonable, the factors listed here should be evaluated to ascertain the true status of the patient.

Unit Options

Some Sao_2 units provide only basic information—that is, a pulse rate and an Sao_2 readout. Even these basic units, however, also have a pulse bar graph to indicate the strength of the peripheral pulse being evaluated. Other models include additional information, such as noninvasive blood pressure (NIBP) monitoring, $ETCO_2$ readings (capnography), and ECG readouts (Fig. 6.14). The more parameters measured by the device, the more information acquired by the anesthetist, but there is also greater potential for machine malfunction.

Troubleshooting

Maintaining an appropriate level of oxygen in the patient's blood is paramount. With a patient attached to the anesthesia machine with 100% oxygen (O_2) running, the Sao_2 reading

TABLE 6.2 Anesthetic Monitoring: Normal Parameters for Cats and Dogs	
Arterial oxygen saturation (Sao_2)	95%–99%
End-tidal carbon dioxide level ($ETCO_2$)	35–45 mm Hg
Blood pressure:	
Systolic	90–160 mm Hg
Diastolic	50–90 mm Hg
Mean arterial pressure (MAP)	
Awake	85–120 mm Hg
Under anesthesia	70–99 mm Hg

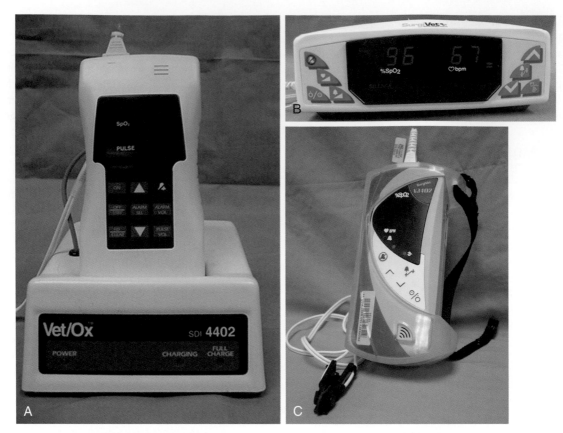

Fig. 6.12 Basic pulse oximeters: A and C, handheld styles; B, tabletop style.

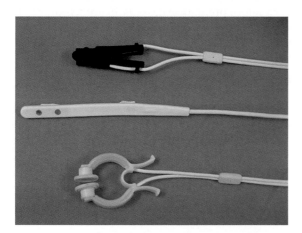

Fig. 6.13 Pulse oximeter sensors. *Top to bottom:* Lingual sensor, reflectance probe, universal C clamp.

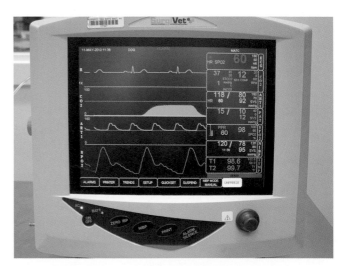

Fig. 6.14 Multiparameter anesthesia monitor.

should be 95% or greater. To prevent the animal from experiencing hypoxia, the veterinary technician needs to evaluate the situation if the reading hits 97% to determine whether the machine is malfunctioning or whether in fact the patient's Sao_2 levels are dropping. Assessing the patient and the equipment quickly is important to correct the problem appropriately. Sometimes the sensor has slipped from its original position, and simply repositioning it may correct the problem. Sometimes with the lingual probe, wetting the tongue with tap water can aid in obtaining a more accurate reading. It has been found

that when the lingual probe is used with felines, folding the tongue can be beneficial. Folding the tongue lengthwise provides a thicker tissue mass and generally a more accurate reading. If the patient is not exchanging gases well even though a normal respiration rate is present, ventilation of the patient may need to be provided manually. Artificial ventilation helps expand the lungs more completely, thereby allowing better gas exchange.

Capnometer or Capnograph

Capnometry is the measurement and evaluation of the level of CO_2 in the patient's exhaled breath, or the $ETCO_2$. This component of anesthesia is important because it can help the anesthetist evaluate the patient's respiratory rate and the quality of the respirations, therefore allowing better interpretation of the patient's depth of anesthesia. An arterial blood gas sample evaluation is the best method to determine blood CO_2 levels, but this is not usually performed in most practices. The alternative, $ETCO_2$ monitoring, is an option that accurately reflects the arterial CO_2 levels.

Measurement

The capnometer can measure $ETCO_2$ by one of two methods (Fig. 6.15). The sensors used are either a mainstream or a sidestream device. A mainstream device evaluates the patient's CO_2 levels as the breath passes through the airway. This sensor requires the patient to be intubated and correlates to the patient's breathing pattern. A sidestream device uses a vacuum to draw a portion of the exhaled breath down a tiny tube to the main unit for evaluation. The delay in the collection of the sample translates into a displayed pattern that is "out of sync" with the patient's breathing pattern. The tubing can also become kinked or clogged leading to incorrect readings. The mainstream unit tends to be bulky and can pull on the ET tube. Both types increase the respiratory dead space.

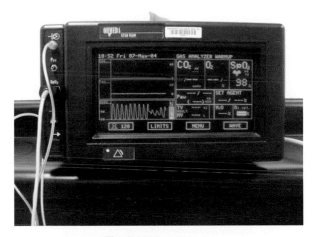

Fig. 6.15 Capnograph.

Display Wave

The display on the capnometer is a digital readout of the $ETCO_2$. The display of a capnograph is in the form of a wave. The incline of the wave indicates the exhaled portion of a breath. The plateau at the peak height of the wave indicates the $ETCO_2$ value. As the patient begins to inhale, the wave begins the decline because inspired CO_2 levels should be close to zero (Fig. 6.16). Some monitoring devices are capnometers, whereas others are capnographs. Either can combine the measurement of $ETCO_2$ with other monitoring parameters to provide the anesthetist with the most complete picture of the patient and the anesthetic episode.

Normal Values

Normal levels of expired CO_2 are 35 to 45 mm Hg for both dogs and cats. Levels that depart from the accepted range require quick, efficient evaluation by the anesthetist to determine the appropriate course of action. Values less than 35 mm Hg, or **hypocarbia**, can be attributed to overzealous artificial ventilation, increased respiratory rate, too light a plane of anesthesia, pain, or hypoxia. Administering analgesics, easing up on ventilation, increasing

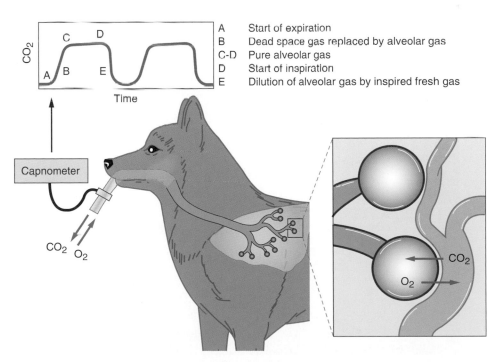

A	Start of expiration
B	Dead space gas replaced by alveolar gas
C-D	Pure alveolar gas
D	Start of inspiration
E	Dilution of alveolar gas by inspired fresh gas

Fig. 6.16 Capnograph tracing. (a), Start of expiration; (b), dead space gas replaced by alveolar gas; (c) and (d), pure alveolar gas; (e), dilution of alveolar gas by inspired fresh gas. *ETCO₂*, End-tidal carbon dioxide. (From Thomas JA, Lerche P: *Anesthesia and analgesia for veterinary technicians*, ed 5, St Louis, 2017, Elsevier.)

anesthesia depth, or treating an underlying hypoxia may help resolve the hypocarbia. Values greater than 45 mm Hg are caused by hypoventilation, which leads to higher levels of CO_2. If more CO_2 is being produced than removed, a dangerous situation can quickly develop. Hypercarbia can be the result of a decreased respiratory rate, decreased respiratory minute volume, exhausted soda lime, malfunction of one of the unidirectional valves on the anesthesia machine, or a kinked endotracheal tube. Elevated CO_2 levels generally imply that some or all of the gas that was just exhaled has been rebreathed. Corrections to lower the CO_2 include checking the machine and increasing ventilation to remove the excess CO_2.

Blood Pressure Monitor

Blood pressure monitors are used to assess a patient that is either awake or under anesthesia. Monitoring the blood pressure

allows for an approximation of tissue perfusion in the anesthetized patient. Blood pressure monitors should be used in conjunction with other devices to enable the anesthetist to provide the best anesthetic care possible.

Indirect Monitoring

In private small animal hospitals, blood pressure is most often monitored by indirect methods (Fig. 6.17). Doppler crystals are placed on the skin over arteries to produce an auditory assessment of pulse quality and blood pressure trends (Fig. 6.18). Common arteries that are used with the Doppler crystal include the coccygeal, dorsal pedal, and digital. Theoretically any artery can be used, but these are usually the most accessible. A sphygmomanometer and a cuff can be added to the ensemble to allow estimated numeric assessment of diastolic and systolic pressures (Fig. 6.19).

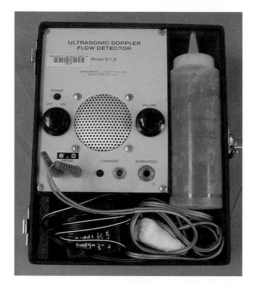

Fig. 6.17 Doppler unit in carrying case.

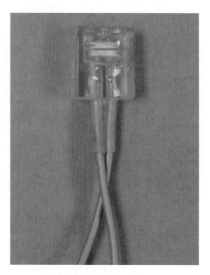

Fig. 6.18 Concave side (the side placed next to animal) of Doppler crystal.

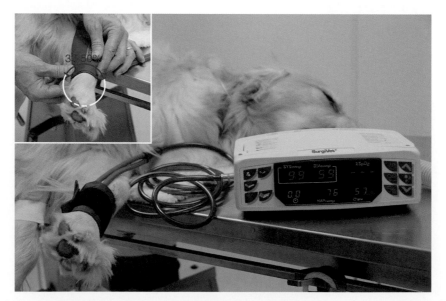

Fig. 6.19 Oscillometric blood pressure monitor with a cuff placed on the metacarpus. The following measurements are indicated: systolic blood pressure (BP), 99 mm Hg; diastolic BP, 59 mm Hg; mean arterial blood pressure (MAP), 76 mm Hg; pulse, 57 beats/min. *Inset:* Selecting an appropriately sized blood pressure cuff, the width of which should be 30% to 50% of the circumference of the extremity.

Noninvasive blood pressure machines (Fig. 6.20), which eliminate the need for a manual sphygmomanometer, are available. The units have cuffs that are placed on the patient, and the cuff inflation line is attached to the machine. See Fig. 6.21 for common cuff placement sites. The machine inflates the cuff at either preset intervals or manually determined intervals, the cuff is deflated, and a blood pressure measurement is acquired. The reliability of the numeric value displayed depends on the use of an appropriately sized cuff. Cuffs that are either too large or too small give inaccurate results. To ensure that the proper-sized cuff is being used, the following guidelines should be used: (1) the cuff width should be 40% of the circumference of the limb on which it is to be used, and (2) the length should be appropriate so as to fall into the securing range indicated on the cuff.

Direct Monitoring

Direct blood pressure monitoring is performed by placing an arterial catheter. The catheter is then attached to an aneroid manometer or to a transducer attached to an oscilloscope. The oscilloscope then displays the information being received through the transducer. Usually, numeric values for diastolic pressure, systolic pressure, and mean arterial pressure (MAP) and a waveform for the pulses are displayed. This procedure is more technically challenging than indirect monitoring and requires more expensive equipment. The advantage of direct monitoring is that a "true" evaluation of the pressure can be made. With indirect monitoring, only trends can be observed because accurate numbers are not available.

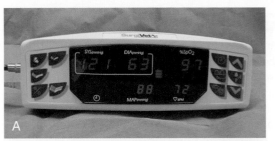

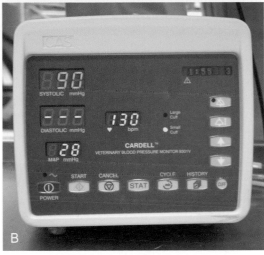

Fig. 6.20 A, Combination unit with blood pressure monitor and pulse oximeter. B, Blood pressure monitoring unit.

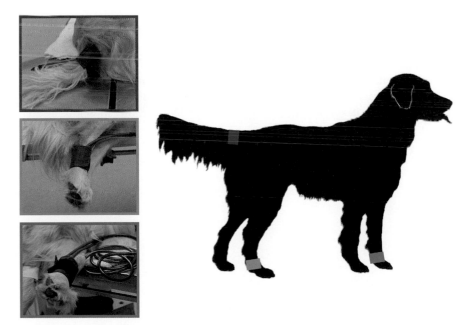

Fig. 6.21 Locations for placement of a blood pressure cuff. *Red*, base of the tail. *Green*, metatarsus. *Blue*, metacarpus. (From Thomas J, Lerche P: *Anesthesia and analgesia for veterinary technicians*, ed 5, St Louis, 2017, Elsevier.)

ELECTROCARDIOGRAPH

Continuous electrocardiograph (ECG) monitoring of anesthetized patients provides valuable information. In addition to providing a heart rate and wave formation tracing, many ECG machines are capable of monitoring other parameters, including pulse oximetry readings, temperature, and respiratory rate. Some electrocardiographs can also provide direct blood pressure monitoring options and tracing printouts. Regardless of the additional functions provided with an ECG unit, the basic ECG tracing (electrocardiogram) is a valuable source of information for the anesthetist. Continuous, or even intermittent, monitoring of the heart rate and rhythm with an ECG can alert the anesthetist to current or impending problems that may be avoided. For example, the appearance of a premature ventricular contraction (PVC) alone may be an isolated incident, but repeated multiple PVCs can be a sign of impending, severe cardiac distress. Other situations, such as atrial dysfunction (evident as changes in the P wave), myocardial hypoxia, and electrolyte disturbances (evident as changes in the T wave), can be observed with continuous ECG monitoring.

▌ KEY POINTS

1. Hands-on monitoring can be more reliable than mechanical device monitoring. Mechanical devices can register incorrect readings. Do not rely exclusively on mechanical monitoring devices.
2. For a full evaluation of the patient's condition and stage of anesthesia, the anesthetist should assess multiple parameters, including reflexes.
3. There is a direct correlation between progression of hypotension and progression of anesthetic depth.
4. To determine a decreasing or increasing trend in body temperature, pulse, and respiratory rate (TPR), the technician must be sure to measure these preanesthetic values of the patient. Preanesthetic TPR is invaluable information.
5. Patients undergoing long surgical procedures may need intraoperative doses of analgesia.
6. Pulse oximeters measure the level of oxygen saturation of the blood.
7. Capnometry is the measurement of the level of exhaled CO_2; a normal reading is 35 to 45 mm Hg.
8. Blood pressure can be monitored by direct or indirect methods.

▌ REVIEW QUESTIONS

1. What monitoring device is used to detect heart arrhythmia?
   a. Capnograph
   b. Electrocardiograph
   c. Doppler blood pressure monitor
   d. Oscillometric blood pressure monitor
2. Agonal breaths occur when the patient
   a. has suffered a cardiac arrest.
   b. is being assisted with ventilation.
   c. is in the surgical plane of anesthesia.
   d. is in the excitatory stage of anesthesia.
3. Assisted ventilation helps to prevent
   a. atelectasis.
   b. ET tube leakage.
   c. rapid respiration.
   d. changes in anesthetic depth.
4. Blue color to mucous membranes suggests
   a. anemia.
   b. pigmentation.
   c. severe blood infection.
   d. poor oxygenation in the body.
5. Which drug will cause a slowing in CRT?
   a. Atropine
   b. Ketamine
   c. Medetomidine
   d. Glycopyrrolate
6. Cardiac insufficiency leads to hypotension due to
   a. dehydration.
   b. excessive blood loss.
   c. excessive vasodilation.
   d. poor pumping action of cardiac muscle.
7. What drug may contribute to the development of malignant hyperthermia?
   a. Ketamine
   b. Atropine
   c. Sevoflurane
   d. Medetomidine
8. What is an automatic response to a stimulus made by a patient without conscious awareness?
   a. Shock
   b. Reflex
   c. Pulse deficit
   d. Hypotension
9. Which reflex is elicited by touching the medial canthus of the eye?
   a. Aural
   b. Pedal
   c. Corneal
   d. Palpebral
10. When a patient has undergone cardiac arrest, you would expect the pupils to be
    a. fully dilated.
    b. mildly dilated.
    c. normal in size.
    d. pinpoint-sized.
11. Which device measures the percentage of oxygen saturation of the patient's hemoglobin?

a. Capnometer
b. Pulse oximetry
c. Electrocardiogram
d. Doppler blood pressure monitor

12. Which device reflects the level of arterial CO_2?
    a. Capnometer
    b. Pulse oximetry
    c. Electrocardiogram
    d. Direct blood pressure monitor

13. Which of these is a normal capnometer reading for a patient?
    a. 40 mm Hg
    b. 60 mm Hg
    c. 75 mm Hg
    d. 100 mm Hg

14. Which stage of anesthesia is the excitement stage?
    a. Stage I
    b. Stage II
    c. Stage III
    d. Stage IV

15. What is a pulse deficit?

16. Define hypercarbia.

17. What is the function of a sphygmomanometer?

18. What is a disadvantage of using a capnometer on a patient?

19. List three alternative places the lingual probe of a pulse oximetry unit can be placed on the patient during a dental procedure.

20. List 3 alternate ways to monitor a patient's vital signs during an entropion surgery.

BIBLIOGRAPHY

Bassert J, Beal A, Samples O: *Clinical textbook for veterinary technicians,* ed 9, St. Louis, 2018, Elsevier.

Muir WW III, Hubbell JAE, Bednarski RM: *Handbook of veterinary anesthesia,* ed 4, St Louis, 2007, Mosby.

Simpson K: Let's talk about capnography. *SurgiVet,* August 2003: Available at http://www.surgivet.com.
https://www.smiths-medical.com/resources/lets-talk-about-capnography

Thomas JA, Lerche P: *Anesthesia and analgesia for veterinary technicians,* ed 5, St Louis, 2017, Elsevier.

Asepsis

Paige Allen

LEARNING OBJECTIVES

After completion of this chapter, the reader will be able to:
- Define asepsis, sterile field, and surgical conscience.
- Maintain asepsis.
- Maintain a sterile field.
- Open sterile packs without contaminating their contents or the sterile field.

- Discuss the correct method of loading and passing a scalpel blade and handle.
- Discuss the techniques used to pass various types of surgical instruments safely to the surgeon.

KEY TERMS

Asepsis
Circulating assistant
Sterile

Sterile field
Strike-through contamination
Surgical conscience

Surgical technician

ASEPSIS

The surgical area is restricted because it needs to be as free of microorganisms as possible. If proper techniques are not followed, a surgical wound could easily become infected. Infections acquired because of lack of attention to aseptic technique can be serious and even fatal. Asepsis (absence of pathogenic microorganisms that cause infection) makes the environment surgically clean but not sterile (absence of all living microorganisms, including spores).

It is the responsibility of the veterinary technician to keep the surgical area as aseptic as possible. This is accomplished by properly cleaning and disinfecting the room. All personnel should adhere to a written dress code and perform proper handwashing and hand scrubbing. In addition, proper patient preparation must occur. All of these will help prevent pathogenic microorganisms from contaminating the environment and entering the surgical wound. Aseptic techniques, along with sterile techniques, are the most important practices to prevent infection in the patient.

Surgical conscience is the commitment of the surgical personnel to adhere strictly to aseptic technique, because anything less could increase the potential risk of infection, resulting in harm to the patient. Any break in aseptic technique is immediately reported and addressed or corrected, whether anyone else is present to observe the violation.

Maintaining Asepsis

Maintaining asepsis in the surgical area is accomplished by practicing aseptic and sterile techniques. The Association of periOperative Registered Nurses (AORN) has listed several "Recommended Practices for Maintaining a Sterile Field." These recommendations should also be followed in the veterinary surgery area (Box 7.1).

Sterile Field

Scrubbed personnel function within a sterile field. The sterile field is defined as any area (person, table, or patient) that has been covered with a sterile barrier. This would include a gown,

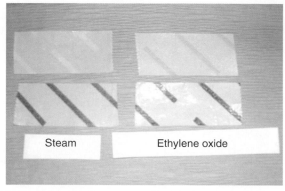

Fig. 7.1 Sterilization indicator tape. *Top left:* Steam sterilization indicator tape before being exposed to steam. *Bottom left:* Steam sterilization indicator tape after being exposed to steam. *Top right:* Ethylene oxide gas sterilization indicator tape before being exposed to ethylene oxide gas. *Bottom right:* Ethylene oxide gas sterilization tape being exposed to ethylene oxide.

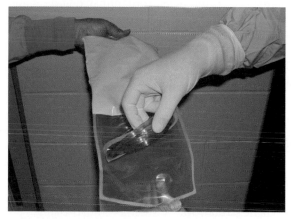

Fig. 7.2 Circulating assistant opens a peel-away pouch to expose the contents for removal by surgical technician.

sterile table cover, or drape. The scrubbed personnel's gown is sterile in front from the chest to the level of the sterile field. The sleeves of the sterile gown are sterile from 2 inches above the elbow to the top of the edge of the cuff. The neckline, shoulders, and cuffed portion of the gown sleeves may become contaminated by perspiration and therefore are not considered sterile. The back of the gown is never considered sterile because a member of the surgical team cannot observe it constantly. The cuffs of the gown are considered contaminated because hands have passed through them.

Sterile drapes should be used to establish a sterile field on the patient. Drapes are barriers that help to prevent microorganisms from passing between sterile and nonsterile areas. The drapes should cover the entire animal, the surgical table, and the equipment that is part of the sterile field. The circulating assistant, or any other non–scrubbed-in personnel, should never reach over the draped, sterile areas. If any drape becomes wet, it is considered contaminated because strike-through will occur. Strike-through contamination occurs when liquids soak through a drape from a sterile area to an unsterile area, and vice versa. A sterile field should be maintained and monitored continuously by the entire surgical team. The sterile field should never be left unattended (Box 7.2).

Opening Items for Use in the Sterile Field

Any item used within a sterile field should be sterile. Before opening any item for use in the sterile field, make sure the package is inspected for sterility. Confirm that (1) there are no tears or holes in the outer package and (2) the item has gone through the proper sterilization by checking the sterile indicators. Indicators are located on the outside of the package such as indicator tape (Fig. 7.1). Check the seal of the package to ensure it is secure and not broken at any point. Check the package itself, and if it looks worn from being handled too much, it should be considered contaminated. A larger surgical pack should have a sterile indicator inside to ensure that the sterilizing agent has penetrated to the center of a thick pack. The expiration date should be checked, although AORN maintains that the sterility of the item is event related and not time related (see Chapter 14). This means that if all the previously described features have been

checked on the package, the time and expiration date of sterilization are not significant.

All items introduced onto a sterile field should be opened, dispensed, and transferred by methods that maintain sterility and integrity. Edges of all sterile wrappers and packages are considered nonsterile. Therefore, when opening an item, be sure all edges are secured so that they do not contaminate the field or the sterile packaged item.

The surgical technician may lift the item straight out of the package, without touching any of the edges of the package (Fig. 7.2). Heavy, sharp, or large items may be opened on a separate table near the sterile field for retrieval by the surgical technician. Sterile supplies are opened by unwrapping the flap farthest away first, the sides next, and the nearest flap last. Never reach across or over a sterile area to open the final flap.

Opening Fluids for Use in the Sterile Field

Irrigation fluids should be poured carefully to prevent any spills onto the sterile field and to avoid splash-back. It is best to have the scrubbed-in person hold the basin away from the field or to place it at the edge of the sterile table. Once the fluids have been

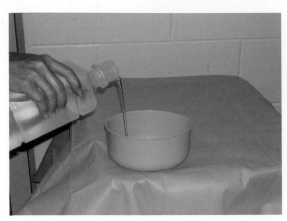

Fig. 7.3 Sterile water being poured into a sterile bowl. Note that the bowl is set in the corner of an empty table to avoid possible contamination if splashing occurs.

opened, the cap is considered contaminated and cannot be replaced onto the bottle, so the remaining fluids must be discarded (Fig. 7.3).

Moving Around the Sterile Field

All personnel moving within or around a sterile field should do so in a manner to maintain the integrity of the sterile field. The surgical team must be aware of the sterile and nonsterile areas in the surgery room at all times. Movement creates air currents, which can be a source of contamination in the surgical room. Movement in the room should be kept to a minimum, and traffic in or out of the room should occur only as necessary.

Scrubbed personnel should not walk away from the sterile field. When scrubbed-in personnel must change positions around the sterile field, they should be a safe distance apart so as not to touch. When they pass each other, they should pass face to face (sterile to sterile) or back to back (unsterile to unsterile).

Unscrubbed (non–scrubbed-in) personnel should always face the surgical field. Unscrubbed persons should not walk between two sterile fields. For example, unscrubbed personnel should not walk between the sterile, draped patient and the sterile equipment table.

The surgical scrub team should not change levels of position—from sitting to standing, and vice versa—during a procedure. The lower portion of the gown is considered contaminated, and when the scrubbed person sits, this portion of the gown is closer to the hands, arms, and the sterile field and therefore could cause contamination.

There should be minimal talking in the surgery room, and the surgery room doors should remain closed as much as possible. All non–scrubbed-in persons should be a safe distance from the sterile field. A limited number of non–scrubbed-in observers should be allowed in the surgery room at one time. The more congested the surgery room, the more difficult it is to monitor the sterile field, and the sterile team has less room to move adequately around the sterile field. The surgical conscience is followed to report any breaks in aseptic or sterile technique. All of the items discussed here are important to protect the sterile field and ultimately the life of the patient.

DUTIES OF THE CIRCULATING ASSISTANT

The **circulating assistant** is the person who opens packs and is a runner for the surgical team. Proper opening of sterile packs is important to maintain a sterile field. All packages must be checked thoroughly for any damage or inadvertent break in the material. Speed should not be a top priority. Although opening items in a timely way is necessary, rushing can cause unnecessary mistakes. Timing is also a factor. If the scrubbed-in person is not ready to receive the item, or if the equipment table is not properly prepared, the circulating assistant should consider delaying opening the item until a later, more convenient time.

Wraps and packages may be sterilized at the hospital or by the manufacturer. Wraps and packages sterilized by the manufacturer are usually disposable items. Packages sterilized at the hospital often do not come with directions on how to open them. This skill comes with knowledge and practice. The manufacturer often supplies directions explaining which end to open first.

Opening Peel-Away Pouches

Many paper or plastic pouches for packaging individual sterile instruments have a side sealed with an arrow (↑) indicating which end to open. Holding the packet at the end with the arrow allows easy opening of this type of seal; with both hands, grasp the package with the thumbs and slowly peel the package open by adducting the thumbs (Fig. 7.4). Do not roll the wrists because doing so may cause the package to not open properly. While peeling the package open, hold the item firmly so that the item is stabilized and does not slide across the nonsterile edges of the package.

The plastic or paper tubing or pouches with a straight seal are opened similarly, except that a constant pull must be maintained on both sides. Instruments and sutures can be either handed to the surgeon or unwrapped to make them available for the surgical team. If necessary, small, sterile items can be opened on a clean, dry, flat, nonsterile surface. Place the item paper side down, hold on to the top sealed edge with a thumb and finger of one hand, and pull the plastic side with the other

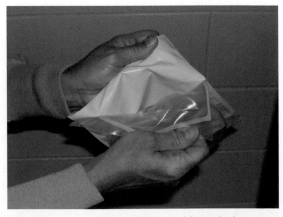

Fig. 7.4 Opening a peel-away pouch by touching only the outer edge of the separated ends, then carefully pulling them apart by adducting the thumbs.

hand. The scrubbed-in assistant can carefully pick the item off the sterile paper and transfer it to the sterile table. Suture can be given directly to a scrubbed-in person by opening the package and allowing the scrubbed-in person to retrieve the inner suture package.

Opening Wrapped Packs

Wrapped sterile packs are opened on a clean, flat, dry surface in the surgery room. Place the sterile pack on a flat surface so that the wrapped edges are uppermost. Remove or tear the indicator tape and open the distant flap first, taking care not to reach over the sterile contents of the pack. Open the side flaps one at a time, taking care to touch only the exposed tabbed corners and no other part of the wrap. Open the nearest flap last. For especially large packs, the circulating assistant may need to walk around the table to avoid reaching over the sterile field. If the package is double wrapped, the scrubbed-in team member can open the inner wrap.

Some wrapped items are small enough to be opened with one hand by the circulating assistant. Opening a pack correctly with one hand allows the circulating assistant to hand the item to the scrubbed-in team member for its removal from the wrap without contaminating the scrubbed-in person. To open a sterile pack with one hand, start by holding the pack in one hand (hand A), then insert thumb of hand A under the taped fold (Fig. 7.5). Then, using hand B, remove the tape and lift the top fold back, tucking the top flap into the grasp of hand A by folding the top flap under the pack. Using hand B, unwrap the two side folds, one at a time, tucking each one into the grasp of hand A underneath the pack. Using hand B, grasp the last corner tab and pull it back to be held by hand A, as the item is carefully removed from the wrap by the scrubbed-in personnel (Fig. 7.6).

Opening Gowns and Gloves

Gowns are opened much like packs. There needs to be a clean, flat, dry surface for both gown and gloves. Remove the gown from the package (if a disposable, sterile gown), and place the gown on a flat surface so that the wrapped edges are uppermost. If a resterilized cloth gown is used, remove the tape from the outer wrap.

Open the distant flap first, taking care not to reach over the sterile contents of the pack. Open the side flaps one at a time, taking care to touch only the exposed tabbed corners and no other part of the wrap. Open the nearest flap last. If the gown is

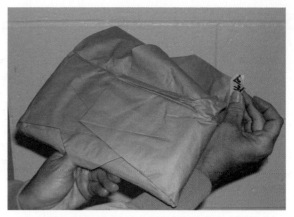

Fig. 7.5 Opening a pack with one hand. The thumb of one hand is slid under the tab of the taped edge, and the pack is held between that thumb and the fingers of that hand while the other hand unwraps the pack.

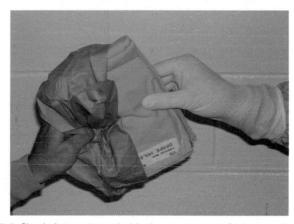

Fig. 7.6 Circulating assistant holds the outer wrap of an opened pack in an extended hand to allow the scrubbed-in person to reach in to remove the pack's contents without breaking sterility.

double wrapped, the scrubbed-in team member can open the inner wrap.

Sterile gloves are removed from the outer package and placed on the table. At the top and bottom of the package are folds. Unfold these ends, taking care to overfold slightly to decrease the memory of the paper. Place hands under the flaps of the side and pull toward the outside. Take care that the top and bottom folds do not come back in and contaminate the gloves. If possible, fold the cuff end of the paper wrap over the edge of the counter.

▎ KEY POINTS

1. Aseptic technique is used to maintain the absence of disease-causing organisms in the surgical environment.
2. Asepsis does not guarantee sterility.
3. Sterile items used in surgery are free of all microorganisms, including spores.
4. A surgical conscience requires acknowledging when a breach in asepsis or sterility has occurred and taking the necessary steps to address and correct it, even if no one else witnesses the breach.
5. The space above and surrounding an open sterile pack is considered part of the sterile field.
6. The sterile field cannot be entered or touched by non–scrubbed-in personnel.
7. If non–scrubbed-in personnel enter or touch the sterile field, it is no longer sterile and is considered contaminated.

REVIEW QUESTIONS

1. The definition of sterile is
   a. absence of all living organisms, including spores.
   b. maintaining a clean environment in the surgical suite.
   c. the absence of pathogenic microorganisms that cause infection.
   d. the commitment of the surgical personnel to adhere strictly to aseptic technique.

2. The sterile field is defined as
   a. the whole operating room
   b. any area covered with a sterile barrier.
   c. the drape covering the patient.
   d. the entire area surrounding the surgery table.

3. What areas of the scrubbed-in personnel's gown are part of the sterile field?
   a. The entire front of the gown
   b. The entire gown—front, back, and sides
   c. The front from the chest to the level of the sterile field
   d. The front and back from the chest to the level of the sterile field

4. When irrigation fluid is used during a surgery, the remaining fluid is
   a. considered contaminated and discarded.
   b. kept to be used for nonsterile procedures.
   c. left in the bottle with the cap replaced and saved for another patient.
   d. considered sterile and may be recapped and stored for up to 10 days.

5. When unscrubbed personnel move in the surgery room, they should face
   a. toward the surgery field.
   b. away from the surgery field.
   c. whichever direction they are walking.
   d. unscrubbed personnel should not move about the surgery room.

6. The commitment of the surgical personnel to adhere strictly to aseptic technique is called
   a. sterility.
   b. aseptic technique.
   c. surgical conscience.
   d. strike-through contamination.

7. Sterile drapes are used during surgery to
   a. make a waterproof barrier.
   b. establish a sterile field on the patient.
   c. allow the surgical field to go unattended.
   d. ensure sterility of instruments used during surgery.

8. A sterile package may be used if
   a. the seal is broken.
   b. there are tears in the package.
   c. the outside indicator tape is activated.
   d. the package looks worn from being handled too much.

9. AORN considers that an item maintains its sterility until
   a. the expiration date on the package.
   b. one year from the sterilization date.
   c. an event occurs that causes sterility to be lost.
   d. one year after the expiration date on the package.

10. Which of these areas of a gown are considered sterile?
    a. Cuffs
    b. Shoulders
    c. Neckline
    d. Forearm

11. How should scrubbed-in personnel pass each other during a surgical procedure?

12. If a gown is double wrapped, who opens the inner wrap?

13. What are the duties of the circulating assistant?

14. Who may touch the sterile field?

BIBLIOGRAPHY

Association of periOperative Registered Nurses (AORN): *Standards, recommended practices, and guidelines: recommended practices for maintaining a sterile field*, Denver, 2004, AORN.

Bassert JM, Thomas JA, editors: *McCurnin's clinical textbook for veterinary technicians*, ed 8, St Louis, 2014, Saunders.

Fairchild S: *Perioperative nursing: principles and practice*, ed 2, Philadelphia, 1996, Lippincott.

Fossum TW, Hedlund CS, Hulse DA, et al.: *Small animal surgery*, ed 3, St Louis, 2007, Mosby.

Spry C: *Essentials of perioperative nursing*, ed 2, Boston, 2004, Jones & Bartlett.

Tobias KM, Johnston SA: *Veterinary surgery: small animal*, St Louis, 2012, Saunders.

Operating Room Personnel

Paige Allen

OUTLINE

LEARNING OBJECTIVES

After completion of this chapter, the reader will be able to:
- Discuss personal preparation for duties as a surgical technician.
- Describe proper attire in the surgical area.
- Define endogenous and exogenous threats to asepsis.
- Explain the general guidelines for personal hygiene of veterinary surgical personnel.
- Describe and perform a surgical hand scrub.

- Explain and perform a surgical hand rub.
- Describe the different types of surgical hand prep solutions.
- Explain and demonstrate the process to aseptically dry hands and arms after performing a surgical hand scrub or rub.
- Describe and demonstrate the procedure for donning a surgical gown.
- Describe and perform open and closed gloving.
- Define and perform assisted surgical gloving.

KEY TERMS

Endogenous contamination
Exogenous contamination
Microbial shedding

Surgical hand scrub
Surgical hand rubs

For the veterinary technician with a passion for surgery, performing duties as the surgical technician (or scrubbing-in) is a coveted job. The technician performs a critical service for the surgeon in providing retraction of tissue, lavaging the surgical field with sterile fluid, and managing (running) the instrument table. For the surgeon, having a skilled, qualified surgical technician can significantly affect the duration and outcome of the surgical procedure.

There are two sources for contamination in the operating room. The first is endogenous contamination. Endogenous contamination comes from the patient itself. It can occur from the patient's skin or if the patient has an underlying, asymptomatic infection. The second source is exogenous contamination, and it comes from the surgical team and from the environment in which the surgery occurs. Exogenous contamination

can be more closely controlled by the veterinary technician; proper attire can assist with this task.

The surgical area should be a restricted, clean area, separate from the rest of the hospital. The surgery area should not be used for clipping patients or any other procedures except for sterile surgery. This restricted surgical environment should be kept as free of microorganisms as possible.

NUTRITION AND HYGIENE

Before scrubbing in, the technician must review some personal considerations. If personnel know in advance that they will be assisting on a surgical case, they should consume a meal of substance, not a candy bar or other sugary food. The technician should also consume plenty of fluids to combat dehydration, as well as be sure to visit the restroom before the case begins.

The closeness of the surgical team and the risk of patient infection require consideration of personal hygiene and appearance. Fingernails need to be kept shorter than the fingertips and free of nail polish. The use of perfume or cologne should be avoided. When working in close quarters, it is respectful to remember that people are becoming increasingly sensitive to smells. More importantly, the smell from perfume or cologne may mask odors from the inhalation gas. It is critical that the anesthetist be able to detect any leaks in the system through odors.

PROPER ATTIRE IN SURGICAL AREA

The physical and emotional stress associated with surgery can compromise the patient's immune system during surgery and during the convalescent period. In addition, the stress may cause surgical patients to be more vulnerable to infection and disease. Proper surgery room attire reduces microbial shedding. Microbial shedding occurs when microorganisms are released into the environment from the body of surgical personnel. These microorganisms are present in sebaceous and sweat glands around the hair follicles of the entire body. Proper attire of surgery room personnel helps decrease the risk of infection for the patient by providing barriers against microorganisms. In the surgery room, proper surgical attire, for the whole team, should include freshly laundered scrub suits, head covers, masks, and possibly shoe covers.

There should be a written surgical dress code that can be easily followed and enforced. This dress code should include the definition of areas where surgical attire must be worn, appropriate attire within those defined areas, and the choice of cover apparel outside the surgical suite. The scrub suit should be covered with clean cover apparel at all times when outside the surgical area and must be removed upon entry into the surgical area. It is important that a dress code for the use of cover apparel in the surgical preparation area be posted to avoid contamination of the scrub suit while personnel are working in this area. The scrub suit covering should be considered when personnel are restraining and clipping the patient for surgery. Guidelines should also be provided for general personal cleanliness, including care of fingernails and the wearing of jewelry when participating in surgical procedures (Box 8.1).

Scrub Suit

Street clothes should never be worn in surgery because they carry dirt, debris, and microorganisms. All personnel should wear clean, freshly laundered scrub suits (scrubs) at the veterinary hospital. Ideally, all scrubs should be laundered in the hospital laundry. Scrubs should not be worn from home to the hospital, nor should they be worn home from the hospital. The scrub suits could bring microorganisms into the hospital and home to infect the surgery personnel's own pets. Only clean scrub suits should be worn in the surgical area. Scrubs should be changed if they become visibly dirty or wet.

BOX 8.1	**Surgical Dress Code**

- A surgical dress code should be written and posted so that it can be easily followed and enforced.
- A dress code should include the defined areas where surgical attire must be worn, appropriate attire within those defined areas, and the acceptable options for cover apparel outside the surgical area.
- The scrub suit should be covered with a clean laboratory coat at all times when outside the surgical area.
- Personnel are not allowed to wear laboratory coats in the surgery room.
- Scrub suits worn in the surgery room should not be worn home.
- Clean, freshly laundered scrub suits should be donned just before entry into the surgery room and should not be worn from home into the hospital.
- Proper surgical attire includes wearing a head cover that completely covers all head and facial hair, surgical masks that effectively cover the mouth and nose, and clean shoes with or without shoe covers.
- Head covers and masks need to be donned before the surgical hand scrub or hand rub is begun.
- Masks must fit properly so that a cough or sneeze is not vented out the side of the mask.

The scrub top should fit the body snugly and be tucked into the scrub pants (Fig. 8.1). This prevents body scurf (epidermal scales) from being shed as a result of friction produced by the body rubbing against the scrub top. The scrub top should be short sleeved so personnel can scrub hands and arms for surgery. When personnel are leaving the surgical area, the scrub suit should be covered by a clean laboratory coat, which is removed when they reenter the restricted area.

Head Covers

Everyone in the surgical area should wear head covers. All hair on the head and face should be covered because hair collects bacteria when left uncovered. The head cover prevents bacteria, dandruff, and other contaminants from falling either onto the scrub suits or into the surgical environment. Several types of head covers are available, including bouffant, hood, and skullcap. The head cover chosen should fit well and should cover all hair. The bouffant covers the hair on the head adequately and is preferred over the skullcap (Fig. 8.2). The hood should be worn if there is facial hair that is not covered by the mask. Skullcaps should be worn only if the hair is very short and there is no hair outside the cap at the side or the nape of the neck. Fig. 8.3 is an example of a poor choice of head covering; this person should not wear a skullcap.

Masks

The mask should be worn in the surgery room when open sterile supplies or scrubbed personnel are present. The mask should be worn over the mouth and nose. Because the mask functions to filter droplets containing microorganisms that come from the mouth and nose, it should be changed frequently. The strings should be tied tightly, and the mask should conform to the face so that no air escapes without being filtered by the mask.

If a sneeze or cough is imminent, without turning the head, the person should step back from the sterile field. If the mask is secured properly, the cough or sneeze should be filtered. If the

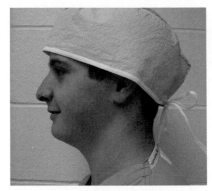

Fig. 8.3 This skullcap does not effectively contain all hair on the head and should not be worn; it cannot effectively prevent hair from falling into the surgical site and contaminating the site.

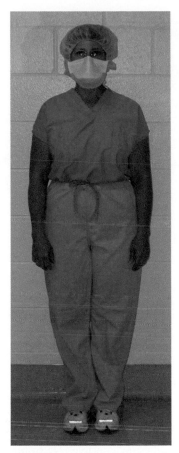

Fig. 8.1 Proper surgical attire includes a clean scrub suit. The scrub top is tucked into the pants. All jewelry and name tags are removed. A head cover, mask, and clean shoes are worn.

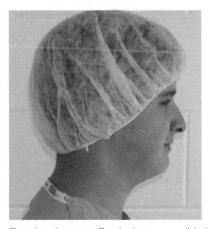

Fig. 8.2 A bouffant head cover effectively covers all hair on the head and prevents hair from falling into the surgical site.

mask is not secured properly, or if the head is turned, the cough or sneeze will be vented out of the side of the mask directly onto the sterile field.

Shoes and Shoe Covers

Shoes worn in the surgery room should be comfortable and cleaned frequently (whether or not shoe covers are worn). Shoes should have enclosed toes and heels to protect personnel from injury if heavy or sharp objects are dropped onto their feet. Shoe covers are optional. If worn, shoe covers should be changed if they become torn, wet, or soiled and when personnel reenter the surgical area. Although it is not imperative that special shoes be worn only in the surgery area, it is common sense to make sure shoes are clean and are not carrying feces or hair into the surgical area. Foot attire has no proven significance in reducing the incidence of postoperative wound infections, and the primary reason for its use is to decrease floor contamination.

Prior to scrubbing, the surgical cap and mask should be applied, and the gown pack and surgical gloves should be opened but kept sterile.

SURGICAL HAND SCRUB AND HAND RUB

The **surgical hand scrub** is defined as the process of removing as many microorganisms as possible from nails, hands, and arms by mechanical washing and chemical antisepsis before a person participates in a surgical procedure. The surgical hand scrub is also designed to maintain the lowest possible microbial counts throughout the surgical procedure.

When performing the surgical hand scrub, it is important to remember that the skin is never made sterile. Skin becomes surgically clean; if there are any holes (detected or undetected) in the surgical gloves or gown, the probability of introducing microbes into the surgical field is reduced. The use of prophylactic antibiotics should never be considered a substitute for a proper hand scrub.

The scrub procedure consists of a mechanical part and a chemical part. The mechanical part is the removal of bacteria and debris by producing friction when rubbing or brushing. This removes dirt, oil, and transient organisms that are loosely attached to the skin. During the chemical part of the scrub, the antiseptic, antimicrobial skin-cleansing agents are used. These agents inactivate or inhibit the growth of microorganisms found on the surface of the skin and in hair follicles, sebaceous glands, and sweat glands.

Two methods of scrubbing procedures can be used. The first is the timed method, and the second is the stroke count method. Both methods should take a minimum of 5 minutes to perform correctly. The surgical hand scrub should always begin with a brief, general hand and arm wash to loosen surface debris and transient microorganisms (organisms that are loosely attached to the skin surface.) This wash is not included in the 5-minute minimum.

The method chosen is not as important as using the same method consistently so that the lowest number of microorganisms remain on the surface of the skin. As a part of either method, it is important to follow an anatomic pattern each time. Fingers have four sides, and the tip, hands, and arms have four sides. Before either method, a nail-cleaning pick should always be used to remove debris from the subungual area of each finger. Stiff brushes are not recommended on the skin because they can cause skin abrasions and may release more resident microbes from the deep layers of the skin, which is counterproductive. Many scrub agents come with disposable, antiseptic-impregnated scrub brushes that have soft brushes, sponge, and nail-cleaning pick included.

The antimicrobial scrub agent or an alcohol-based hand rub should be chosen from the U.S. Food and Drug Administration (FDA) product category defined as hand scrubs or alcohol-based rubs. Avagard (3M, St Paul, MN) is an example of a scrubless, brushless, waterless antiseptic hand preparation product referred to as a rub. The agent selected should be nonirritating and fast acting and should have a prolonged depressant effect on residual bacteria. It should cover a broad spectrum of bacteria. The length of scrub time varies according to the manufacturer's recommendations and written directions for use.

The brushless technique (alcohol rub), with or without water, consists of rubbing an antimicrobial agent on the hands and arms. Brushless rubbing agents typically are alcohol based, with the addition of moisturizing emollients and surfactants that help clean the skin. Some agents are combinations of alcohol and other antimicrobial agents, such as chlorhexidine gluconate, or alcohol with preservatives.

Whichever FDA-approved antimicrobial scrub agent or alcohol-based rub is chosen, a standardized protocol should be established and written for each surgical hand procedure according to the manufacturer's recommendations for the particular scrub or rub agent used. A copy should be posted in the scrub room. Every person scrubbing for a procedure should be familiar with these instructions.

Before the surgical hand scrub (or rub) is performed (Box 8.2), the patient should be properly clipped, prepped, moved into the surgery room, and positioned on the table correctly for the surgical procedure. The surgery room should be set up with the proper pack and instrumentation (Fig. 8.4).

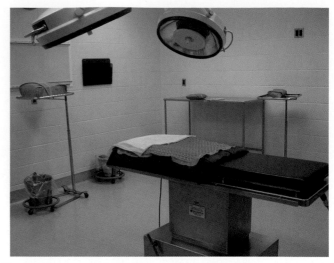

Fig. 8.4 The operating room is arranged with the appropriate surgical packs before the surgical hand preparation is performed. The circulating warm-water pad on the surgery table, and the kick buckets are lined with plastic liners. The surgery room is free of clutter, and only those items needed for the specific procedure to be performed are in the surgery room.

Types of Scrub Solutions

In the choice of an antimicrobial (antiseptic) detergent, several desirable characteristics are recommended for the surgical scrub product: (1) FDA compliant, (2) broad spectrum of activity, (3) fast acting and effective, (4) nonirritating, and (5) with persistent effects and cumulative activity. Whatever type of scrub agent is chosen, it is important to follow the manufacturer's written directions for use. These include the scrub time, whether the use of a brush is recommended, and whether it is a brushless, alcohol-based surgical rub.

Several types of antimicrobial skin-cleansing agents are available. The following agents are discussed: chlorhexidine gluconate, iodophors, alcohol (Table 8.1), and the brushless rub.

Chlorhexidine gluconate (4%) is a broad-spectrum antimicrobial agent. It is more effective against gram-positive bacteria than gram-negative organisms. Chlorhexidine gluconate is a fair inhibitor of fungi. It is active against enveloped viruses and has minimal action against tubercle bacillus. Organic matter minimally affects it. Most importantly, chlorhexidine gluconate 4% is persistent (has the ability to stop microbial regrowth with repeated use). The residual effect is maintained for more than 6 days.

Iodophors (7.5%) are complexes consisting of iodine and a carrier. Iodophors have a wide range of activity against gram-positive and gram-negative bacteria, tubercle bacilli, fungi, viruses, and some spores. Iodophors are neutralized rapidly in the presence of organic materials. These agents have minimal residual effect and can cause skin irritation and damage.

Alcohol (60%–90%) is an agent with rapid antimicrobial properties against organisms, but it does not have residual activity. It has excellent bactericidal activity against gram-positive and gram-negative bacteria and good activity against tubercle bacillus as well as many fungi and viruses. It is not sporicidal. It aids in removing oils from the skin. The disadvantages of alcohol are its

TABLE 8.1 Characteristics of Selected Antimicrobials Used in Surgical Scrub Solutions

Spectrum of Activity*	Fungi	Viruses	Tubercle Bacilli	Affected By Organic Matter	Speed of Action	Disadvantages	Advantages
Chlorhexidine Gluconate 4%							
Broad spectrum (more effective against gram positive than gram negative)	Fair	Enveloped viruses	Minimal	Minimal	Intermediate Significant immediate antimicrobial effect	Eye irritant	Persistent; ability to stop microbial growth with repeated use Residual effect maintained for more than 6 days
Iodophors 7.5% (Complexes That Consist of Iodine and Carrier)							
Broad spectrum (some spores)	Yes	Yes	Yes	Neutralized rapidly	Significant immediate antimicrobial effect	Odor, staining, tissue irritation	Persistent for 4–6 hours
Alcohol							
Broad spectrum (not sporicidal)	Many	Many	Yes	Conflicting evidence No residual activity	Rapid	Drying effect Volatile and flammable	Lacks persistence

*Including against gram-positive and gram-negative bacteria.

BOX 8.3 Ideal Antiseptic Properties

- Nonirritating to skin
- Fast acting
- Broad spectrum
- Has good residual effect

---

drying effect on the skin and its flammability, so it needs to be stored carefully.

Brushless rubs (with or without water) have gained some popularity in veterinary medicine (e.g., Avagard). This brushless technique has an alcohol base with an antimicrobial ingredient such as chlorhexidine gluconate or triclosan. These agents reduce bacterial counts on hands more rapidly than antimicrobial soaps or detergents. Combining alcohol (for rapid reduction of microbial growth) and chlorhexidine (for persistent and cumulative effect) prevents microbial regrowth. The advantages of the brushless rub are that the scrub time is shorter than with other agents and techniques and damage to the skin from brushes is avoided (Box 8.3).

Prescrubbing Guidelines

In preparation for scrubbing, the technician should remove all rings, watches, and jewelry. Jewelry may harbor microorganisms that routine handwashing cannot remove, and earrings, necklaces, and body-piercing objects could fall into the surgical field. Pens, name tags, and other items should be removed from scrub top pockets.

Fingernails should be well manicured. They should be short, clean, and healthy. Healthy nails are desired because any small cuts or torn cuticles can harbor microorganisms. Fingernails should not extend past the fingertips because they could cause tears in the surgical gloves, which could be a source of infection to the patient. Artificial nails are unacceptable because they harbor microorganisms, especially fungi. Nail polish should not be worn because polished nails, if chipped, harbor more microorganisms than unpolished nails.

If eyeglasses are worn, they must be clean and thoroughly dry. Elastic bands are recommended to hold eyeglasses in place, thus preventing them from falling into the surgical field. The cap and mask should be applied, making sure all hair is covered by headgear and that the mask is snug and comfortable. To prevent eyeglasses from fogging up because of the mask, tape can be put over the upper edge of the mask, or specially designed masks can be purchased. Hands should be thoroughly washed with an antimicrobial soap and water and towel dried. The sterile gown and gloves, as well as any other sterile equipment that needs to be opened, should be opened in the surgery area if the circulating assistant (nonsterile assistant) is not available.

Surgical Hand Scrub Using Antimicrobial Scrub Agent

A traditional, standardized, surgical hand scrub procedure is important and should become second nature to the **surgical technician.** It is important to follow the guidelines from the manufacturer, which should include, but may not be limited to, the following actions.

Wash hands and forearms to the elbows with antimicrobial scrub and running water immediately before beginning the surgical scrub (Fig. 8.5). Make sure to thoroughly cover all areas with the scrub because contact time is important for most agents to work properly. Clean the subungual areas of both hands under running water using a disposable nail-cleaning pick (Fig. 8.6). Rinse hands and forearms under running water. Keep the hands above the elbows, and allow water to run off at the elbows. Remember to always hold the hands higher than the elbows and away from surgical attire.

Dispense the approved antimicrobial scrub agent according to the manufacturer's written directions. Do not touch anything with your hands. Apply the antimicrobial agent to wet hands and forearms. Some manufacturers may recommend using a soft, nonabrasive sponge (Fig. 8.7).

Visualize the surfaces of the fingers, hand, and arm as having four sides with the additional tip of the fingers. Begin by brushing the fingertips of the first hand 10 times, making sure the

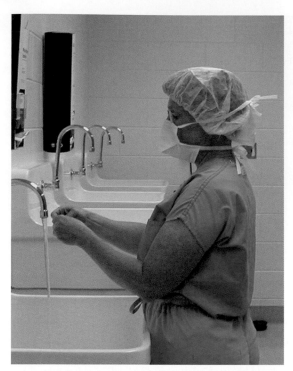

Fig. 8.5 The hands and forearms are washed with soap and water before the official surgical hand preparation is performed. The head cover and mask are already on before the hand prep begins. The gown and glove pack should be opened before the hand prep is started.

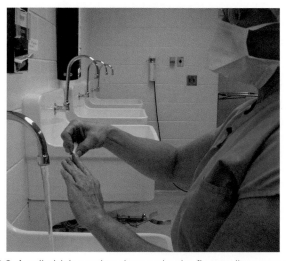

Fig. 8.6 A nail pick is used to clean under the fingernails as part of the surgical hand prep.

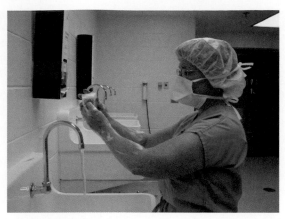

Fig. 8.7 In this surgical hand prep, a soft sponge is used. Note that the hands are held above the elbows throughout the scrub.

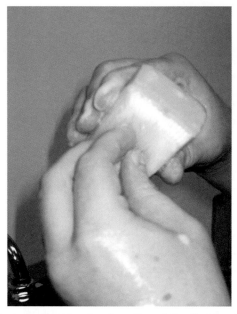

Fig. 8.8 Begin by brushing the fingertips of the first hand 10 times, making sure the brush also goes under the fingernails.

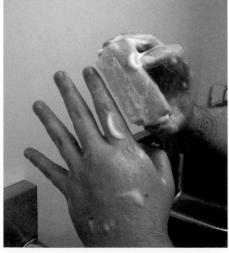

Fig. 8.9 Move to the lateral side of the index finger and scrub from the tip to the base of the finger 10 times.

brush also goes under the fingernails (Fig. 8.8). Move to the lateral side of the index finger and scrub from the tip to the base of the finger 10 times (Fig. 8.9). Repeat the 10-time scrubbing process on the other 3 sides of the index finger. Make sure that the brush and antimicrobial scrub also contact the webbing between fingers. Move to the other four fingers, and repeat the process on all sides of each finger. When scrubbing the lateral side of the last finger, make sure to scrub the lateral side of the hand in the same motion (Fig. 8.10).

Move the brush to the palm of the hand and scrub 10 times (Fig. 8.11). Move to the thumb side of the hand and scrub the outside of the thumb and the side of the hand in one motion

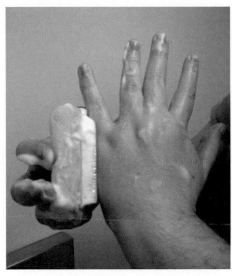

Fig. 8.10 When scrubbing the lateral side of the last finger, make sure to scrub the lateral side of the hand in the same motion.

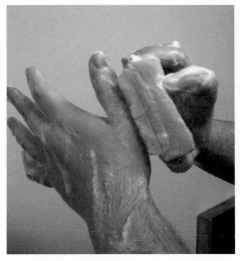

Fig. 8.12 Move to the thumb side of the hand and scrub the outside of the thumb and the side of the hand in one motion.

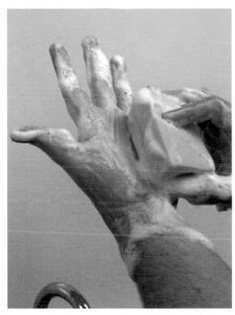

Fig. 8.11 Move the brush to the palm of the hand and scrub 10 times.

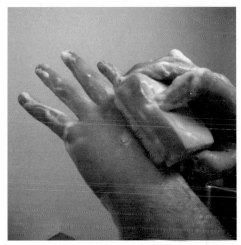

Fig. 8.13 Move to the back of the hand and scrub from the base of the fingers to the wrist using 10 strokes.

(Fig. 8.12). Complete the three remaining sides of the thumb. Move to the back of the hand and scrub from the base of the fingers to the wrist using 10 strokes (Fig. 8.13). Scrub the arm from the wrist to the elbow in the same manner, using 10 strokes on each of the four sides of the arm (Fig. 8.14). Leaving the antimicrobial scrub on the first arm, proceed to the second arm and follow the same process.

When the scrub on both arms is complete, rinse the first arm, beginning at the fingertips. Make sure to keep the hands above the elbows and allow water to run off the elbow. Do not allow the any part of the hands or arms to touch anything (sink, scrub top, etc.) (Fig. 8.15). Rinse the brush and rescrub the first arm. Rinse the second arm in the aforementioned fashion. Repeat this process on each hand and arm to make sure that manufacturer's contact time requirements are met. It is important to avoid splashing surgical attire.

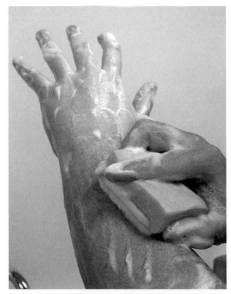

Fig. 8.14 Scrub the arm from the wrist to the elbow in the same manner, using 10 strokes on the four sides of the arm.

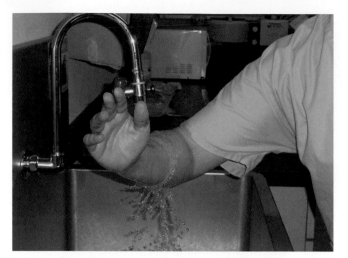

Fig. 8.15 When the scrub on both arms is complete, rinse, beginning at the fingertips. Make sure to keep the hands above the elbows and to allow water to run off the elbow. Do not allow any part of the hands or arms to touch anything (sink, scrub top, etc.).

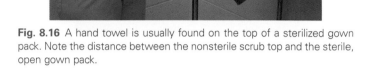

Fig. 8.16 A hand towel is usually found on the top of a sterilized gown pack. Note the distance between the nonsterile scrub top and the sterile, open gown pack.

Surgical Hand Rub Using Antimicrobial Rub Agent

A standardized protocol for alcohol-based surgical hand rubs should follow the manufacturer's written instructions.

Begin by washing hands and forearms with soap and running water immediately before beginning the surgical hand antisepsis procedure. Clean the subungual areas of both hands under running water using a nail-cleaning pick. Rinse the hands and forearms under running water. Dry the hands and forearms thoroughly with a paper towel. Dispense the manufacturer-recommended amount of surgical hand rub product. Apply the product to the hands and forearms, following the manufacturer's written directions. The rub should always start with the fingers, proceed to the hands, and continue up the arms to the elbow. The rub process will follow the same procedure as the traditional scrub. This means to apply the rub to all sides of the hand, fingers, and arm. Some manufacturers may require the use of water as part of the process. Rub thoroughly until dry. Repeat the product application process as indicated in the manufacturer's written directions.

Drying the Hands

After completing the surgical hand scrub, or rub, the hands and arms need to be thoroughly dried with a sterile towel. From the sterile gown and towel pack, pick up the towel by the corner (Fig. 8.16). Be careful not to drip water on the gown pack. Step back from the sterile table, always being aware of the sterile items in the environment to prevent contamination. Open the towel full length, using one end of the towel to gently rub the fingers, hand, and arms (in that order) of the first hand and arm (Fig. 8.17). Do not rub back and forth; instead, rub circumferentially beginning at the wrist and moving to the elbow. Bend at the waist slightly so that the towel does not brush against the scrub suit. When ready to dry the second hand and arm, bring the first, dry hand to the opposite end of the towel and repeat (Fig. 8.18). When drying is completed, drop the towel onto the

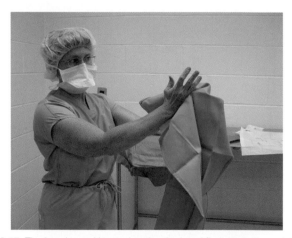

Fig. 8.17 The hand towel is used to dry the hand first, then the wrist, and then the forearm. Once the towel leaves the hand, it cannot go back up to the hand. It is important to bend slightly at the waist and extend the arms to prevent the sterile towel from touching the nonsterile scrub top.

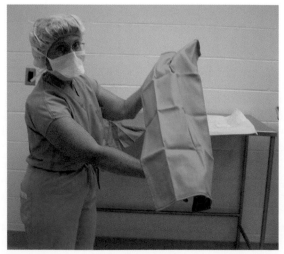

Fig. 8.18 Use the opposite end/side of the hand towel to dry the second hand and arm.

floor with the hand that is currently holding it, without allowing either hand to fall below waist level.

Gowning

The purpose of gowning and gloving is to create a barrier between the sterile and nonsterile areas. Gowns and gloves cover the surgical team members' skin to prevent it from being a possible contaminant.

Gowns and gloves should be opened prior to scrubbing on a dry, flat surface away from other sterile supplies so that dripping water from the scrub person's arms will not contaminate them.

Gowns are folded inside out in the packs. Grasp the whole gown, and lift the folded gown out of the package. Step away from the table, making sure there is adequate space to gown without contaminating anything (Fig. 8.19). After locating the neckline and armholes, hold the gown by the neckline (Fig. 8.20) and allow it to unfold (do not shake it). Keep the inside toward the body and the hands in the armholes. Slide both arms into the sleeves of the gown by reaching and extending both arms at the same time (Fig. 8.21). The circulating assistant will continue to pull the gown onto the scrubbed-in

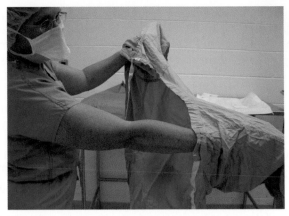

Fig. 8.21 Both arms are advanced into the sleeves simultaneously, but the hands are not allowed to pass all the way through the cuffs in order to allow for closed gloving.

person, carefully bringing the gown over the shoulders, fastening the neck of the gown, and tying the waistline, all while standing behind the person gowning and touching only the hem of the collar and back of the gown. If the gown is not fitting comfortably, the circulating assistant may grasp the gown by the hem at the bottom of the gown and pull downward. This may help the gown fit more comfortably. After the scrubbed person has gloved, the neck fastening may need to be adjusted to remove excess slack in the sleeve area of the gown. The scrubbed person's hands remain inside the cuffs and must not be exposed outside the gown to perform the closed-gloving technique.

If the surgical gowns used are the wraparound style, the front tie should not be touched until sterile gloves have been donned by the surgical technician. On reusable gowns the wraparound ties are tied in the front of the gown by a single bow-tie knot. On disposable gowns, a disposable paper tag covers the end of the ties. This gown can be properly donned with the help of a nonsterile circulating assistant. Both these gowns cover the back of the body, thereby reducing the chance of contamination because most of the body is covered. The back of the gown or the body is never considered sterile. If either tie drops on the reusable gown or the disposable gown, the circulating assistant retrieves both ties and fastens them behind the scrubbed person's back.

Gloving

There are three methods of gloving: (1) closed gloving, (2) open gloving, and (3) assisted gloving. Both open gloving and closed gloving enable the scrubbed personnel to glove themselves. Closed gloving is the preferred method for the surgical team. Assisted gloving requires the assistance of another scrubbed-in team member.

Closed Gloving

Closed gloving provides assurance against contamination because no bare skin is exposed in the process. The following technique is used for the closed-gloving technique. Remember to always keep the hands within the cuffs of the gown.

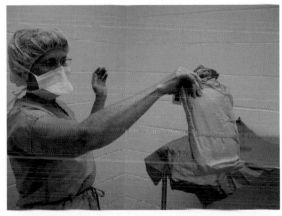

Fig. 8.19 As the gown is removed from the table, the person steps back away from the table to prevent the gown from touching any non-sterile items as it unfolds.

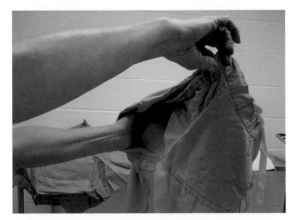

Fig. 8.20 The neckline is identified and held while the armholes are found, and the gown is allowed to open.

With the left hand, pick up the right glove from the inner wrapper of the glove package by the folded cuff (Fig. 8.22). Extend the right hand (still within the cuff) with the palm facing upward. Place the palm of the glove palm down against the palm of the hand with the thumb and fingers of the glove facing the body. (The thumb side should be underneath on the same side as the thumb of the right hand facing upward.) When performing closed gloving, remember the saying, "Palm to palm, thumb to thumb, fingers of glove facing the elbow."

Through the gown cuff, grasp the back of the glove cuff with the right hand (Fig. 8.23). With the left hand, pull and lift the cuff up and over the gown cuff and the right hand (Fig. 8.24). The hand is still inside the sleeve. With the left hand, grasp both the top of the right glove cuff and the gown cuff, and pull toward the elbow while pushing the hand through the gown cuff and

into the glove. Be sure the cuff of the glove completely covers the cuff of the gown (Fig. 8.25). Glove the left hand using the same technique (Figs. 8.26 to 8.28).

Open Gloving

Open gloving is another method that enables the scrubbed personnel to glove themselves. The open-gloving method should not be used routinely for surgical gloving. The closed or assisted technique is preferred, but the open method is used if one glove becomes contaminated in surgery and an assistant is not available to perform assisted gloving. Open gloving is also used when only the hands need to be sterile and no gown is needed, such as for minor surgical procedures, bone marrow biopsies, or catheterizations. For open gloving in surgery, instead of leaving the hands in the sleeves of the surgical gown,

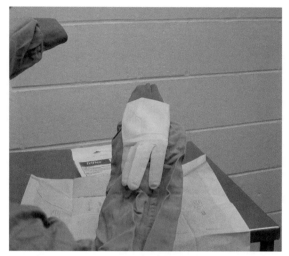

Fig. 8.22 When performing the closed-gloving technique, "palm to palm, thumb to thumb, and fingers face the elbows" means that the palm of the hand covered by the cuff of the gown is facing up and the palm side of the glove is facing down toward the palm of the hand. The thumb of the hand covered by the cuff of the gown is directly beneath the thumb of the glove. The fingers of the glove are lying over the wrist of the gown-covered hand, facing toward the elbow of the gown-covered arm.

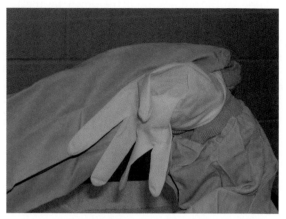

Fig. 8.24 The cuff of the glove is extended over the cuff of the gown to perform closed gloving.

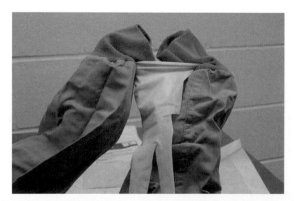

Fig. 8.23 During closed gloving, the hands remain within the cuffs of the gown until the gloves are secured over the cuffs of the gown, and then the hand can be extended out of the gown and into the glove. This requires manipulating the gloves through the material of the gown.

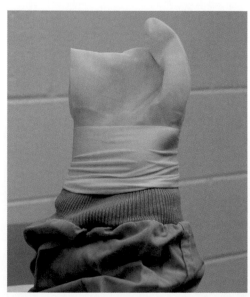

Fig. 8.25 The cuff of this glove needs to be unfolded and pulled down to cover the entire cuff of the gown; this will assist placement of the fingers and thumb into the glove.

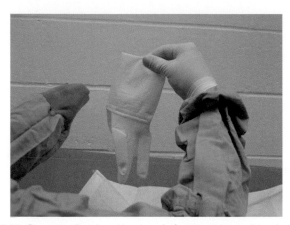

Fig. 8.26 Once the first hand is gloved, that hand is used to place the second glove palm down onto the extended left hand covered by the cuff of the gown. Note that the palm of the left hand covered by the cuff of the gown is facing up.

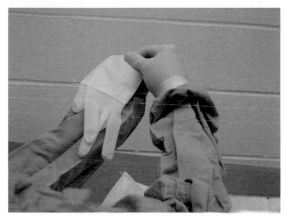

Fig. 8.27 The thumb of the glove is directly above the thumb of the left hand covered by the cuff of the gown, and the fingers of the glove are facing the elbow of the left arm. "Palm to palm, thumb to thumb, and fingers facing the elbow."

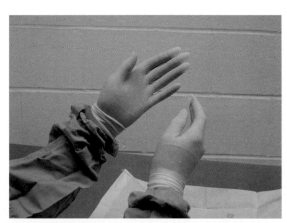

Fig. 8.28 Once the hand is extended into the glove, the cuff of the glove needs to be unfolded and pulled down to cover the entire cuff of the gown.

the hands are extended all the way through the cuff and the sleeves. The hands are entirely exposed. The following technique is used for the open-gloving technique.

With the left hand, pick up the right glove by grasping the cuff on the "future" inside surface (nonsterile surface) of the fold only (Fig. 8.29). Gently guide the fingers into the glove, leaving the cuff well turned over the hand. Keep the thumb in the palm of the hand until it is well inside the glove. Do not adjust the cuff (Figs. 8.30 and 8.31). Place the gloved fingers of the right hand under the everted left glove cuff, on the sterile side of the left glove (Fig. 8.32). Slide the fingers of the left hand into the glove, keeping the thumb inside the palm of the hand, until inside the glove. Pull the glove on all the way (Figs. 8.33 and 8.34). With the left hand, slide the fingers under the outside edge of the right cuff and unfold it by stretching it up the wrist. Avoid touching any bare, exposed skin (Fig. 8.35).

Assisted Gloving

Assisted gloving is used when a sterile team member helps another scrubbed-in team member glove. If a glove is contaminated during surgery, it needs to be changed. The contaminated

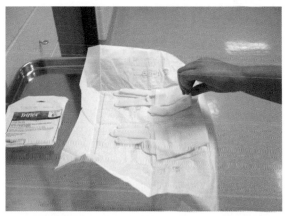

Fig. 8.29 Only the "skin surface" of the glove being put on during open gloving can be touched. This means that only the folded cuff of the first glove can be touched.

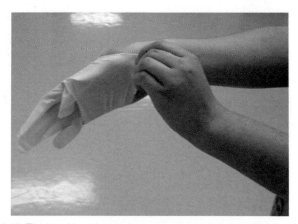

Fig. 8.30 The hand is extended into the glove, and the cuff is pulled up the wrist.

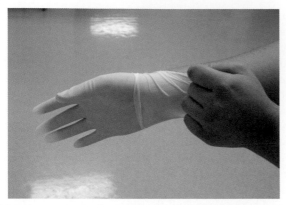

Fig. 8.31 Even when the fingers are all the way into the glove, the cuff is not unfolded yet.

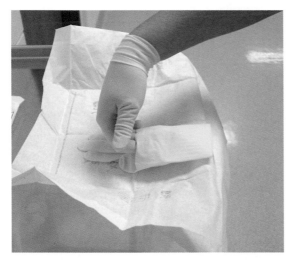

Fig. 8.32 The gloved hand carefully reaches under the folded cuff of the second glove to pick it up. The second glove is put on before the cuff of the first glove is unfolded up the wrist.

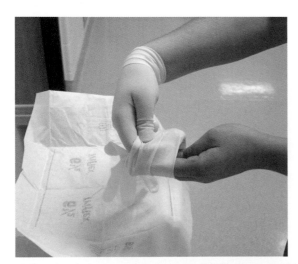

Fig. 8.33 Care is taken not to touch the exposed skin of the hand being gloved with the sterile glove already donned. This would contaminate the first glove.

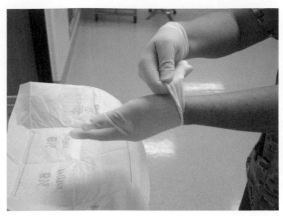

Fig. 8.34 Pulling the cuff of the second glove up the arm and away from the wrist prevents the gloved hand from touching the exposed skin and assists in finishing the step of pulling on the second glove.

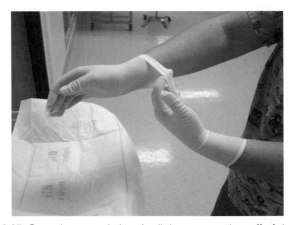

Fig. 8.35 Once the second glove is all the way on, the cuff of the first glove can be unfolded and extended up the arm. Only the fingers (not the thumb) of the second hand to be gloved are used to unfold the cuff. This prevents the thumb from touching the exposed skin on the arm.

person should step away or at least keep the contaminated hand away from the sterile field. The circulating assistant grasps the outside of the glove cuff, but below the top of the glove, to ensure the sterile gown is not touched. The glove is pulled off inside out. The cuff of the gown should not be pulled over the hand because the cuff is contaminated with skin cells and scurf. The hands are extended all the way through the cuffs and sleeves. Assisted gloving is the best method to use to reglove. If this is not possible, open gloving away from the sterile field is necessary.

The following technique is used for the assisted gloving technique. The already gloved, sterile team member picks up the sterile glove, then places fingers from both hands under the cuff on the sterile sides of the glove. The palm of the glove is held toward the person being gloved (Fig. 8.36). The cuff of the glove should be stretched widely open so that the hand can be placed in the glove without touching the surgical technician. The surgical technician can avoid touching the hand to be gloved by holding the thumbs out (Fig. 8.37). As the person slips into the glove, pull up on the glove to assist with the entrance of the hand into the glove (Fig. 8.38). Make sure to bring the cuff of the glove over the cuff of the sleeve. Repeat for the other hand.

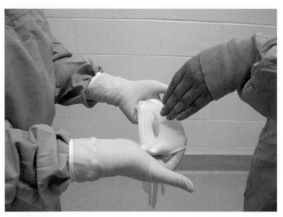

Fig. 8.36 Assisted gloving requires the help of another scrubbed-in and gloved person. The palm of the glove being placed is held toward the person needing the glove.

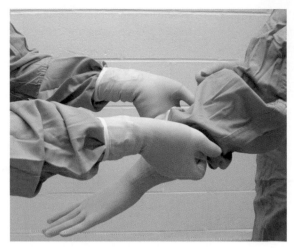

Fig. 8.38 The assistant pulls the cuff of the glove over the cuff of the gown as the hand is pushed into the glove. Note that the assistant's thumbs are still held away from the glove.

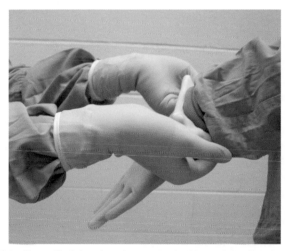

Fig. 8.37 The cuff of the glove is stretched wide, and the thumbs of the assistant are not used to hold the glove. This prevents the assistant from accidentally touching the exposed hand of the person needing the glove.

The person being gloved can assist by using the one gloved hand to hold open the cuff of the other sterile glove being donned, while the surgical technician's thumbs are kept under the glove's cuff until the glove is donned.

Contaminated Gown

If a gown becomes contaminated during surgery, it must be removed. The contaminated person steps away from the sterile field. The circulating assistant opens new sterile gloves and gown. The circulating assistant unfastens the gown and pulls it off inside out. The contaminated person then removes the gloves by grabbing the cuff of the glove (not the gown) and pulling the glove off inside out.

Rescrubbing is not required to regown and reglove. If only a sleeve has been contaminated, sterile sleeves may be used to cover the contaminated area.

RESPONSIBILITIES

Once the surgical technician is scrubbed in, maintaining sterility and assisting the surgeon are the primary concerns. In addition, the surgical technician needs to manage the instrument table (i.e., arrange the instruments on the table, count instruments and gauze squares [sponges] before opening and closing a body cavity), pass instruments to the surgeon, retract and moisten tissues, and maintain hemostasis. With all these duties, it is easy to forget to be considerate of the technician's own body. To avoid becoming weak in the knees or nauseated during surgery, it is important to avoid locking the knee joints while assisting and to eat before scrubbing in. Slowly shifting the weight from leg to leg and slightly bending the knees helps surgery personnel to prevent blood from pooling and to stay alert.

▌ KEY POINTS

1. A surgical dress code should be written and posted so that it can be easily followed and enforced.
2. The dress code should include the defined areas where surgical attire must be worn, appropriate attire within those defined areas, and the acceptable options for cover apparel outside the surgical area.
3. The scrub suit should be covered with a clean laboratory coat at all times when outside the surgical area.
4. Personnel are not allowed to wear laboratory coats in the surgery room.
5. Scrub suits worn in the surgery room should not be worn home from the hospital.
6. Clean, freshly laundered scrub suits should be donned just before going into the surgery room and should not be worn from home into the hospital.
7. Proper surgical attire includes wearing a head cover that completely covers all head and facial hair, surgical masks that effectively cover the mouth and nose, and clean shoes with or without shoe covers.

8. Proper surgical attire requires the removal of all jewelry; this includes wedding bands, body-piercing objects, and watches.
9. Fingernails need to be well manicured and cannot extend beyond the tips of the fingers. Fingernails cannot be covered with nail polish.
10. The purpose of the surgical hand scrub or hand rub is to remove as many microorganisms as possible from the nails, hands, and arms.
11. All jewelry, name tags, and pens need to be removed before beginning the surgical hand scrub or hand rub.
12. Head covers and masks need to be donned before beginning the surgical hand scrub or rub.
13. Sterilized gown and glove packs need to be opened before beginning the surgical hand scrub or rub.
14. When using an antimicrobial detergent, it is important to follow the manufacturer's directions regarding the scrub time and whether or not a scrub brush should be used.
15. Closed gloving is the best gloving technique to guard against contamination because no bare skin is exposed in the process.

REVIEW QUESTIONS

1. An example of endogenous contamination would be
   a. a hole in the surgeon's glove.
   b. the patient's hair on the surgical site.
   c. the surgeon's hair on the surgical site.
   d. the anesthetist touching the surgical drape.
2. Which of these procedures may be done in the surgical area?
   a. Clipping hair
   b. Nail trim
   c. Final surgical scrub of incision
   d. Surgeon surgical hand scrub
3. A duty of the surgical assistant is
   a. managing instruments.
   b. opening suture material for the surgeon.
   c. monitoring the patient while it is under anesthesia.
   d. providing extra packs of instruments when needed.
4. A short sleeve scrub top should be worn to
   a. prevent overheating of the surgical personnel.
   b. allow scrubbing of hands and arms.
   c. prevent staining of sleeves with surgical scrub agents.
   d. minimize contamination of scrub top at home.
5. When surgical personnel who are scrubbed in have to sneeze, they should
   a. scrub out of surgery.
   b. turn their head to the side.
   c. step back from the sterile field.
   d. turn their back to the surgery table.
6. Which of these are acceptable qualities of a scrub brush?
   a. Stiff bristles, soft sponge
   b. Stiff bristles, FDA-approved antiseptic
   c. Soft bristles, FDA-approved antiseptic
   d. Soft bristles with alcohol as scrub agent
7. Which of these is a quality of chlorhexidine gluconate 4%?
   a. Neutralized rapidly in the presence of organic material
   b. Active against enveloped viruses
   c. Minimal residual effect
   d. May be irritating to skin
8. A disadvantage of using an alcohol-based scrub is
   a. flammability.
   b. removes oils from skin.
   c. good activity against tubercle bacillus.
   d. less bactericidal activity for gram-negative bacteria.
9. When applying a rub-based scrub, how should the hands be dried?
   a. Use a sterile towel to dry the hands.
   b. Rub hands and arms until they are dry.
   c. Air dry after thorough application of scrub.
   d. Use hand and arm motion to decrease drying time.
10. Open gloving is used for
    a. all routine elective surgeries.
    b. minor surgical procedures where no gown is worn.
    c. regloving during surgery due to contamination of a glove.
    d. when a sterile team member helps another scrubbed-in team member glove.
11. List 2 ways to avoid becoming nauseated during surgery.
12. List 3 qualities of a scrub agent.
13. Skullcaps should only be worn if:
14. When should a hood be worn as headwear in surgery?
15. What are the advantage of using a brushless scrubs?

BIBLIOGRAPHY

Association of periOperative Registered Nurses (AORN): *Standards, recommended practices, and guidelines*, Denver, 2004, AORN.

Fairchild S: *Perioperative nursing principles and practice*, ed 3, Philadelphia, 1996, Lippincott.

Fossum T, Hedlund CS, Hulse DA, et al.: *Small animal surgery*, ed 3, St Louis, 2007, Mosby.

Gruendemann BJ, Bjerke N: Is it time for brushless scrubbing with an alcohol based agent? *AORN J* 74:859, 2001.

Paulson D: Comparative evaluation of five surgical hand scrub preparations. *AORN J* 60:246, 1994.

Phillips N: *Berry & Kohn's operating room technique*, ed 10, St Louis, 2004, Mosby.

Slatter D: *Textbook of small animal surgery*, ed 3, Philadelphia, 2003, Saunders.

Spry C: *Essentials of perioperative nursing*, ed 2, Boston, 2004, Jones & Bartlett.

Surgical Assisting—Duties During Surgery

Paige Allen

LEARNING OBJECTIVES

After completion of this chapter, the reader will be able to:
- Discuss the role of the sterile surgical assistant as related to care of the surgical field.
- Discuss the correct method of loading and passing a scalpel blade and handle.
- Describe the techniques used to pass various types of surgical instruments safely to the surgeon.
- Discuss the desired method of handling tissue to avoid trauma.
- Describe the procedure for performing an instrument count.
- Describe the procedure for performing a sponge count.
- Describe the various methods of maintaining hemostasis on the operative field.
- Describe the correct procedure for draping a surgical patient.
- Discuss the various options for administering/introducing drugs onto the operative field and surgical site.
- Recognize common suture patterns.
- Describe the proper procedure for removing sutures.

KEY TERMS

Bone wax
Fenestration

Hemostasis
Pronation

Supination

INSTRUMENT HANDLING AND PASSING

Accepting sterile packs and equipment from a circulating assistant is a critical responsibility of the surgical technician. For a double-wrapped pack, the outer wrap should be properly unfolded by the circulating assistant and then offered to the surgical technician. Care must be taken so that the surgical technician does not contaminate himself or herself when taking the pack. When taking a peel-packed item from the circulating assistant, it is equally important that the surgical technician be aware of the nonsterile portions of the packaging and avoid touching those areas. The surgical technician needs to be attentive to the situation when taking any sterile item from the circulating assistant. Miscommunication, a quick movement, or not securely grabbing the item can result in disaster. Dropping the equipment or contaminating the equipment or

supply would require a flash sterilization procedure. Worse yet, dropping the equipment or supply and having it break or be damaged as it hits the floor is a catastrophe in the operating room.

The surgical technician is responsible for properly passing the instruments to the surgeon, maintaining the instrument table, and ensuring the working order of the instrumentation throughout the procedure. Setting up and managing the instrument table allows the technician to assist the surgeon more efficiently. An organized table makes it easier for the technician to find the requested instrument quickly. Instruments should be laid out so that the ring handles (or shafts) of the instruments are closest to the surgical technician. Where the technician stands in relation to the table and patient dictates which direction the instruments should face.

Technicians scrubbed into a procedure may have the sole responsibility of managing the instrument table (e.g., for cardiovascular procedures, total hip replacements). Procedures involving extensive instrumentation and equipment greatly benefit from having a technician "run the table." Properly passing the instruments to the surgeon is a skill that must be mastered not only for efficiency in movement but for safety as well. The shape and purpose of the instrument determines the method used to pass it safely and properly to the surgeon.

At other times the technician may be required to scrub in to assist the surgeon with the procedure. Assisting in the procedure may entail tissue retraction, hemostasis, or any other assistance needed by the surgeon. A technician scrubbed in to assist with surgery will increase intraoperative efficiency and decrease surgery and anesthesia time, which all are beneficial to the health of the patient.

Scalpel Blades and Handles

Scalpel blades should be handled with the greatest respect. Needle holders are the only instrument that should be used to attach and remove the blade from the scalpel handle. The use of any other instrument or device (e.g., hemostat, finger) is inappropriate and can be dangerous. Needle holders are designed to hold metal and therefore can withstand the stress of clamping a metal blade and then placing it on the handle. Hemostat tips are designed to grasp tissue or vessels and will be damaged if used to place a blade on a scalpel handle.

To load a handle with a scalpel blade, the needle holder should firmly grasp the blade on the noncutting edge and slip it onto the handle (Fig. 9.1). Once loaded, the handle and blade should be passed to the surgeon in a specific manner. The technician should hold the scalpel handle with the blade facing away from the hand, with the point toward the technician (Fig. 9.2). The thumb and index finger should be holding the handle with the hand in a supinated position. **Supination** (or *supinated*) indicates that the palm of the hand is facing upward or outward. Pronation of the technician's hand follows as the handle is passed into the waiting hand of the

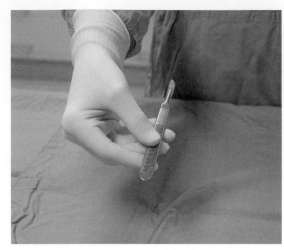

Fig. 9.2 Step 1 in properly passing a loaded scalpel handle. The scalpel blade is pointed toward the assistant, with the cutting edge of the blade away from the assistant's hand.

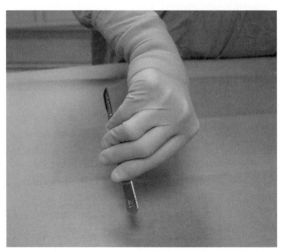

Fig. 9.3 Step 2 in properly passing a loaded scalpel handle. The assistant pronates the hand and places the handle firmly in the waiting hand of the surgeon.

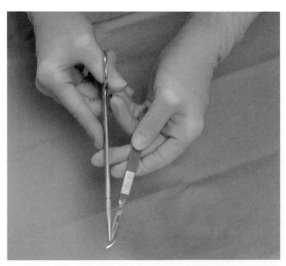

Fig. 9.1 Loading the scalpel blade onto the scalpel handle.

surgeon (Fig. 9.3). **Pronation** is the rotation of the hand and forearm so that the palm faces backward or downward. As the surgeon grasps the handle, the technician should maintain the forward momentum of the hand so as not to contact the cutting edge of the blade. This method of passing the instrument allows the cutting edge of the blade to face away from the assistant as well as the surgeon for optimal safety and handling.

Passing Ring-Handled and Other Instruments

When passing an instrument to the surgeon, it is important to remember to place the instrument firmly in the palm of the waiting hand to decrease the chance that the instrument will be dropped. The surgeon must know that the instrument is in hand without having to look up from the field.

The first ratchet of a ring-handled instrument should be closed before the instrument is passed. The ring handles should be facing the floor and the tip of the instrument facing the ceiling (Fig. 9.4). The box lock should be held between the surgical technician's thumb and index finger, with the shaft of the instrument stabilized by the remaining fingers of the delivering hand (Fig. 9.5).

The technician should hold an instrument with a curved tip with the curve facing the thumb holding the instrument (Fig. 9.6). When held in this fashion, after being passed to the surgeon, the instrument is positioned for immediate placement on the tissue.

When passing an instrument without ring handles, such as a thumb tissue forceps, the technician should hold it with the tips facing the floor. The other end of the instrument should be held firmly with the thumb and index finger while the remaining fingers stabilize the instrument (Fig. 9.7). When held in this manner, once placed in the hand of the surgeon, the instrument is ready to be used.

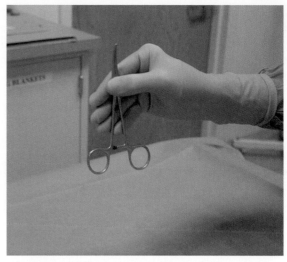

Fig. 9.6 Proper technique for passing a curved-tipped instrument.

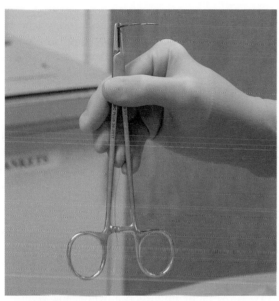

Fig. 9.4 Proper hand position for passing a loaded needle holder. The needle is loaded for a right-handed surgeon.

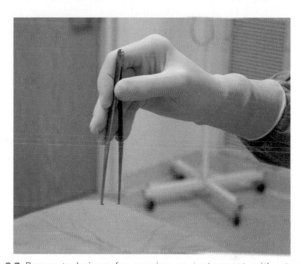

Fig. 9.7 Proper technique for passing an instrument without a ring handle.

TISSUE HANDLING

The careful handling of tissue in the surgical field is an extremely important responsibility of the surgical technician. Healthy tissue needs to be handled appropriately so as not to cause trauma. Unhealthy tissue requires extreme care in handling so as not to compromise its viability further. The surgical technician must be aware of the status of the tissue in the field and must be familiar with appropriate methods of tissue retraction. Healthy tissue may withstand the pressure of a hand-held retractor, but too much pressure may cause vascular tissue damage. If too little retraction is provided, however, the surgeon will not be able to see clearly, and the procedure may be compromised. Communication between the surgeon and the veterinary technician is essential to the patient's health and recovery.

When a self-retaining retractor (e.g., Balfour retractor for abdomen, Finochietto retractor for chest) is used, a moist lap pad is generally placed between the blades of the retractor and the tissue. The lap pad acts as a cushion to alleviate excessive

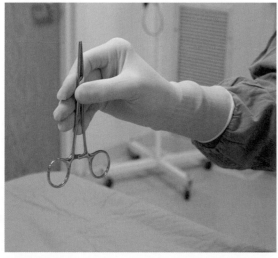

Fig. 9.5 Proper technique for passing a straight-tipped instrument.

pressure on the tissue and helps keep the tissues moist. For some situations the surgeon may choose to place stay sutures in an organ to facilitate retraction or manipulation of the organ. Surgical technicians holding stay sutures must be careful not to hold them too firmly because of the risk of ripping the suture from the tissue.

Another situation that requires careful tissue handling is during an enterotomy or anastomosis. Often the surgeon has the technician use his or her fingers as "clamps." After milking as much intestinal content away from the proposed intestinal incision site as possible, the surgical technician will use the index and middle fingers to clamp the tissue. Care must be taken to provide adequate stabilization of the tissue without putting excessive pressure on the delicate structure.

Keeping Tissues Moist

Another important duty of the surgical technician is to keep the exposed tissues moist. Systemic hydration should be achieved and maintained through the infusion of intravenous (IV) fluids, but the tissue must be kept moist topically as well. Generally, an isotonic solution such as lactated Ringer's solution or 0.9% normal saline is used as a lavage fluid. Depending on the surgical procedure, an antibiotic may be added to the solution for topical application.

One of the most important guidelines in surgical assisting is that *moist tissue is happy tissue.* If the tissues are kept moist, rather than allowed to dry out, the circulation is less compromised and tissue function remains intact. The heat from lights and exposure to room air makes tissue vulnerable to adverse conditions.

A bowl on the sterile field can be filled with warm isotonic solution. A single gauze square can be soaked in this lavage solution and then squeezed while suspended above the exposed tissues to drip the lavage solution onto the tissues. It is important to avoid wiping or rubbing the gauze sponge on the tissue directly. The friction created even with gentle wiping or rubbing irritates the tissue and promotes the formation of adhesions between the irritated surface of the affected tissue and other abdominal organs or body tissues. Adhesions may become problematic for the patient, requiring more surgery later to correct. The bowl containing the warm lavage solution should be kept at the back of the instrument table, preferably on a separate tray, so that if spillage does occur, there is no contamination of the sterile field. Any spilled solution remains on the tray and does not soak the covering on the table.

Maintaining Hemostasis

Maintaining hemostasis (the stopping of blood flow) on the surgical field is also an important duty of the scrubbed-in surgical technician. If vessels are cut, the technician should be ready to pass the necessary hemostat. Blotting the hemorrhaging site before the surgeon places the hemostat helps the surgeon place the clamp on the vessel without including excessive tissue in the hemostat. It is important to remember that bleeding tissue should be blotted, not wiped, when trying to achieve hemostasis. Wiping with a sponge may cause coagulation already initiated to be wiped away. Firm, but not excessive, pressure blotting is more

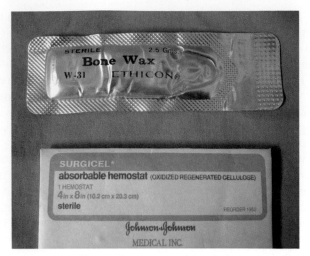

Fig. 9.8 Bone wax and Surgicel.

effective. The blood-soaked sponge count can serve as an estimate of blood loss. A 3 × 3–inch sponge holds approximately 6 mL of blood. A 4 × 4–inch sponge holds approximately 10 mL of blood. Ideally, only radiopaque sponges should be included in surgical packs. Less expensive, nonradiopaque sponges can be used for routine external use.

Other items available for controlling hemostasis are products such as absorbable gelatin or cellulose sponge (Gelfoam®, Pfizer, New York; Surgicel®, Johnson & Johnson Ethicon, Somerville, NJ) and bone wax (Fig. 9.8). Gelfoam is gelatin sponge material that is absorbent and, when placed in a tissue defect (e.g., a punch biopsy site on the liver), encourages hemostasis by swelling to fill the defect. Surgicel is a cellulose product that, when laid on a tissue surface, promotes hemostasis by enhancing clot formation. Although Surgicel is absorbable, some sources suggest its removal after achievement of hemostasis because the product may inhibit callus formation and encourage infection. Bone wax, as the name implies, is a hemostatic agent made of beeswax and a softening agent that is used on a cut bone surface to assist with hemorrhage control. It is a poorly absorbed product and thus should be used sparingly.

Hemostasis may also be achieved by the use of electrocautery. The technician, at the direction of the surgeon, may cauterize tissue or a vessel or may elevate the hemostat that is on the vessel so that the surgeon can activate the cautery.

EQUIPMENT COUNT

Instrument Count

The first duty that the surgical technician should perform is an instrument count. An instrument count documents how many instruments are present at the outset of the procedure. Before the surgical site is closed, a second count of the instruments should be done. Most anesthesia logs have a space to record the initial surgical instrument count and the instrument and sharps count at closure. The circulating assistant helps the surgical technician keep track of how many instruments (if any) were removed from the sterile field and how many sharps were used.

Sponge Count

Next, the surgical technician should perform a sponge count. Only radiopaque sponges should be used in surgical situations (Fig. 9.9). These gauze sponges have a radiopaque string woven into the fiber that is visible on a radiograph if a sponge is inadvertently left in a patient.

The initial quantity of sponges in the pack is counted before any sponges are used. As the sponges are used, they should be discarded in a dedicated sponge bowl or kick bucket. The sponge bowl should be a basin located off the sterile field or a back table. As the sponges are discarded, the circulating assistant can unfold and count each sponge. It is important to unfold the sponges in case two or more sponges are stuck together. All sponges, whether gauze squares or laparotomy ("lap") pads (Fig. 9.10), subsequently added to the sterile field must be accounted for as well.

Before the surgical site is closed, the sponges on the sterile field must be counted (by the surgical technician) and the number of discarded sponges counted (by the circulating assistant), then totaled. The sum of these two groups of sponges must equal the number of sponges documented as entering the sterile field. If the numbers do not agree, the hunt for the missing

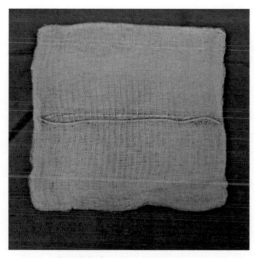

Fig. 9.9 A radiopaque sponge.

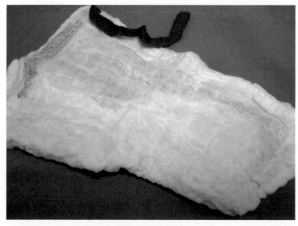

Fig. 9.10 A laparotomy pad.

sponge begins. First, other trash receptacles in the room should be checked to see whether a sponge was discarded in an inappropriate place. If the missing sponge is not found there, the sterile team should evaluate the surgical field. Sponges may accidentally become tucked between the folds of the drapes. If the missing sponge is still not recovered, an intraoperative radiograph should be taken. If radiology is not an option, the wound should be closed and a radiograph taken in the immediate postoperative period. Using only radiopaque sponges intraoperatively aids in identifying sponges left in the patient. The incident must be thoroughly documented in the medical record in the event the sponge is not recovered.

DRAPING—BASIC PRINCIPLES

Surgical technicians are often involved with draping the patient, if not entirely responsible for this task. Draping materials can be quite varied. Some surgeons may prefer to use cloth hand towels as the ground drape, or first layer, when draping a patient. Other larger top sheets can also be made of cloth or paper. Fenestrated drapes can be of the cloth variety or paper, but the paper option requires the surgeon to make the **fenestration** (an opening in a drape through which surgery is performed) once the drape is opened on the sterile field. The use of ground drapes (towels) and then four top sheets is highly preferable to the use of a fenestrated drape. Linen drapes are advantageous because they can assist with patient thermal regulation better than the lightweight paper drapes. Linen drapes require laundering and refolding, a service that can be provided by an outside company or completed by the veterinary technician or veterinary assistants in the practice. Paper drapes are available on bulk rolls and can be cut to custom fit the patient. Commercially prepared paper or paper/plastic combination drapes are also available. Regardless of the manufacturer, paper drapes are intended to be used as disposable, one-time-use items and should not be cleaned or laundered and reused. The type of procedure to be performed as well as the surgeon's preference influence the choice of cloth or paper. Surgical procedures expected to be very messy (cesarean section, enterotomy, etc.) may be better served by the use of disposable paper drapes.

Foundational principles regarding draping can be applied to most surgical procedures. The edges where hands are holding ground drapes should be turned over to protect sterile gloves from being contaminated by the patient's skin or hair. Sterile personnel placing drapes must also be careful to not contaminate gown sleeves or the front of the gown on the surgical table or anesthesia equipment or cables that may be near the patient. Ground towels, if used, should be placed on the patient in a specific order. The first drape is placed on the side of the patient that is closest (nearest) to the person draping. The drape for the opposite side of the patient should be placed second. A sterile person must never reach across a nonsterile field; therefore, the second drape can be placed after the sterile person walks to the other side of the table. After the two lateral drapes are placed, the cranial drape is placed. Placement of the drapes in relationship to the proposed incision site depends on the veterinarian's preference and the procedure being performed. A general rule of thumb is to place the edge of the drape ½ to ¾ inch from the incision line.

Once the cranial drape is in place, penetrating towel clamps must be used to secure the towels (Fig. 9.11). Proper use and handling of the surgical instrument is imperative. The surgical technician's ring finger and thumb should be placed in the ring handle of the instrument. This position allows the index finger to be extended to stabilize the box lock, thereby easing the task of placing the towel clamp properly (Fig. 9.12). Penetrating towel clamps are designed to pierce the skin and secure the drapes to the patient (Fig. 9.13). Care must be taken to ensure that the towel clamp points have penetrated through the drape material and into the patient's skin. Towel clamps should be placed close to the intersecting corner of the two towels to avoid bunching of the drape. The fourth and final ground drape, the caudal drape, can be placed once the other three towels are secured. When placing cranial and caudal towels, in most cases, the person performing the draping must stand on the long side of the surgical table and rotate the waist and shoulder to place the towel. The habit of draping from the short end of the table should be avoided because often access to that end is blocked by equipment (e.g., anesthesia machine) or the instrument table.

After the ground drapes have been secured, the top drape(s) should be placed. There are two options at this point for continuing the draping process. If a single fenestrated paper drape is to be used, the fenestration must be created before the drape is laid on the patient. Once the drape touches the patient, the underside is considered nonsterile and should not be manipulated. It is impossible to cut the fenestration after the drape is on the patient without contaminating the sterile field. To avoid this scenario, the fenestration should be cut, based on the size of the opening created by the ground towels, before the drape is opened and placed on the patient. Once the drape (paper or linen) is on the patient, nonpenetrating towel clamps are used to secure the paper/top drape to the towels underneath. Nonpenetrating towel clamps should clamp around the neck of the penetrating towel clamp located under the paper drape (Fig. 9.14). The second option for top drapes is to use four paper or linen large drapes and place them on the patient in exactly the same order the ground towels were placed. As with the fenestrated drape, these top sheets are secured to the towels underneath with the nonpenetrating towel clamps (Fig. 9.15). The margins for draping a patient depend on the procedure being performed, the surgeon's preference, and the potential for extended incisions or alternate surgical

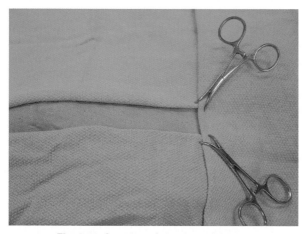

Fig. 9.11 Securing of the ground drapes.

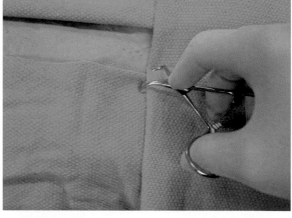

Fig. 9.13 Placement of the penetrating towel clamp.

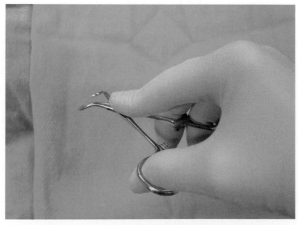

Fig. 9.12 Proper holding of the towel clamp.

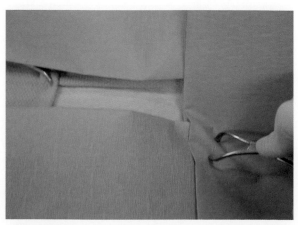

Fig. 9.14 Placement of the nonpenetrating towel clamp.

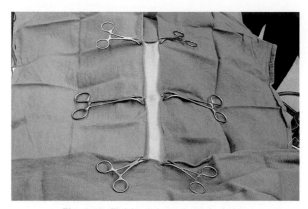

Fig. 9.15 Finished draped surgical site.

sites. Communication between the technician and the surgeon is imperative to guarantee a properly draped patient.

DRUG ADMINISTRATION

Administration of systemic drugs is not usually a task that is handled by the surgical technician. A nonsterile member of the team, such as the circulating assistant or the anesthetist, is usually responsible for this task. Additional analgesics, antibiotics, and cardiac medications are all examples of types of drugs that could be administered intraoperatively. A surgical technician may be involved with drug administration if it is a medication that needs to be administered via the surgical site. Infusion of a local anesthetic and addition of an antibiotic to lavage fluid are examples of intraoperative drug administration. If a medication is to be administered by syringe and needle in the sterile field, the circulating assistant must aseptically open the desired size of syringe and needle onto the sterile field. The circulating assistant then holds the bottle of medication upside down. A sterile member of the team then takes the assembled sterile syringe and needle and inserts it into the bottle. After the sterile member withdraws the desired amount of medication, it is a good idea to recap the needle, have the circulating assistant take that needle off the syringe, and open another sterile needle to be used.

SUTURE-RELATED RESPONSIBILITIES

There are several suture-related responsibilities for the surgical technician. One responsibility is cutting the sutures once the veterinarian has completed the suture placement. The length to cut the suture depends on the type of sutures used (absorbable versus nonabsorbable) and the placement of the suture (internal or external). Absorbable sutures are generally cut quite short, leaving only ⅛ to ¼ inch of suture beyond the knot. Minimal amounts of absorbable suture are left in the patient to reduce the possibility of complications. Nonabsorbable suture is generally cut so that the suture ends extend about ½ inch beyond the knot. Suitable length is necessary to facilitate suture removal in 10 to 14 days.

Another suture-related responsibility is running the suture when the surgeon is placing a continuous pattern. The technician's responsibility is to keep the suture out of the incision and

out of the way of the surgeon. If the path is clear, all the surgeon needs to do is place the stitches. Running the suture significantly reduces anesthesia time because the surgeon can suture much faster.

The third responsibility involving suture is recognizing suture patterns. Although closing wounds and placing sutures is not typically a skill that veterinary technicians need to master, some state Practice Acts do allow technicians to perform suturing. It is, however, essential that veterinary technicians are qualified to recognize suture patterns for various reasons. The technician must not only know what a suture line should look like but also be able to identify whether or not a suture line has been compromised (loosened sutures, missing sutures, etc.). It is also important to know the different suture patterns to appropriately remove the suture once the wound has healed.

Common Suture Patterns

Suture patterns are categorized by either the way they appose tissue edges (appositional, everting, inverting) or by the tissue layer where they are placed (subcutaneous, subcuticular, skin). Suture patterns are also named by the method of placement (interrupted or continuous).

Subcuticular versus Subcutaneous

A *subcutaneous suture pattern* is placed in the subcutaneous tissue layer. This pattern brings the skin edges into apposition but generally does not appropriately close the skin. This pattern is often used to decrease dead space in a wound, with skin sutures still being needed.

A *subcuticular suture pattern* is placed in the subcuticular space just under the skin. Often subcuticular patterns are placed to eliminate the need for skin sutures. The skin edges are close enough in apposition that further external sutures are unnecessary. This pattern may be used with canine castration incisions or cesarean section incisions or for animals that may chew at skin sutures. Most often these two patterns are placed in a continuous manner, but sometimes an interrupted pattern is indicated.

Continuous Patterns

The most commonly used continuous pattern is a *simple continuous*. Fig. 9.16 shows an example of a simple continuous pattern. There is a knot at either end of the suture line and continuous suture in between. Simple continuous patterns can be employed in subcutaneous space, subcuticularly, as a skin suture on muscle layers on the linea alba, or in any other area where a relatively air-tight, fluid-tight apposition is needed.

The *Ford interlocking* pattern (Fig. 9.17) is another continuous pattern. Though not used as often in small animal surgery as it is in large animal surgery, it creates a very strong suture line.

Other types of continuous patterns are Lembert and horizontal mattress. A Lembert pattern is an inverting pattern generally used to close a hollow organ (stomach, urinary bladder, intestine, etc.). These patterns can be placed to appose tissue edges but, if pulled more tightly, create an inverting pattern. A continuous horizontal mattress pattern can be placed in a continuous pattern but is more often used in an interrupted fashion.

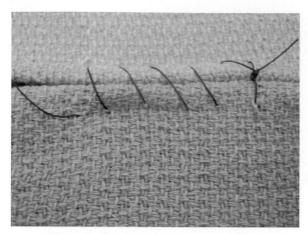

Fig. 9.16 Simple continuous suture pattern.

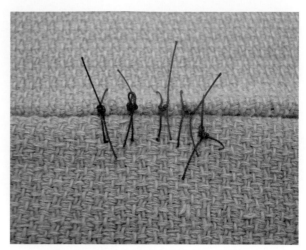

Fig. 9.18 Simple interrupted suture pattern.

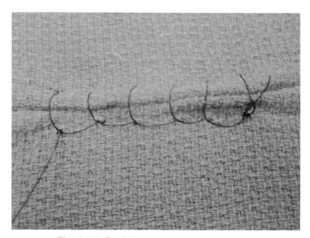

Fig. 9.17 Ford interlocking suture pattern.

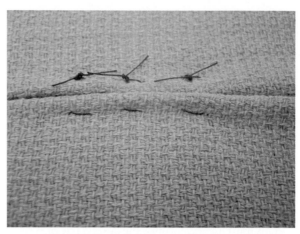

Fig. 9.19 Horizontal mattress suture pattern.

Interrupted Patterns

The *simple interrupted pattern* is a common suture pattern used in veterinary surgery (Fig. 9.18). It is an easy, quick, and versatile pattern to place. It is often used to close the skin, linea alba, muscle layers, subcutaneous space, and so on. It is also the pattern used to secure implants such as Penrose drains. The simple interrupted pattern results in appositional tissue edges unless excessive tension is used, in which case it results in an inverting pattern. Wound healing is poor with an inverting pattern, so care must be taken to ensure that the edges remain in apposition.

The disadvantages to using the simple interrupted pattern include that it is time consuming and that it results in having foreign material (suture) in the wound.

Another interrupted pattern is the *horizontal mattress,* seen in Fig. 9.19. The horizontal mattress pattern is time consuming to place but is ideal in areas of tension. If pulled too tightly, it will result in an everting pattern, so care must be used to keep the tissue edges appositional if that is the intention. A *cruciate pattern* (Fig. 9.20) is a modification of the horizontal mattress. Once placed, it results in an X over the wound edges.

A *vertical mattress* pattern (also called "far-far, near-near" because of how the needle is passed through the tissue) is a stronger suture pattern in areas of tension but is also time

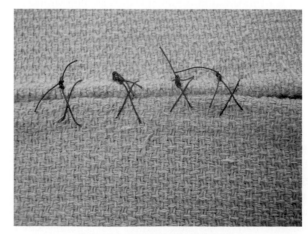

Fig. 9.20 Cruciate suture pattern.

consuming to place. Its advantage over the horizontal mattress is that there are fewer incidences of unintentional everting of wound edges (Fig. 9.21).

Suture Removal

When removing sutures from a wound, the following instruments should be employed: a suture (stitch) removal scissors and a

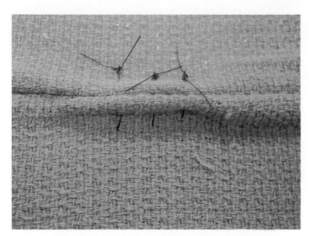

Fig. 9.21 Vertical mattress suture pattern.

thumb tissue forceps. Some people like using a hemostat instead of a thumb tissue forceps, but because hemostats are intended for holding vessels, it is an inappropriate use of the instrument to have it grab suture. However, if the hemostat is not used in a surgical situation and is labeled as such ("exam room only"), then its use is permitted for suture removal. Sutures are generally removed 10 to 14 days postoperatively. If any medication has been administered that may delay healing, the suture removal date will need to be delayed. Before removal of any sutures, the incision must be inspected to ensure that healing has occurred. There should be no gaps in the incision, nor any drainage, redness, or swelling.

When removing the suture from an interrupted pattern, use the thumb tissue forceps to grab one of the suture ends (tags) and gently apply tension away from the wound. Then place the hooked blade of the suture removal scissors beside the knot. With one quick motion, cut the suture and pull it out of the skin. This same method is employed until all sutures have been removed. Some veterinarians prefer a slightly altered method of suture removal designed to prevent exposed suture from being dragged beneath the skin as it is removed. Rather than applying tension on the suture tags, utilize the tissue forceps to immobilize the knot. Next place the suture removal scissors as close to the skin as you can before cutting and use the forceps to remove the suture material. If there is some scabbing on the wound, there will be increased discomfort for the patient. Also, if sutures have been allowed to remain in place longer than the recommended 10 to 14 days, the skin can begin to grow over the sutures and bury the stitch. Removal of these sutures can be very uncomfortable for the patient and, depending on the amount of over growth, may require sedation of the patient.

For a continuous pattern, the removal process begins in the same fashion. Using a thumb tissue forceps, grab the free end of the suture at one end of the suture line and, using the hook blade of the suture removal scissors, cut the suture just next to the knot. It is unwise to pull the entire suture line through the wound because it may introduce bacteria to the entire wound. Therefore every third or fourth stitch of the continuous pattern should be snipped and then the shorter piece of suture pulled out. This method is also less uncomfortable for the patient. When the entire line of sutures has been removed, the final stitch of the continuous pattern needs to be removed like an interrupted stitch.

KEY POINTS

1. It is usually the surgical technician's responsibility to perform both an instrument count and a sponge count before the procedure begins and again before the incision is closed.
2. Proper technique, for safety and efficiency reasons, must be used when passing various types of surgical instruments to the surgeon.
3. Tissue handling is a delicate process and must be properly performed by the surgical technician.
4. Keeping exposed tissues moist intraoperatively is an essential task of the surgical technician.
5. Effectively assisting the surgeon includes providing hemostasis on the surgical field.
6. The use of ground drapes and then four top sheets is highly preferable to the use of a fenestrated drape.
7. The edges of ground drapes where the hands are holding them should be turned over to protect the sterile gloves from being contaminated by the patient's skin or hair.
8. A sterile person must never reach across a nonsterile field; therefore, the second drape can be placed after the sterile person walks to the other side of the table.
9. Proper use and handling of the surgical instruments are imperative.
10. Communication between the technician and the surgeon is imperative to guarantee a properly draped patient.
11. If a medication is to be administered by syringe and needle in the sterile field, the circulating assistant must aseptically open the desired size of syringe and needle onto the sterile field.
12. The technician's responsibility is to keep the suture out of the incision and out of the way of the surgeon.
13. Suture patterns are categorized by either the way they appose tissue edges or by the tissue layer where they are placed.
14. Sutures are generally removed 10 to 14 days postoperatively.

REVIEW QUESTIONS

1. Benefits of having a surgical technician scrubbed in to assist in surgery include
   a. decreased surgery and anesthesia time.
   b. increased surgery and anesthesia time.
   c. increased charges to the client.
   d. decreased charges to the client.
2. Which instrument is used to attach and remove the scalpel blade from the scalpel handle?
   a. Needle holders
   b. Thumb forceps
   c. Mosquito forceps
   d. This is placed without the aid of an instrument.
3. Proper passing of a ringed instrument to a surgeon includes which steps?
   a. Close the first ratchet of the instrument, and point the tip toward the ceiling.
   b. Open the ratchet of the instrument, and point the tip toward the ceiling.
   c. Close the first ratchet of the instrument, and point the tip toward the floor.
   d. Open the ratchet of the instrument, and point the tip toward the floor.
4. The reason to lavage tissue during surgery is to
   a. hydrate the patient.
   b. promote hemostasis.
   c. retain tissue function.
   d. promote adhesion formation.
5. During surgery, it is best to place the bowl of lavage solution
   a. on a separate tray.
   b. next to the sterile field.
   c. in the surgical technician's hands.
   d. at the front of the instrument tray.
6. A 3 × 3–inch sponge gauze holds how approximately much blood?
   a. 3 mL
   b. 6 mL
   c. 10 mL
   d. 15 mL
7. A 4 × 4–inch sponge gauze holds how approximately much blood?
   a. 3 mL
   b. 6 mL
   c. 10 mL
   d. 15 mL
8. Which product used for hemostasis acts by swelling to fill the defect?
   a. Gelfoam
   b. Surgicel
   c. Bone wax
   d. Hemostat
9. The first duty that the surgical technician should perform is
   a. draping the patient.
   b. counting the instruments.
   c. blotting the incision site.
   d. preparing the electrocautery for use.
10. What is an advantage of using a paper drape?
    a. Easy to clean and reuse
    b. Comes pre-fenestrated
    c. Conserves patient's body heat
    d. Provides for easy clean up in messy procedures
11. A subcuticular suture pattern is what type of suture pattern?
    a. Everting
    b. Inverting
    c. Appositional
    d. All of the above
12. Which suture pattern is used for areas of tension?
    a. Ford interlocking
    b. Horizontal mattress
    c. Simple interrupted
    d. Simple continuous
13. Describe the best way to use a sponge to aid in hemostasis and explain why this is best.
14. How should instruments be laid out on the instrument table?
15. Define hemostasis.
16. Describe what a surgical technician does when they are "running the suture."
17. Why is it important to do a sponge count before and after surgery?

BIBLIOGRAPHY

Bassert JM, McCurnin DM, editors: *McCurnin's clinical textbook for veterinary technicians*, ed 9, St Louis, 2017, Saunders.

Fossum TW, Hedlund CS, Hulse DA, et al.: *Small animal surgery*, ed 5, St Louis, 2018, Mosby.

Surgical Procedures

Susan Burcham

OUTLINE

LEARNING OBJECTIVES

After completion of this chapter, the reader will be able to:
- Understand and give a description of each surgical procedure discussed.
- Properly position patients for specific surgical procedures.
- Drape the patient for specific surgical procedures.
- Discuss the advantages and disadvantages of specific surgical procedures.
- Identify surgical instruments and supplies that may be used for specialized surgical procedures.
- Discuss surgical options for various ophthalmic conditions.
- Discuss surgical options for aural hematomas.

- Identify and prevent common complications that may arise during surgical procedures.
- Properly identify the bones and joints of the dog and cat.
- Identify different types of fractures.
- Identify the different types of fixation devices related to fracture repair.
- Discuss the different repair options for cruciate ligament rupture.
- Identify specific biopsy instruments and understand tissue preservation techniques for biopsy samples.
- Discuss minimally invasive options to general surgery, such as endoscopy, laser surgery, and laparoscopy.

KEY TERMS

Abdominocentesis
Ablation
Aerophagia
Anastomosis
Anuria
Blepharospasm

Celiotomy
Coaptation
Conjunctivitis
Cryptorchid
Cystotomy
Cystourethrogram

Dehiscence
Disarticulation
Dysuria
Endotoxemia
Enophthalmos
Enterotomy

Entropion	Laparotomy	Septicemia
Evisceration	Lavage	Splenectomy
Gastrectomy	Ligate	Stenosis
Gastritis	Malunion	Stranguria
Gastropexy	Neoplasia	Trichobezoar
Gastrotomy	Nonunion	Trocar
Hematuria	Nosocomial infection	Urethrotomy
Herniation	Orchiectomy	Uroabdomen
Ileus	Onychectomy	Urolith
Insufflation	Osteomyelitis	Urolithiasis
Intussusception	Percutaneous	Uveitis
Ischemia	Peritonitis	Volvulus
Keratitis	Photophobia	
Lacrimation	Pollakiuria	

INTRODUCTION

Surgical procedures are included in this textbook because well-educated veterinary technicians need to be knowledgeable of the common procedures they will be participating in with the surgeon. From aseptic preparation of the correct part of the patient, appropriate sterilization of the instruments, correct suture and instrumentation, positioning of the patient, and surgical assisting, the veterinary technician is an integral part of all surgical procedures. This chapter includes the common procedures a technician is likely to encounter in small animal general and emergency practice, from elective spays and neuters to intestinal resections and anastomoses, as well as common orthopedic procedures.

RESPONSIBILITIES OF THE SURGICAL TECHNICIAN

When performing a surgical procedure, the veterinarian's complete attention needs to be directed to the procedure being performed. Even the simplest of procedures can take a turn for the worse if the veterinarian is forced to shift focus. The job of the veterinary technician is to ensure the veterinarian does not become distracted or shift focus. As outlined in previous chapters, the technician must perform careful preplanning, including instrumentation selection, patient preparation, and attention to positioning and aseptic preparation of the surgical site. The technician should also strive to make sure that all equipment that could be required is accessible in the surgery suite before moving the patient into the surgery suite.

Intraoperative duties usually involve assisting the surgeon as a sterile surgical technician or a circulating assistant. The sterile surgical technician scrubs in, wearing a gown and gloves. The duties of the surgical technician may include retraction of tissues, assistance with fracture reduction, sponging of incisions or wounds, applying suction, and manual hemostasis. As a circulating assistant, he or she may participate in nonsterile activities, such as opening the surgical pack and passing instruments or suture material aseptically. In many practices the technician may also be responsible for monitoring the anesthetized patient while acting as a circulating assistant.

Being a competent surgical technician requires (1) proficient knowledge of the surgical procedure, the surgical instruments, and aseptic and sterile techniques and (2) anticipation of the surgeon's needs.

There are too many surgical procedures to list them all in the confines of this text. The goal of this chapter is to discuss common procedures, arranged by anatomic location. General information regarding preparation, instrumentation, intraoperative concerns, and postoperative considerations will be outlined. Specific surgeries with unique criteria will then be discussed at the conclusion of each section. At the end of the chapter, laparoscopic, endoscopic, and laser procedures are covered in more depth.

ABDOMINAL PROCEDURES

Instruments

A routine surgical instrument pack is adequate for most abdominal procedures (Fig. 10.1). A Balfour abdominal retractor, a self-retaining abdominal retractor, should be previously

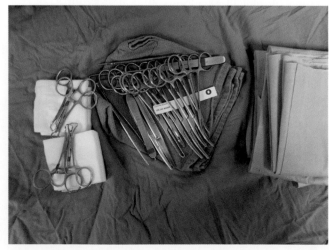

Fig. 10.1 Soft tissue pack.

sterilized and accessible (Fig. 10.2). The Balfour retractor holds the abdomen open and allows for better visualization of abdominal contents. Balfour retractors are available in different sizes, and selection of the appropriate size is based on the size of the patient. Additional special instruments may be needed, depending on the results of the abdominal exploratory surgery.

Sterile laparotomy sponges (Fig. 10.3) should be available. Heated lavage fluid and suction may also be indicated.

Patient Positioning and Preparation

For most abdominal procedures the patient should be positioned in dorsal recumbency to allow for a ventral midline approach. The ventral abdomen should be clipped from just above the xiphoid process to the pubis. Adequate hair clipping is important to allow extension of the incision cranially or caudally for better exposure. Unless otherwise indicated, the bladder should be expressed before the patient is transported into the surgical suite.

Patient Draping

For any abdominal procedure, a four-quarter draping method should be considered (Fig. 10.4).

General procedure. A blade is used to incise the skin and then the subcutaneous tissues. The abdominal wall should be tented to make a sharp incision into the linea alba and through the peritoneum. The incision is expanded cranially and caudally to allow access to the abdominal organs. The sterile surgical assistant can moisten laparotomy sponges and place them on either side of the incision. Exposure to the air and surgical lights cause the abdominal organs to become dry, which can lead to impaired healing. Care should also be taken to ensure any exposed organs remain moist by covering them with sterile laparotomy sponges. The sterile surgical assistant should also take care when handling the exposed viscera; gloves or sponges used should be moistened to reduce tissue damage.

Abdominal Wall Closure

Surgical closure, including suture material, is the veterinarian's preference, but the technician should have the material prepared. There are typically three layers of closure:
1. Linea alba, for strength and closure of abdominal compartment
2. Subcutaneous layer, to reduce dead space
3. Skin

The linea alba is usually closed in a simple interrupted or simple continuous pattern, using an absorbable suture material. Absorbable suture material is also used for the subcutaneous layer and is generally performed in a simple continuous pattern.

Skin can be closed according to the preference of the surgeon. The choices are a simple interrupted pattern with a nonabsorbable suture, a continuous appositional suture pattern with an absorbable suture material, or skin staples (see Chapters 1 and 9). The information on suture type, pattern, and the layers closed should be included in the surgery report.

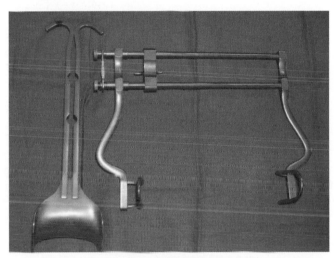

Fig. 10.2 Balfour retractor.

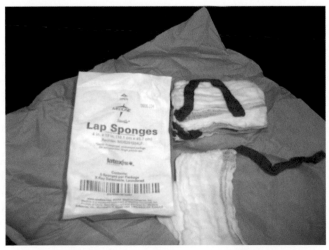

Fig. 10.3 Sterile laparotomy (lap) sponges.

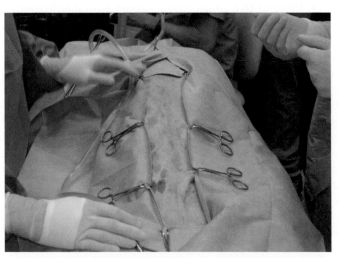

Fig. 10.4 Four-quarter draping technique.

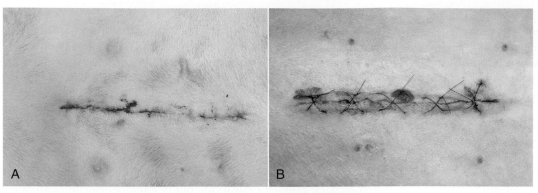

Fig. 10.5 These photographs were taken 4 hours after surgery. A, A celiotomy incision after routine ovario-hysterectomy. B, A celiotomy incision after severe traction on the skin during surgery for exposure. Note the minimal redness, swelling, and drainage from incision in A compared with that in B. (From Bassert JM, Thomas, JA, editors: McCurnin's clinical textbook for veterinary technicians, ed 8, St Louis, 2014, Elsevier.)

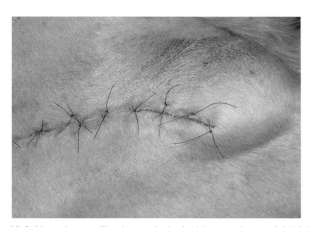

Fig. 10.6 Note the swelling beneath the incision on the cranial thigh of this dog. The swelling was nonpainful, and the dog's vital signs were normal. The swelling was diagnosed as a seroma. (From Bassert JM, Thomas, JA, editors: McCurnin's clinical textbook for veterinary technicians, ed 8, St Louis, 2014, Elsevier.)

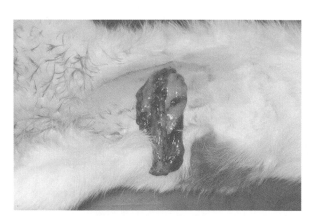

Fig. 10.7 Complete dehiscence of an abdominal incision. Note the intraabdominal contents protruding through the incision. (From Bassert JM, Thomas, JA, editors: McCurnin's clinical textbook for veterinary technicians, ed 8, St Louis, 2014, Elsevier.)

Postoperative Considerations and Instructions

The incision should be checked at least once a day for redness, swelling, or discharge; twice-daily checks would be optimal (Figs. 10.5 and 10.6). This careful examination should continue until the sutures or staples are removed, or for 10 to 14 days postoperatively. Complications from a laparotomy procedure include dehiscence, evisceration, and sepsis. Dehiscence, separation of all layers of an incision or wound, may occur because trauma to the sutures by the animal or as a result of suture breakage or knot slipping or untying. The sooner the problem is detected, the less likely more severe problems will occur. Dehiscence of all layers of the incision can lead to evisceration, which is exposure of the abdominal organs (Fig. 10.7). Evisceration can result in sepsis and blood loss as a result of self-mutilation of the exposed intestine and may lead to resection and anastomosis of the affected intestine.

If dehiscence with or without evisceration occurs, the situation must be attended to immediately.

Manipulation of the viscera during surgery is necessary but can lead to ileus and/or pancreatitis postoperatively. The affected patient may exhibit vomiting or inappetence. If vomiting or anorexia persist 24 to 48 hours postoperatively, intravenous fluid therapy and additional diagnostic work may be necessary.

Surgery Report

A surgery report should be completed for each surgical procedure performed at the hospital. The report is valuable part of the medical record and aids in maintaining surgical history for any future procedures that may be performed on the animal as well as any legal issues that could arise. The surgery report provides patient information as well as protection for the hospital. The surgery report should consist of the date of the surgery; the hospital's name; the owner's name, address, and phone number; and the patient's name, date of birth (DOB), species, breed, and hospital identification number, if applicable. A complete record of the procedure performed should be recorded on this form and placed in the animal's record. Box 10.1 shows an example of a surgery report for an abdominal exploratory procedure.

BOX 10.1 Surgery Report: Celiotomy

Animal Hospital Name
Owner: John Doe
Address: 555 Sterling Lane
Jupiter, NY 55555
Phone number: 555-5555
Animal Name: Sasha
Animal #: 65656501
Species: Canine
Breed: Labrador
DOB: 05/05/10
Date of Surgery: 01/03/2011
Primary Surgeon: Dr. Vet
Assistant: Technician Scrub
Diagnosis or Preoperative Signs: Persistent vomiting and lethargy.
Surgical Procedure: Exploratory celiotomy.

Description of Surgical Procedure
Surgical Approach: A ventral midline skin incision was made extending from approximately 2 cm below the xiphoid process to approximately 6 cm cranial to the pubis. Subcutaneous tissue was bluntly dissected to expose the linea alba. The linea alba was incised to expose the abdominal cavity and viscera.

 Surgical Pathology: No perforations or necrosis of the stomach were noted. All other organs were grossly unremarkable.

 Surgical Procedure: The abdominal cavity was thoroughly explored for any gross abnormalities or perforations in the gastrointestinal tract. The abdominal cavity was lavaged with 3 L of warm saline and closed routinely.

 Closure:
Gastric mucosa and submucosa: 3-0 PDS in simple continuous suture pattern.
Gastric seromuscular layer: 3-0 PDS in Cushing pattern.
Linea alba: 2-0 PDS in simple continuous suture pattern.
Subcutaneous tissue: 3-0 PDS in simple continuous suture pattern.
Subcuticular layer: 3-0 Monocryl in simple continuous suture pattern.
Skin: Skin staples.

SPECIFIC ABDOMINAL PROCEDURES

Abdominal Exploratory Surgery
Definition

Abdominal exploratory surgery refers to surgical exploration of the abdominal cavity. Related terms include the following:
Celiotomy: Surgical incision into the abdominal cavity
Laparotomy: Flank incision into the abdominal cavity

Indications

Exploratory surgery may be indicated for a variety of reasons. Most often an exploratory procedure is indicated for diagnostic or curative purposes. Diagnostic purposes include obtaining surgical biopsy specimens of abdominal organs for analysis because of a chronic disease process. Curative surgery may be required because of an *acute abdomen,* which is a sudden onset of clinical signs associated with the abdomen. Some causes of acute abdomen can be life threatening and may require an emergency exploratory laparotomy. Common indications for abdominal exploratory surgery are abdominal masses, traumatic injury to the abdomen, or suspected foreign body ingestion.

Abdominal Exploratory Procedure

The Balfour retractor may be placed to allow full exposure of the abdominal cavity. When placing a Balfour retractor, the assistant should visualize the insertion on the side of the surgeon, and the surgeon should visualize the insertion on the side of the assistant. Visualization assures organs are not entrapped within the Balfour retractor.

The surgeon then performs a systematic exploration of the entire abdomen and its contents. Most surgeons have a preferred system for exploring the abdomen and conduct the exploration the same way each time they perform the procedure. Such an approach ensures that all organs and structures are observed, and a disease process is not overlooked. The circulating technician should note any abnormalities seen within the abdominal cavity and record the findings in the pathology section of the surgery report (Box 10.2). A postoperative sponge count should take place before closure of the abdominal incision to ensure no sponges are left in the abdomen.

Gastric Foreign Bodies and Gastrotomy
Definition

A gastric foreign body is any ingested foreign object that becomes lodged in the stomach and is unable to be digested; it may also be referred to as a gastric obstruction. A distinction is made between *gastric foreign bodies,* which are found in the stomach, and *intestinal foreign bodies,* which are found anywhere in the intestines (duodenum, jejunum, ileum, or large intestine). *Linear foreign bodies* are usually objects such as string or thread and are seen most often in felines. A linear

---

BOX 10.2 Systematic Exploration of the Abdominal Cavity

1: Explore the Cranial Quadrant
 • Examine the diaphragm (including the esophageal hiatus) and the entire liver (palpate the liver).
 • Inspect the gallbladder and biliary tree; express the gallbladder to determine its patency.
 • Examine the stomach, pylorus, proximal duodenum, and spleen.
 • Examine both pancreatic limbs (palpate gently), the portal vein, hepatic arteries, and caudal vena cava.
2: Explore the Caudal Quadrant
 • Inspect the descending colon, urinary bladder, urethra, and prostate or uterine horns.
 • Inspect the inguinal rings.
3: Explore the Intestinal Tract
 • Palpate the intestinal tract from the duodenum to the descending colon and observe the mesenteric vasculature and nodes.
4: Explore the "Gutters"
 • Use the mesoduodenum to retract the intestine to the left and examine the right "gutter." Palpate the kidney, and examine the adrenal glands, ureter, and ovary.
 • Use the descending colon to retract the abdominal contents to the right. Examine the left kidney, adrenal gland, ureter, and ovary.

From Fossum TW, Cho J, Dewey C, et al: Small animal surgery, ed 5, Philadelphia, 2019, Elsevier.

foreign body is complicated because a part of the foreign object may become lodged under the tongue or in the stomach, while the rest of the object continues through the intestines. Linear foreign bodies may cause *plication* (pleating or folding) of the intestines due to the tension across the foreign material (Fig. 10.8).

Indications

A primary reason to perform a **gastrotomy** (incision into the stomach) is to remove a foreign body. Dogs tend to be indiscriminate eaters and eat or swallow an assortment of objects. Some commonly ingested items are rocks, bones, corncobs, and toys. Another indication to perform a gastrotomy is for the retrieval of full-thickness gastric biopsy specimens or removal of **neoplasia**. Common gastric neoplastic conditions in dogs and cats include adenocarcinoma, lymphosarcoma, leiomyosarcoma, and leiomyoma.

Common foreign bodies in cats are **trichobezoars** (hairballs), string, yarn, and thread. In cats, linear foreign bodies are often affixed under the tongue or at the pyloric sphincter and may cause intestinal plication. If a linear foreign body is suspected, the base and underside of the tongue should be inspected for the presence of a foreign object prior to surgery. Foreign bodies are more common in younger animals because of their curiosity, but an animal of any age can have a gastric or intestinal foreign body. Patients at higher risk for foreign bodies are those with a history of foreign body ingestion or who have medical conditions that predispose them to *pica* (craving for unnatural articles of food).

The most common clinical sign associated with a gastric obstruction is vomiting. Vomiting may be intermittent, and some animals may otherwise act normal. Vomiting may be absent if the object is in the fundus of the stomach rather than obstructing the pyloric sphincter. Other clinical signs are lethargy, abdominal pain, anorexia, and depression. Clinical signs worsen if the foreign body has perforated the stomach leading to **peritonitis** (inflammation of the peritoneum).

Diagnostic testing for gastric foreign bodies should include radiographs of the abdomen. Radiopaque foreign bodies may be apparent on survey radiographs. Many foreign bodies are radiolucent and therefore may require contrast medium to identify. One common contrast study is the barium study. Barium is administered to the patient orally, then a series of films are taken at predetermined intervals. Either the foreign body becomes highlighted by the surrounding barium or the barium ceases to move through the gastrointestinal (GI) tract. The time required for the barium to move through the stomach and into the intestines is compared with normal gastric emptying time. If a delay in gastric emptying is noted, a gastric foreign body may be suspected.

Radiographs should be taken immediately before surgery to verify the location of the foreign object. It is possible for the object to exit the stomach and enter the intestines or even travel as far as the colon, especially in cases where the surgery is temporarily delayed. In that case, unless the object has sharp edges, it is usually allowed to exit the GI tract naturally, without intervention. If the object has moved to the colon and needs intervention to be removed, endoscopy is the preferred procedure for removal.

Special Instruments

A Balfour abdominal retractor and sterile laparotomy sponges should be available. Heated lavage fluid and suction may also be indicated.

The technician should ensure that all instruments used within the stomach are kept away from the rest of the surgical instruments. The technician and surgeon must avoid contaminating the sterile abdomen with bacteria from the stomach. A good way to approach this situation is to have a sterile towel on which all gastric instruments can be placed during the gastrotomy. Once the gastrotomy is complete, the surgeon and assistant(s) (scrub team) should change gloves. The instruments contaminated by gastric contents should be removed from the instrument table and replaced with new, sterile instruments.

Patient Positioning

The patient should be positioned in dorsal recumbency for a ventral midline incision. The patient should be clipped and prepared for an abdominal procedure.

Patient Draping

A four-quarter draping method should be considered.

Gastrotomy Procedure

The surgeon should inspect the abdominal contents before proceeding with the foreign body removal. The stomach should be identified and isolated. The surgical assistant can isolate the stomach by packing it off from the rest of the abdominal

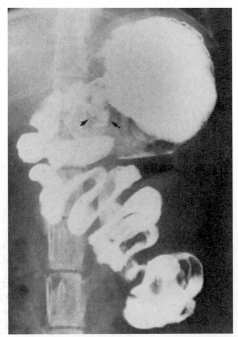

Fig. 10.8 Contrast radiograph detailing a linear foreign body. (From Thrall DE: Textbook of veterinary diagnostic radiology, ed 5, St Louis, 2007, Saunders.)

contents with moist laparotomy sponges. The surgeon then locates the area of the stomach to incise (Fig. 10.9). Stay sutures are placed on either side of the proposed incision site (Fig. 10.10). Stay sutures allow for manipulation of the stomach and prevent leakage of gastric fluid into the abdomen. A stab incision is made with a new scalpel blade (not the same blade used to make the initial skin incision) between the stay sutures, in a hypovascular region of the ventral stomach, generally between the greater and lesser curvatures. The surgical technician should have the suction ready to place into the stab incision to drain the gastric fluid. The surgeon then extends the incision with Metzenbaum scissors. An Allis tissue forceps can generally be used to grasp the foreign body and remove it from the stomach (Fig. 10.11).

Stomach and Abdominal Wall Closure

The stomach can be closed in two layers. The first layer is a simple continuous pattern of a 2-0 or 3-0 absorbable suture. This suture pattern provides apposition. The second layer is a continuous inverting pattern of 3-0 absorbable suture. It may be beneficial to perform a local lavage of the gastric incision site to help dilute any pollutants. The gloves of the scrub team

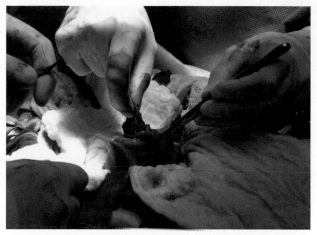

Fig. 10.11 Removal of gastric foreign body (peach pit)

should be changed, and all instruments that were exposed to gastric contents should be removed from the table. Instruments used to close the abdomen should be instruments that were not exposed to the stomach during surgery. A warm lavage of the entire abdomen maybe performed, and the abdomen is closed routinely.

Postoperative Considerations and Instructions

One postoperative goal for gastrotomy patients is to correct any prior fluid loss or electrolyte imbalance. If the patient continues to vomit after surgery, food and water should be withheld and intravenous fluids should be continued. A centrally acting antiemetic can be administered to help control the vomiting. In the absence of vomitus, a bland diet can be introduced 12 to 24 hours postoperatively. Prognosis for the gastrotomy patient should be considered good if there were no perforations in the stomach from the foreign body. If perforations were evident and peritonitis was present, the prognosis may be considered guarded. Box 10.3 shows an example of a surgery report for a gastrotomy.

Intestinal Foreign Bodies and Enterotomy
Definition

Foreign bodies of the intestines are any intraluminal obstruction of intestinal contents caused by an ingested object or objects; these foreign bodies may also be referred to as *intestinal obstructions.*

Indications

A primary indication to perform an **enterotomy** (incision into the intestines) is to remove a foreign body. Some foreign bodies will pass through the esophagus and stomach but are too large to pass through the intestines. The objects found in dogs and cats as gastric foreign bodies can also be found in the intestines (e.g., corncobs, balls, bones, peach pits, linear objects such as string). Intestinal foreign bodies may cause a partial or complete obstruction of the intestinal bowel. Some foreign bodies may slowly make their way through the intestinal tract, causing damage or perforations along the way.

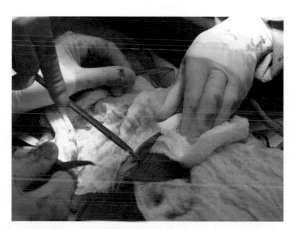

Fig. 10.9 Placement of stay sutures in the gas-distended stomach of a dog with a gastric foreign body.

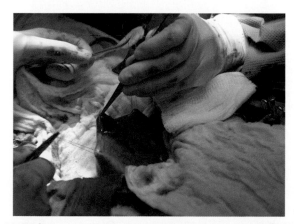

Fig. 10.10 Gastrotomy incision is made between the stay sutures. Note that stay sutures are gently lifted upward to avoid leakage of gastric fluid.

BOX 10.3 Surgery Report: Gastrotomy

Animal Hospital Name
Owner: John Doe
Address: 555 Sterling Lane
Jupiter, NY 55555
Phone number: 555-5555
Animal Name: Sasha
Animal #: 65656501
Species: Canine
Breed: Labrador
DOB: 05/05/10
Date of Surgery: 01/03/2011
Primary Surgeon: Dr. Vet
Assistant: Technician Scrub
Diagnosis or Preoperative Signs: Gastric foreign body.
Surgical Procedure: Gastrotomy.

Description of Surgical Procedure
Surgical Approach: A ventral midline skin incision was made extending from approximately 2 cm below the xiphoid process to approximately 6 cm cranial to the pubis. Subcutaneous tissue was bluntly dissected to expose the linea alba. The linea alba was incised to expose the abdominal cavity and viscera.

Surgical Pathology: Foreign bodies (tennis ball remnants) were present in the stomach. No perforations or necrosis of the stomach was noted. All other organs were grossly unremarkable.

Surgical Procedure: The abdominal cavity was thoroughly explored for any gross abnormalities or perforations in the gastrointestinal tract. Stay sutures were placed in the stomach using 3-0 PDS. The stomach was gently retracted from the abdominal cavity, where an incision approximately 5 cm long was made over a relatively avascular area of the gastric body between the greater and lesser curvatures of the stomach. All foreign material was removed from the stomach. The abdominal cavity was lavaged with 3 L of warm saline and closed routinely.

Closure:
Gastric mucosa and submucosa: 3-0 PDS in simple continuous suture pattern.
Gastric seromuscular layer: 3-0 PDS in Cushing suture pattern.
Linea alba: 2-0 PDS in simple continuous suture pattern.
Subcutaneous tissue: 3-0 PDS in simple continuous suture pattern.
Subcuticular layer: 3-0 Monocryl in simple continuous suture pattern.
Skin: Skin staples.

may include lethargy, intermittent anorexia, and intermittent vomiting.

Linear foreign bodies can manifest any or all of these clinical signs. A portion of the linear foreign body may become embedded at the base of the tongue or pylorus, while the rest of the object moves down the intestinal tract as a result of peristaltic movement. Continuous peristalsis causes *plication* of the intestines (folding or bunching up of the intestines on themselves along the length of the linear foreign body), which can cause the linear foreign body to be pulled tightly. The tension on the string may cause it to act as a knife along the compromised intestinal tissue; the string may cut into the mucosa of the intestines, causing perforations along the way. The damage to the mucosa and the perforations can result in peritonitis as well as considerable abdominal pain. When abdominal palpation is performed on a patient with plicated intestines and peritonitis, the abdominal muscles often tighten, indicating abdominal pain.

Another indication to perform an enterotomy is collection of a full-thickness biopsy specimen from an intestinal segment. Malignant intestinal tumors are common and can cause partial or complete obstruction. The different types of intestinal neoplastic conditions are mentioned in the following section on intestinal resection and anastomosis.

Special Instruments

A general use soft tissue surgery pack in conjunction with Doyen intestinal clamps will be needed for an enterotomy. The Doyen clamps allow the surgeon to clamp the intestines on either side of the incision site (Fig. 10.12). Doyen clamps are considered nontraumatic and prevent intestinal contents from leaking into the abdomen while the procedure is performed. If Doyen clamps are unavailable, the fingers of the assistant can serve the same purpose. If manual clamping with the assistant's fingers is employed, it is important to make sure that the technician's gloves are moist to prevent tissue trauma. Sterile

Others may become lodged in a segment of intestine where they cause a complete obstruction. A complete obstruction prevents intestinal chyme (intestinal contents) from proceeding beyond the obstruction. A partial obstruction may allow some intestinal contents to move beyond the point of the foreign object.

Common clinical signs associated with an intestinal foreign body include abdominal pain, vomiting, diarrhea, depression, anorexia, and weight loss. The location in the intestinal tract (proximal vs. distal), type (partial vs. complete), and duration of the obstruction impact the severity of clinical signs. Complete obstructions cause more acute and produce more serious clinical signs. More proximal obstructions may cause persistent vomiting and dehydration. Clinical signs of distal small intestine (e.g., ileum) and partial obstructions

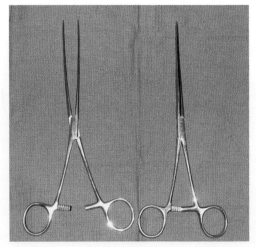

Fig. 10.12 Doyen clamps. These intestinal clamps are considered nontraumatic to the intestines.

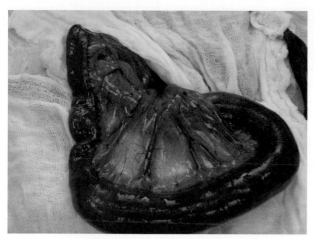

Fig. 10.13 Midjejunal intestinal foreign body in a dog.

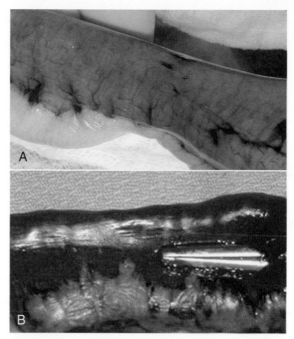

Fig. 10.14 The normal intestine is pink with visible vessels and motility. Note the difference in color between the normal intestine (A) and the devitalized segment of bowel (B). (From Bassert JM, Thomas, JA, editors: McCurnin's clinical textbook for veterinary technicians, ed 8, St Louis, 2014, Elsevier.)

laparotomy sponges should be available. Heated lavage fluid and suction may also be indicated.

The surgical technician must ensure that all instruments used within the intestines are kept away from the rest of the surgical instruments. This practice aids in avoiding contamination of the abdomen with intestinal bacteria. All instruments exposed to the intraluminal contents of the intestines should be placed on a sterile towel during the enterotomy and then removed from the instrument table once the intestines are closed. The other option is to have an instrument set solely used for the GI tract, then substitute a clean set after the intestinal closure. Once the enterotomy is complete, all scrubbed personnel should change gloves, and a new set of instruments can be introduced for closure of the abdomen. A Balfour retractor should also be available for better exposure of the abdomen.

Enterotomy Procedure

A full exploratory procedure should be performed before an enterotomy is begun. The GI tract should be examined completely. Once the intestinal foreign body is located (Fig. 10.13), the affected intestine can be isolated from the abdomen by being packed off with laparotomy (lap) sponges.

The surgeon needs to decide, from an analysis of the intestine, whether an enterotomy or a resection and *anastomosis* should be performed. If necrosis or perforations of the intestinal segment are absent, an enterotomy may be sufficient (Fig. 10.14). The intestinal contents should be milked away from the foreign body site. Doyen clamps or the fingers of a technician can be placed a few centimeters away on either side of the proposed enterotomy. The enterotomy incision should be made just distal to the foreign body on the *antimesenteric border* (the side of the intestine without the attached mesentery) of the intestine (Fig. 10.15), along the long axis. This region is selected because the viability of the intestines proximal to the foreign body is more likely to be compromised, and it is preferable to suture healthy intestine. The incision may need to be extended with Metzenbaum scissors to allow the

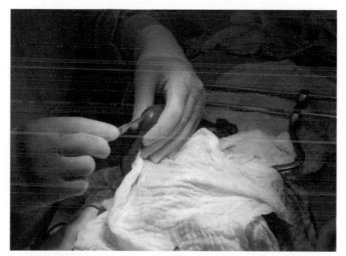

Fig. 10.15 Enterotomy incision performed at the antimesenteric border of the jejunum. The incision is made over the distal aspect of the foreign body.

removal of the foreign body (Fig. 10.16). Forceps or gloved fingers may be useful in grasping and slowly removing the object.

Intestine and Abdominal Wall Closure

Once the foreign body is removed, the enterotomy incision can be closed (Figs. 10.17 and 10.18). An absorbable monofilament taper point suture in a simple interrupted suture pattern may be used to close the incision. Multifilament suture should never be

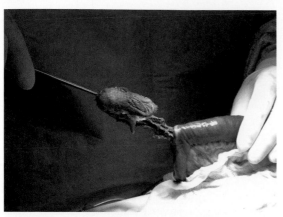

Fig. 10.16 Removal of an intestinal foreign body (cloth) in jejunum of a dog.

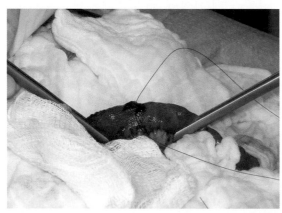

Fig. 10.17 Partial-thickness closure of a jejunal enterotomy site in a dog.

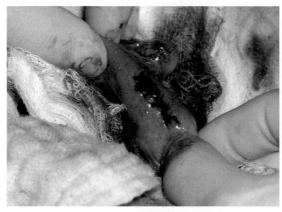

Fig. 10.18 Complete closure of the jejunal enterotomy site using absorbable suture material in a simple interrupted suture pattern.

used in the GI tract; the braid of the suture can act as a wick for bacteria. A local lavage of the enterotomy site is warranted, and a warm abdominal lavage of the entire abdomen may be considered. All scrubbed personnel should change gloves, and the instruments used to perform the enterotomy should be placed aside. Clean instruments (those not used in the intestines) should be used to close the layers of the abdominal cavity. The abdominal cavity can be closed routinely, as previously described.

BOX 10.4   Surgery Report: Enterotomy

Animal Hospital Name
Owner: John Doe
Address: 555 Sterling Lane
Jupiter, NY 55555
Phone number: 555-5555
Animal Name: Sasha
Animal #: 65656501
Species: Canine
Breed: Labrador
DOB: 05/05/10
Date of Surgery: 01/03/2011
Primary Surgeon: Dr. Vet
Assistant: Technician Scrub
Diagnosis or Preoperative Signs: Intestinal foreign body.
Surgical Procedure: Enterotomy.

Description of Surgical Procedure
Surgical Approach: A 15-cm ventral midline incision was made from the umbilicus to the pubis through the skin, subcutaneous tissues, and linea alba.
  Surgical Pathology: All abdominal organs were examined. A foreign body was palpable at the proximal jejunum region. All other organs were unremarkable.
  Surgical Procedure: A 4-cm incision was made through the antimesenteric border of the proximal jejunum at the distal end of the foreign body. The area was packed off with lap sponges to protect the abdomen from any intestinal spillage. A stocking material (approx. 12 cm long) was removed through the enterotomy incision. The incision was closed with 3-0 PDS in a simple interrupted appositional suture pattern. The abdomen was lavaged with warm sterile saline. The enterotomy site was surrounded with omentum and replaced into the abdomen.
  Closure:
  Linea alba: 2-0 PDS in simple interrupted suture pattern.
  Subcutaneous: 3-0 Monocryl in simple continuous suture pattern.
  Skin: 3-0 nylon in simple interrupted suture pattern.

Postoperative Considerations and Instructions

One postoperative goal for enterotomy patients is to correct any previous fluid loss or electrolyte imbalances. The owner should be informed of possible complications that could arise postoperatively. Complications include necrosis and perforations of the bowel, as well as leakage and dehiscence of the intestines. All these complications can lead to peritonitis. The prognosis for a patient with peritonitis may be considered guarded. If a simple enterotomy was performed and the bowel appeared healthy intraoperatively, a good prognosis can be given. Early identification of an intestinal foreign body generally improves the outcome. Box 10.4 shows an example of a surgery report for an enterotomy.

Intestinal Resection and Anastomosis
Definition

Intestinal resection and anastomosis (R and A) is the excision of a segment of bowel followed by the reestablishment of the two remaining segments.

Indications

A primary indication for performing an intestinal resection and anastomosis is to remove a section of dead or diseased bowel. Box 10.5 lists the characteristics of devitalized intestinal tissue. Causes of devitalized bowel include foreign bodies, neoplasia, intussusception, necrosis, and ischemia. Ischemia or necrosis of the intestines can lead to peritonitis and a poor prognosis. Peritonitis is an inflammatory process that involves the serous membrane of the abdominal cavity. Leakage of GI contents is a main cause of peritonitis.

As previously mentioned, common clinical signs associated with foreign bodies of the intestinal tract include vomiting, lethargy, abdominal pain, anorexia, and depression. Common clinical signs of neoplasia of the intestinal tract include anorexia, vomiting, weight loss, flatulence, and melena. If an intestinal leakage occurs and peritonitis is present, common clinical signs include abdominal pain, vomiting, fever, and clinical signs of shock, such as tachycardia.

Diagnostic tests should include radiographs and ultrasound, if available, of the abdomen as well as a complete blood analysis. If peritonitis is suspected and an abdominal effusion is identified in the abdomen, an abdominocentesis (puncture of abdominal cavity to obtain fluid) or diagnostic peritoneal lavage should be performed to determine the type of fluid present. If the results of the abdominal fluid analysis reveal the presence of bacteria, a GI leak is suspected.

Special Instruments

Instrumentation is the same as for intestinal foreign body and enterotomy surgery.

Intestinal Resection and Anastomosis Procedure

A full examination of the GI tract should be performed. The segment of diseased bowel should be identified, exteriorized, and packed off with lap sponges (Fig. 10.19).

The surgeon needs to assess the viability of the intestinal segment in question. The presence of peristalsis, vascular pulses, and intestinal color are considered to determine intestinal viability. If the intestinal segment is questionable, it may be the surgeon's preference to resect that region. Neoplasia and necrosis of the intestines are conditions that require resection. The blood vessels from the mesentery to the intestinal segment need to be ligated and transected. The intestinal contents (chyme) should be milked away from the area of the

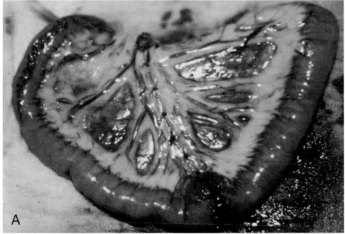

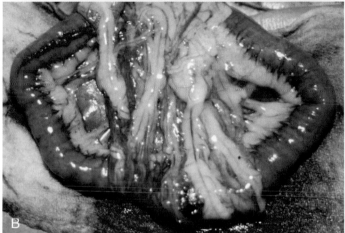

Fig. 10.19 A, Completed jejunal intestinal resection and anastomosis. B, Completed resection and anastomosis wrapped in omentum. (From Tobias K, Johnston S: Veterinary surgery: small animal, St Louis, 2012, Saunders.)

intestine to be resected. The diseased region can be clamped with a crushing forceps (e.g., Carmalt). The area of the intestines to remain in the body can be clamped with Doyen clamps, which are considered nontraumatic and should be gentle on the intestinal tissues. If Doyen clamps are unavailable, the moistened fingers of an assistant will provide the same function.

The surgeon then transects the intestines with a scalpel blade along the outside of the Carmalt forceps, and the intestinal segment, along with the forceps, is removed. A few millimeters of healthy tissue should be removed with the diseased segment to ensure that the anastomosis site is closed with healthy sections of intestine (Fig. 10.20).

Intestine and Abdominal Wall Closure

The technician holds the two segments of intestine close to each other so that they are aligned correctly. A single-layer, simple interrupted suture pattern is often used for an end-to-end anastomosis because it produces minimal stenosis (narrowing) or leakage and heals rapidly. A 3-0 or 4-0 monofilament absorbable suture should be used for the anastomosis site.

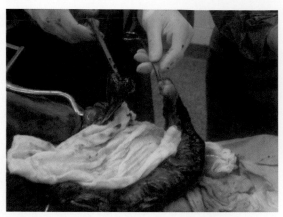

Fig. 10.20 The two segments of bowel are held appositional to each other to begin the anastomosis.

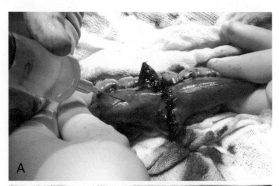

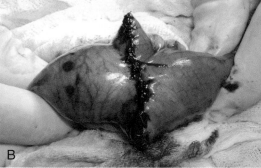

Fig. 10.21 A, To check for leaks after intestinal anastomosis, the intestine is occluded on either side of the incision and the occluded segment of intestine is filled with sterile saline. B, The incision is checked for leakage while the segment is filled with saline. (From Bassert JM, Thomas, JA, editors: McCurnin's clinical textbook for veterinary technicians, ed 8, St Louis, 2014, Elsevier.)

After the anastomosis has been completed, sterile saline can be injected into the surgical site to check for any leakage from the suture site (Fig. 10.21). The intestines should be moderately distended with the sterile saline while maintaining intestinal occlusion. Additional sutures should be placed if leakage occurs. The mesenteric defect should then be closed in a simple continuous or interrupted suture pattern (Fig. 10.22). If peritonitis was present, a closed suction drain may need to be placed to allow drainage of the abdominal cavity. A local lavage of the anastomosis site is performed. In the event of leakage of intestinal contents during

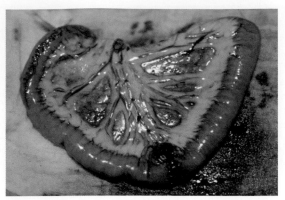

Fig. 10.22 Completed anastomosis of the jejunum.

the procedure, a full abdominal lavage with warm saline should be performed. If peritonitis was present, specimens for bacterial culture of the abdomen should be obtained before closure. The anastomosis site is wrapped with omentum before closure. The scrub team needs to change gloves and the instrument pack to close the abdomen. The abdomen should be closed routinely.

Postoperative Considerations and Instructions

Animals found to have peritonitis during the procedure are usually more critical cases and will need more supportive postoperative care. If the patient is debilitated, intravenous (IV) nutrition may be warranted. IV antibiotics and fluids should be continued. Peritonitis has a high rate of morbidity; this should be explained to the owner. The patient's clinical signs should be closely monitored postoperatively. Any signs of depression, vomiting, fever, abdominal pain or tenderness, or discharge from the incision site could be the result of a dehiscence of the intestinal suture and the presence of peritonitis. Other complications associated with intestinal surgery are leakage of the surgical site, stenosis of the intestinal lumen, intestinal perforation, and death.

A large intestinal resection can lead to short-bowel syndrome. The clinical signs of short-bowel syndrome include malnutrition, weight loss, and diarrhea. Treatment of short-bowel syndrome is based on the clinical signs but includes correction of fluid loss and electrolyte imbalances.

Nutritional support must be provided until the intestines adapt. Prognosis for the patient receiving an intestinal resection and anastomosis can be considered good if peritonitis was absent and removal of large amounts of intestine was averted. The healing process of the intestines is generally rapid but can be interrupted by associated factors, such as debilitation of the patient. Prognosis of the patient with peritonitis should be considered guarded. Box 10.6 shows an example of a surgery report for an intestinal resection and anastomosis.

Gastric Dilation and Volvulus
Definition

Gastric dilation and volvulus (GDV) is the swelling (specifically gaseous distension) and rotation of the stomach on its mesenteric axis. *Dilation* is the stretching of an organ beyond its normal

BOX 10.6 Surgery Report: Intestinal Resection and Anastomosis

Animal Hospital Name

Owner: John Doe

Address: 555 Sterling Lane

Jupiter, NY 55555

Phone number: 555-5555

Animal Name: Sasha

Animal #: 65656501

Species: Canine

Breed: Labrador

DOB: 05/05/10

Date of Surgery: 01/03/2011

Primary Surgeon: Dr. Vet

Assistant: Technician Scrub

Diagnosis or Preoperative Signs: Intestinal foreign body.

Surgical Procedure: Intestinal resection and anastomosis, exploratory laparotomy.

Description of Surgical Procedure

Surgical Approach: A 20-cm ventral midline incision was made through the skin from the xiphoid process to the pubis. The incision was carried through the underlying subcutaneous tissues and linea alba.

Surgical Pathology: A purulent and serosanguinous discharge oozed out of the tissues when the incision was made. Approximately 200 mL of serosanguinous fluid was removed from the abdominal cavity. The mesentery and omentum were grossly inflamed. A foreign body was located midjejunum. The region of intestines where the foreign body was located was inflamed and thickened. Perforations were evident at the mesenteric border of the jejunum. The rest of the bowel and the abdomen were unremarkable.

Surgical Procedure: The abdomen was explored and the entire length of bowel examined. The affected portion of the jejunum was exteriorized and the abdominal cavity packed off with lap sponges. Approximately 5 cm of grossly normal jejunum was resected proximal and distal to the abnormal segment. First, the appropriate jejunal mesenteric vessels were double-ligated with 3-0 PDS and divided between the ligations. Intestinal contents were milked away from the surgical site. Crushing forceps was placed across the small intestines about 2 cm from the proposed site of transection of the intestine. The intestine was transected between each set of crushing and Doyen forceps with a scalpel. The mesentery attached to the resected portion of the bowel was incised, and the abnormal jejunum was completely removed from the surgical site. The bowel edges were apposed with 4-0 PDS in a simple interrupted suture pattern, beginning first at the mesenteric border and taking bites through the submucosal layer. The mesentery was apposed with 4-0 PDS in a simple continuous suture pattern. The abdomen was thoroughly lavaged with sterile saline. Aerobic and anaerobic cultures were collected of the abdomen. A closed suction drain was placed through the skin and into the cranial abdomen. The external portion was attached to the skin with 3-0 nylon. The abdomen was closed routinely.

Closure:

Linea alba: 0 PDS in simple interrupted suture pattern.

Subcutaneous tissues: 2-0 PDS in simple continuous suture pattern.

Subcuticular layer: 3-0 Monocryl in simple continuous pattern.

Skin: 3-0 nylon in simple interrupted suture pattern.

BOX 10.7 General Treatment of Gastric Dilation and Volvulus

1. Decompression of the stomach.
2. Correction of fluid and electrolyte imbalances, correction of arrhythmias, and treatment for shock in most cases.
3. Correction of the malpositioned stomach and partial gastrectomy of devitalized tissue if warranted.
4. Gastropexy procedure, which involves surgically attaching the stomach to the body wall to prevent future gastric dilation and volvulus (does not prevent future bloat).

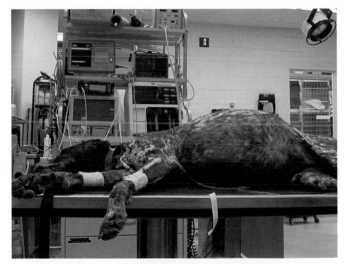

Fig. 10.23 Nine-year-old German shorthair pointer with gastric dilation and volvulus. Note the severely distended abdomen that protrudes past the rib cage.

dimensions. Volvulus refers to the rotation of an organ. A small animal patient can have gastric dilation without the volvulus, commonly referred to as a *simple gastric dilation*. The generic term *bloat* does not distinguish between a simple gastric dilation and gastric dilation with a volvulus.

Indications

GDV is considered a true surgical emergency. Box 10.7 summarizes the common treatment for GDV.

GDV usually occurs in deep-chested, large-breed animals but is sometimes seen in smaller breeds and rarely in cats. GDV may occur at any age but is generally noted in middle-aged to older dogs. The precise etiology of GDV is unknown, but many cases occur after ingestion of a large meal followed by strenuous exercise. Diet, amount of food ingested, frequency of feeding, feeding behavior, and exercise after a meal may all be contributing factors to the development of GDV. Other contributing factors include anatomic predisposition, ileus, trauma, primary gastric motility disorders, vomiting, and stress. The classic clinical sign of GDV is severe abdominal distension, extending past the rib cage (Fig. 10.23). Other signs include restlessness, hypersalivation, abdominal pain, nonproductive attempts to vomit (retching, dry heaving), and signs of shock.

The first step in the correction of GDV is to stabilize the patient and reverse shock. Compression of vessels by the distended abdomen decreases venous return to the heart (effectively reducing vascular volume) and cardiac output, leading to shock; if left untreated, these animals will die from cardiac collapse. Two large-bore IV catheters should be placed in either the cephalic or jugular veins. Venous return is compromised in the caudal half of the animal so catheter placement in the pelvic limbs will not be useful. IV fluids should be administered if shock is present. Oxygen should be available and should be administered if respiratory distress is evident.

The second step in the correction of GDV is to decompress the stomach to allow gas to escape. The gas is most likely associated with one of the following: **aerophagia** (habitual swallowing of air), bacterial fermentation (with associated carbon dioxide production), or metabolic reactions. The gastric gas is unable to escape through normal physiologic means, such as vomiting or eructation, because the esophageal and pyloric sphincters are often twisted or rotated closed. The technician needs to choose an appropriately sized orogastric tube in correlation with the animal's size. The tube should be measured from the point of the nose to the xiphoid process (Fig. 10.24). Tape can be applied to the tube to mark the appropriate length. A roll of tape placed between the upper and lower canine teeth can be used as a mouth gag to hold the patient's mouth open for placement of the stomach tube (Fig. 10.25). Lubricant is applied to the end of the tube for easier passage. The tube is placed through the hole of the tape roll and down the esophagus (Fig. 10.26). Sedation may be required to help keep the animal relaxed and manageable. Damage to the esophagus can occur if the tube is aggressively forced down the esophagus.

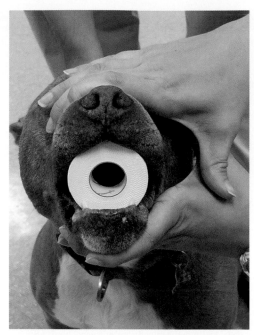

Fig. 10.25 A roll of tape (pictured) or a mouth gag can be used to hold the mouth open while a stomach tube is passed. The assistant should hold the mouth gag in place by holding the mouth shut around the gag.

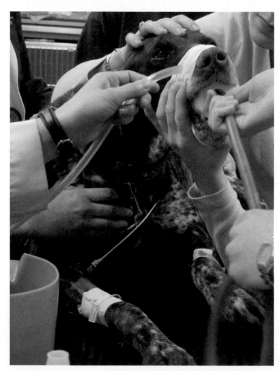

Fig. 10.26 Placement of orogastric tube in a German shorthair pointer with gastric dilation and volvulus. Note the roll of tape between the upper and lower jaws for easier placement of the tube.

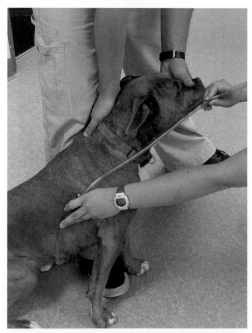

Fig. 10.24 Before a stomach tube is passed, the length of tube to be passed is marked by measuring from the nose to the last rib.

Once air has been removed from the stomach, the stomach should be lavaged with warm water to help remove any gastric contents. If attempts to pass the stomach tube are unsuccessful, **percutaneous** decompression with a **trocar** can be attempted. The small area of the body wall over the distended stomach is clipped and prepped and a 14-, 16-, or 18-gauge needle or catheter can be inserted through the body wall and into the stomach. This allows the evacuation of gas and relieves pressure on the vessels.

When gastric lavage is complete, it is imperative to pinch the gastric tube before removing it; failure to do so can result in leakage from the tube and aspiration of stomach contents by the patient.

The patient should be taken to surgery to correct the position of the stomach as soon as stabilization has been accomplished. The volvulus of the stomach hinders gastric blood flow and can lead to necrosis of the stomach tissue. Timely treatment of GDV can produce survival rates approaching 85%.

Special Instruments

A general use soft tissue surgical pack should be sufficient for GDV surgery. A Balfour abdominal retractor, Army-Navy retractors, and extra towel clamps should be available. An appropriately sized orogastric tube should be available for intraoperative decompression of the stomach. Sterile laparotomy sponges should be available. Heated lavage fluid and suction may also be indicated.

Patient Positioning

The patient is placed in dorsal recumbency and the entire abdomen should be clipped to allow a full abdominal exploratory surgery. The lateral aspects of the abdomen should be clipped as well, in case placement of a gastric feeding tube is warranted.

Procedure for Treatment of Gastric Dilation and Volvulus

Upon entry into the abdominal cavity, the first structure noted is the greater omentum, which usually covers the dilated stomach during a GDV. Blood may be evident in the abdomen, usually due to rupture of the short gastric vessels, which have been stretched during the GDV. An orogastric tube should again be passed through the mouth, down the esophagus, and into the stomach to allow decompression of gas and the release of gastric contents. A warm gastric lavage should be performed until the contents from the stomach are emptied and the lavage water collected is clear.

The surgeon then attempts to rotate the stomach back to its original position. Most stomachs twist or rotate in a clockwise direction and can rotate 90 to 360 degrees (Fig. 10.27). Correction of the malpositioned stomach usually involves rotation in a counterclockwise direction. The stomach should be explored for necrosis. If necrosis is evident, a partial **gastrectomy** may need to be performed. A full exploratory laparotomy should be conducted to be sure no damage has occurred to other abdominal organs. Due to the proximity of the spleen and stomach, the spleen often follows the path of the stomach, and a splenic torsion may be apparent. The spleen should be observed for damage, and a **splenectomy** performed, if warranted. A gastropexy procedure must be done to prevent future GDV.

Permanent Gastropexy Procedures

A **gastropexy**, often termed a pexy, permanently affixes the stomach to the body wall and prevents recurrence of GDV. Many educated owners of large-breed dogs may decide to have an

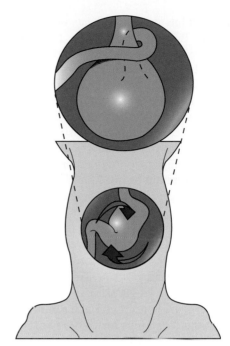

Fig. 10.27 The stomach of a dog with gastric dilation and volvulus generally rotates in a clockwise direction. (From Fossum TW, Hedlund CS, Hulse DA, et al: Small animal surgery, ed 4, St Louis, 2013, Mosby.)

elective gastropexy performed on their pets. This procedure can be done, for example, when a large-breed pet is admitted for an elective ovariohysterectomy (OHE). If available, a less invasive gastropexy procedure can be performed laparoscopically. A variety of pexy procedures can be performed, although they vary on rates of dependability as well as frequency of surgical complications. The goal of all these procedures is to create a permanent adhesion between the gastric serosa and the peritoneal surface of the abdominal wall. For a permanent adhesion to form, the gastric muscle must be in contact with the body wall muscle. Gastropexy procedures include the following types:
- Tube gastropexy
- Circumcostal gastropexy
- Muscular flap gastropexy
- Belt-loop gastropexy
- Incisional gastropexy

Incisional gastropexy is a general term and is not necessarily specific to any of the techniques referenced.

Abdominal Wall Closure

After the gastropexy, the abdomen should be reevaluated. If all or a portion of the spleen appears nonviable, it should be removed. The abdomen should be flushed and then closed routinely.

Postoperative Considerations and Instructions

Dogs can have many complications after GDV repair. Cardiac arrhythmias are common and can continue for 2 to 3 days postoperatively. The arrhythmias are usually ventricular in origin. Treatment of the arrhythmias involves correction of electrolyte imbalances and maintenance of a normal hydration state. If the arrhythmias are more severe and interfere with cardiac output or the animal exhibits premature beats or a sustained cardiac rate greater than 160 beats per minute, IV drug intervention may be necessary. Lidocaine may be administered by constant-rate infusion. The animal should be monitored for muscle tremors, vomiting, and seizures, which are signs of lidocaine toxicity. If side effects are noted, another antiarrhythmic, such as procainamide or sotalol, should be used.

Gastritis may occur secondary to gastric mucosal ischemia. Vomiting should be monitored and can be treated with antiemetics. If no vomiting is reported, water can be offered 1 day after surgery, and food can be introduced in small quantities 24 to 48 hours after surgery. Fluid therapy should be maintained until oral intake is adequate.

Devitalized stomach tissue must be resected to avoid possible septic peritonitis. Gastric viability at surgery is subjective, and postoperative necrosis and perforation can occur postoperatively despite careful assessment. Timely correction of GDV is imperative for a good prognosis. The prognosis may be considered guarded if gastric necrosis was evident. Box 10.8 shows an example of a surgery report for GDV repair.

REPRODUCTIVE PROCEDURES

Ovariohysterectomy

Definition

Ovariohysterectomy (OHE), also called spay or neuter, refers to the surgical excision of the ovaries and uterus.

Indications

The primary indication for OHE is an elective procedure to sterilize the animal. Other indications are as follows:

- Neoplasia of reproductive tract (ovaries, uterine horn, uterine body)
- Treatment of neoplasia elsewhere in the body influenced by reproductive hormones (e.g., mammary tumors)
- Trauma or injury to reproductive tract
- Dystocia (difficult birth)
- Uterine torsion
- Abolition of heat cycle
- Stabilization of other systemic diseases (e.g., diabetes)
- Congenital abnormalities

The OHE is one of the most common surgical procedures performed in small animal practice. Clients may inquire about OHEs more than any other surgical procedure. The veterinary technician should be able to communicate to clients the advantages and disadvantages of having their pets spayed or neutered. Clients may have preconceived notions about spaying their pets, and the technician may be responsible for explaining to the client the importance of OHE and correcting any misconceptions. It is currently recommended that cats should be spayed by 5 months of age to control the excess feline population. The age at which canine OHE is performed is currently controversial and is based on risk factors and benefits to the patient. Clients should be encouraged to discuss the age of spaying (and neutering) of their dog with the veterinarian.

BOX 10.8   Surgery Report: Gastric Dilation and Volvulus

Animal Hospital Name

Owner: John Doe
Address: 555 Sterling Lane
Jupiter, NY 55555
Phone number: 555-5555
Animal Name: Sasha
Animal #: 65656501
Species: Canine
Breed: Labrador
DOB: 01/05/08
Date of Surgery: 12/03/2011
Primary Surgeon: Dr. Vet
Assistant: Technician Scrub
Diagnosis or Preoperative Signs: One-day history of retching, abdominal distension; gastric dilation and volvulus.
Surgical Procedure: Gastric dilation and volvulus (GDV) correction and incisional gastropexy.

Description of Surgical Procedure

Surgical Approach: The patient was placed in dorsal recumbency. A skin incision approximately 25 cm long was made from the xiphoid process to the pubis. The incision was continued through the fascia and linea alba, and the abdomen was entered. A large amount of falciform fat was resected.

Surgical Pathology: The stomach was rotated 270 degrees, grossly distended, and hypermotile. The pylorus was located ventrally and to the left of the fundus.

There was no evidence of devitalized tissues. There was minimal hemorrhage in the abdomen.

Surgical Procedure: Moist laparotomy sponges were placed along the incision, and a Balfour retractor was placed. On entering the abdomen, the omentum was seen covering a gas-distended stomach that was rotated 270 degrees clockwise. The stomach was decompressed with an 18-gauge needle and suction. The stomach was then repositioned by pulling up on the pylorus to rotate the stomach counterclockwise back to its correct anatomic position. A stomach tube was passed and revealed a moderate amount of brown, malodorous fluid. The stomach was lavaged with warm water until the fluid leaving the stomach was clear. The entire surface of the stomach was inspected and appeared healthy. The abdomen was explored routinely. Next, an incisional gastropexy was performed; an incision was made into the seromuscular layer of the stomach in the region of the pyloric antrum. A second incision was made into the right ventrolateral abdominal wall, exposing the abdominal muscles. The edges of the gastric incision were sutured to the abdominal wall incision using two suture lines and a simple continuous pattern. The abdomen was lavaged with 2 L of sterile saline, and the body wall was closed routinely.

Closure:
Incisional gastropexy: 2-0 PDS in two lines of simple continuous patterns.
Linea alba: 0 PDS in simple continuous pattern.
Subcutaneous tissue: 2-0 PDS in simple continuous pattern.
Subcuticular tissue: 2-0 Monocryl in continuous suture pattern.
Skin: Skin staples.

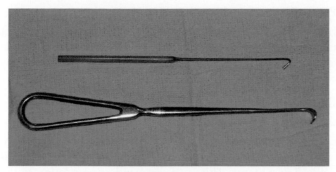

Fig. 10.28 Spay hooks.

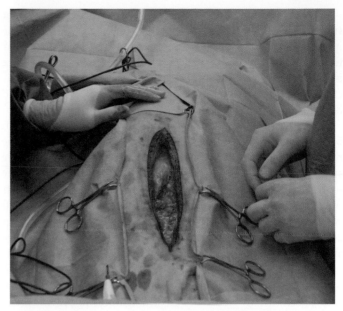

Fig. 10.30 Abdominal incision through the subcutaneous tissue and linea alba.

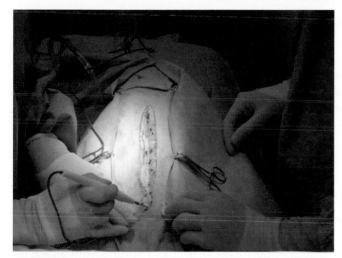

Fig. 10.29 Abdominal skin incision. Electrocautery is used for hemostasis of small vessels.

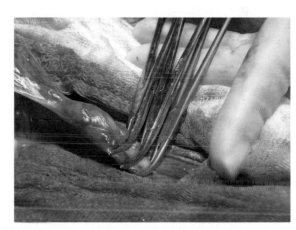

Fig. 10.31 Three-clamp technique of uterine horn. Note ovary caudal to hemostats.

Special Instruments

Surgeons may or may not use a spay hook (Snook hook) for OHE. The hook is used to exteriorize the uterine horn, allowing the surgeon to make a smaller abdominal incision if desired. Spay hooks come in an assortment of sizes; the technician should pick the size appropriate for the animal (Fig. 10.28).

Patient Positioning

Most patients are positioned in dorsal recumbency for OHE. This positioning is best suited for a ventral midline incision. Some surgeons may prefer a lateral (flank) approach to the abdomen for an OHE, which requires positioning the patient in lateral recumbency. The ventral abdomen should be clipped and aseptically prepared from the xiphoid process to the pubis.

Canine and Feline Ovariohysterectomy Procedures

In dogs the start of the incision can be made 3 to 6 cm caudal to the umbilicus. In cats the incision should be started 3 to 4 cm caudally. An incision should be made through the skin (Fig. 10.29) and the subcutaneous tissue and linea alba (Fig. 10.30). The length of the incision is the surgeon's preference.

The left abdominal wall is raised, and the spay hook is slid down against the abdominal wall, with the hook facing laterally. The hook should be turned 180 degrees to trap the uterine horn, and the hook and uterine horn are then elevated from the abdomen. In dogs, the suspensory ligament should be torn or stretched without tearing the ovarian vessels; this maneuver allows exteriorization of the ovary. Tearing the suspensory ligament is generally not necessary to exteriorize a cat's ovary. Plucking of the ligament is the most painful portion of the procedure, and the patient's heart rate and respiratory rate generally increase at this time. Once the pedicle has been ligated, the heart rate and respiratory rate should return to normal anesthetized levels. The method of ligation and transection of the pedicle is the surgeon's preference. Surgeons may decide to use clips, the two-clamp method, or the three-clamp method (Fig. 10.31). Carmalt, Kelly, or Crile forceps may be used for clamping the pedicles. The forceps used depends on the size of the pedicle. Two clamps should be placed across the ovarian pedicle, proximal (deep) to the ovary, and one clamp across the ovarian ligament to allow handling of the uterine horn and ligation of the pedicle.

The technician should be knowledgeable about what type of suture the surgeon will be using and have it ready for use on the instrument table before it is needed. An absorbable suture material is usually used for pedicle ligation. The size of the suture is the surgeon's preference and depends on the size of the pedicle and the patient. If clips are being used, the technician should have the clip applicator loaded and accessible for the surgeon.

The surgeon then places a ligature proximal to the ovarian pedicle clamp and securely ties the ligature. One clamp may be removed or flashed (unclamped and then reclamped) while the surgeon tightens the ligature. Flashing is done to compress the pedicle and secure the ligature so that it is less likely to slide off once the pedicle is transected. If the ligature is not secure and slides off the pedicle, the pedicle will bleed, and the patient could lose a significant amount of blood and die. If the ligature slides off, the pedicle must be isolated (this may require extending the incision more cranially) and the ligature replaced. A second ligature is placed proximal to the first (therefore flashing is not necessary to secure the second ligature) to provide additional security in preventing hemorrhage. The pedicle can then be transected at the level of the third clamp, between the clamp and the ovary. The procedure is then repeated on the opposite uterine horn and ovary.

The body of the uterus should then be exteriorized. Breaking down the broad ligament is usually done to allow the uterus to be fully exteriorized. A two-clamp or three-clamp method can be used. The clamps are placed onto the uterine body, proximal to the cervix. A ligature is placed distal (caudal) to the clamps, toward the cervix (Fig. 10.32). A second suture is then placed distal (caudal) to the first. The surgeon then transects the uterine body with the scalpel blade, between the clamp and the ligatures. The uterine stump should be checked for hemorrhage prior to replacement into the abdomen. Excessive bleeding can occur if the ovarian pedicle and the uterine stumps are not properly ligated. The abdominal cavity should be carefully inspected for hemorrhage before closure.

Abdominal Wall Closure

The abdomen may be flushed in a nonelective OHE. Routine closure of the abdominal wall is common in OHE procedures.

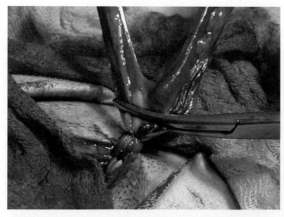

Fig. 10.32 Double ligation of the uterine body, cranial to cervix.

Postoperative Considerations and Instructions

Intraabdominal hemorrhage can occur postoperatively; if not treated, it can be fatal. If ligation of a bleeding stump is attempted without proper visualization, renal dysfunction may occur secondary to ureteral ligation.

Cesarean Section
Definition

Cesarean section, also referred to as cesarotomy or hysterotomy, is delivery of a fetus or fetuses by incision through the abdominal wall and uterus. The word *cesarean* has no relation to the birth of Julius Caesar, as some believe; it takes its name from the Latin word *caedere,* to cut.

Indications

The primary indication for a cesarean section is *dystocia* (difficult birth). Dystocia can develop from issues with the dam or the fetus. Problems with the dam that cause dystocia are
- small pelvic canal size of dam,
- previous pelvic trauma of dam,
- insufficient dilation, and
- uterine inertia (lack of contractility of uterus; can result from overstretching of uterus, toxemia, obesity, or exhaustion). Problems with the fetus that cause dystocia are
- maldeveloped fetuses,
- oversized fetuses, and
- malpositioned fetuses.

The objective of a cesarean section is to remove all the fetuses from the uterus as swiftly as possible. Although it may be performed as an intervention in an emergency, cesarean section is often planned for brachycephalic breeds (e.g., boxers, bulldogs, Pekingese, pugs) or animals with a history of dystocia and/or previous cesarean section.

Special Instruments

A general use soft tissue surgery pack should provide the surgeon with the necessary instruments needed for a cesarean section. Extra hemostats should be available. Extra personnel will also be needed to help warm and resuscitate the puppies or kittens.

Patient Positioning

The animal should be rapidly anesthetized in the surgery room, and a final surgical prep should be performed while the surgeon and scrub assistant are preparing for surgery.

Cesarean Section Procedure

See Box 10.9 for an overview of three different methods of performing a cesarean section.

Neonatal Care

The care of the neonates generally is the responsibility of the assistant or technician. This job can be extremely rewarding, especially if the neonates are resuscitated successfully and can leave the hospital with their mother. If the neonates are transferred still in the uterus (en bloc OHE, which is OHE with cesarean section), the technician needs to incise the uterus by

---

BOX 10.9   Cesarean Section Procedures

Cesarean Without an Ovariohysterectomy

The owner may elect not to spay the animal. The veterinarian should inform the owner of the possibility of future dystocia in this pet. In addition, the client should be made aware that the surgeon may open the abdomen, inspect the uterus, and discover that it has deteriorated to such an extent that leaving it in the abdomen is no longer an option.

Cesarean Followed by an Ovariohysterectomy

An indication to perform this procedure may be to prevent the animal from having dystocia in the future.

En Bloc Resection (radical resection of the uterus and ovaries; neonates removed after resection of uterus)

En bloc removal of the uterus may be optional or essential because of possible fetal compromise or uterine viability.

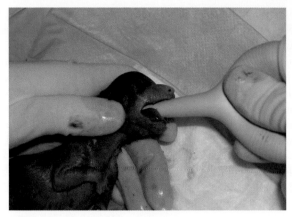

Fig. 10.34 Aspiration of fluid from the oropharynx using an infant suction bulb.

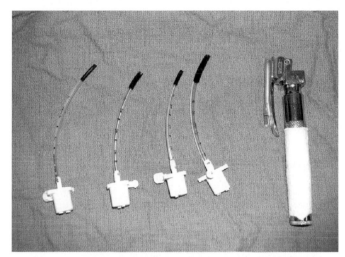

Fig. 10.35 Various neonatal endotracheal tubes and pediatric laryngoscope.

tenting the uterus and using Metzenbaum scissors. Extreme caution must be used when incising the uterus so as not to injure the neonates. The amniotic sac of each neonate needs to be broken as the neonates are removed from the uterus.

The technician should have a warm, dry area prepared for the neonates prior to surgery. The area should include some or all of the following: plenty of clean, warm towels; a radiant lamp; a hair dryer; and circulating warm-water heating pads. Drugs that should be available include naloxone (opioid antagonist), doxapram (respiratory stimulant), and epinephrine (adrenergic agonist). Suture and scissors should also be available to ligate the umbilical cords. The neonates should be dried off immediately with warm towels (Fig. 10.33). A heating unit should be used to aid in the warming process, since the dam will be unavailable to aid in warming the neonates. The neonates should be briskly rubbed to initiate spontaneous respiration.

The technician also must ensure that the clamp on the umbilicus is secure and there is no unnecessary pulling on the umbilicus. Strain on the umbilical cord can cause abdominal herniation from the umbilical site. An infant suction bulb can be used to help aspirate fluid from the oropharynx and nares (Fig. 10.34). If an opioid was used as a premedication for the

dam, a drop of naloxone can be placed under the tongue of each neonate to reverse the effect of the opioid on the neonates. If respiratory efforts of the neonate are slow to commence, a drop of doxapram placed under the tongue can be used to aid in respiratory stimulation. If the newborn has an appropriate heart rate (120–150 beats/min) but is still having respiratory-related issues, tactile stimulation and administration of oxygen by mask may aid in instituting respiration. If respiratory efforts do not commence within about 30 seconds, or if bradycardia occurs, the technician may need to administer positive pressure ventilation by mask. The newborn may need to be intubated and ventilated until it starts to take breaths on its own (Fig. 10.35).

Once respiration has been achieved, cardiovascular stability must be addressed, especially if the patient is bradycardic or has a weak heartbeat. If no heartbeat can be identified, chest compressions should be administered by fingers across the lateral chest wall at a rate of 1 to 2 compressions/second. If chest compressions appear unsuccessful, epinephrine can be administered under the tongue.

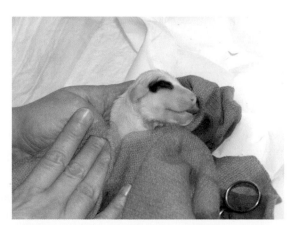

Fig. 10.33 Initiation of tactile stimulation for a neonate.

Some neonates never achieve respiration or a heartbeat once retrieved from the uterus, but every attempt should be made to revive them. A newborn's survival can depend on each individual situation. How long the fetus was wedged in the canal or how long the dam was in labor can determine the outcome. Whimpering and crying sounds from the newborns are always a good sign.

Once the newborn has been stabilized with an adequate respiratory rate and an adequate heart rate, the umbilical cord can be ligated and transected (distal to the ligation) approximately 1 to 2 cm from the body (Fig. 10.36). The newborns should be kept in a warm environment (about 90°F) until the mother's surgery is complete; oxygen supplementation may be a necessary part of a successful resuscitation (Fig. 10.37).

Postoperative Considerations and Instructions

The mammary glands of the dam should be cleaned after surgery to remove any surgical prep solutions and blood. The newborns should be reunited with their mother, and nursing should commence as soon as possible. The mother's behavior toward the newborns should be observed during the first few hours. Care should be taken not to return the newborns to their mother too soon. She could inadvertently injure them if she is still dysphoric from anesthesia. Some mothers may reject or kill their young, so careful observation is important.

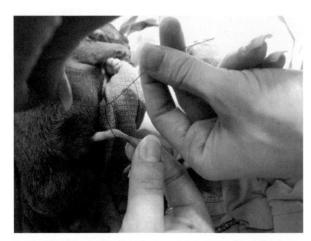

Fig. 10.36 Ligation of the umbilical cord 1 to 2 cm from the body wall.

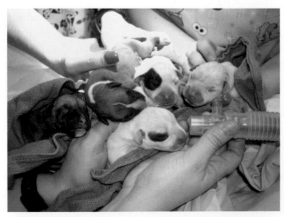

Fig. 10.37 Successful resuscitation of five puppies.

BOX 10.10	Surgery Report: Cesarean Section

Animal Hospital Name
Owner: John Doe
Address: 555 Sterling Lane
Jupiter, NY 55555
Phone number: 555-5555
Animal Name: Sasha
Animal #: 65656501
Species: Canine
Breed: Labrador
DOB: 05/05/09
Date of Surgery: 1/05/2011
Primary Surgeon: Dr. Vet
Assistant: Technician Scrub
Diagnosis or Preoperative Signs: Dystocia.
Surgical Procedure: Cesarean section.

Description of Surgical Procedure
Surgical Approach: A ventral midline skin incision was made cranial to the umbilicus and extended caudally 10 cm.
   Surgical Pathology: Three neonates were removed from the uterus.
   Surgical Procedure: An incision was made through the subcutaneous tissue and linea alba into the peritoneal cavity. The fetus-distended uterus was identified, exteriorized, and packed off with moistened lap sponges. A 5-cm longitudinal incision was made into the ventral aspect of the uterine body, and three puppies were milked out one by one. A hemostat was placed on the umbilical cords, and the umbilical cords were transected. The puppies were handed to the assistants. The remaining placenta was grasped with forceps and removed from the uterine body. The uterus was closed, and the abdomen was lavaged with sterile saline before closure of the peritoneal cavity. Hemostasis was maintained throughout the surgery with the aid of monopolar cautery.
   Closure:
   Uterine body: 3-0 PDS in two continuous layers.
   Linea alba: 2-0 PDS using simple interrupted suture pattern.
   Subcutaneous tissue and subcuticular layer: Each closed with 2-0 PDS using simple continuous suture pattern.
   Skin: Tissue adhesive was applied to the skin.

To reduce stress and exposure to pathogens and **nosocomial infections**, the bitch and the newborns should be released from the hospital as soon as possible. The incision should be closely monitored due to the nursing newborns and the enlarged mammary glands.

Box 10.10 shows an example of a surgery report for a cesarean section.

PYOMETRA

Definition

Pyometra is the accumulation of purulent material (pus) in the uterus. The condition is more prevalent in dogs than cats but can be seen in both species. The condition can be referred to as either open or closed, depending on the cervix. In an open pyometra, the cervix is open, allowing the purulent discharge to drain. With an open pyometra, the purulent discharge will be visible in the vulva and/or externally. Both types are considered serious; as the purulent material accumulates, uterine rupture can occur.

Indication

An OHE is the standard of care for treatment of pyometra. Owners may wish to elect medical management of the condition if the animal is a valuable breeder. This should be discouraged because it is associated with severe complications. The adage "Never let the sun set on a pyometra" has its merits. A pyometra can rupture at any point, releasing all the purulent material into the abdominal cavity and leading to septicemia or endotoxemia. In addition, the rate of recurrence of pyometra after medical therapy is as high as 77%.

They typical signalment of a patient with pyometra is intact females, 6 years of age or older. It is possible for a condition known as *stump pyometra* to develop in a previously spayed female if ovarian tissue was left behind during the original procedure. The remnants of the uterus left near the cervix can become infected. Clinical signs are seen within 4 to 8 weeks after the last estrus (heat) and can include decreased appetite, lethargy, increased thirst and urination, and in some but not all cases, foul-smelling vaginal discharge. A fluid-filled uterus may be detected on abdominal radiographs or ultrasound examination (Fig. 10.38). Additionally, an elevated white blood count is commonly seen on the patient's complete blood count (CBC) results.

Pyometra Surgery

A routine OHE is performed (see previous discussion). Care must be taken because the uterus is typically engorged and friable (Fig. 10.39). The surgeon may require an assistant to scrub in to help lift and remove the uterus.

Postoperative Considerations and Instructions

The animal should be monitored postoperatively as it would be for an OHE. IV antibiotics are typically given until the animal is considered stable. Oral antibiotics should continue for 7 to 10 days postoperatively at the veterinarian's discretion. Antibiotic choice may be based on a culture and sensitivity of the purulent material from the uterus.

Canine and Feline Castration

Castration may also be referred to as a *neuter*, *alter*, or orchiectomy.

Routine Canine Castration

Definition. *Canine castration* refers to the surgical removal of the testicles in the dog.

Indications. The primary indication for performing a canine castration is for sterilization of the dog; this is considered an elective castration. Other indications include the following:

- Prevention of roaming
- Prevention of aggressive behavior or fighting
- Prevention of urine marking
- Correction of congenital abnormalities
- Treatment of scrotal or testicular neoplasia
- Treatment of scrotal abscess, infection, or trauma
- Treatment of hormone-related disease elsewhere in the body (e.g., prostatic disease, perineal hernias, perianal tumors)

Instrumentation. A general use soft tissue surgical instrument pack should be adequate for canine castration.

Patient positioning. The canine patient should be placed in dorsal recumbency for castration. The scrotum should be examined and palpated for the presence of both testicles before

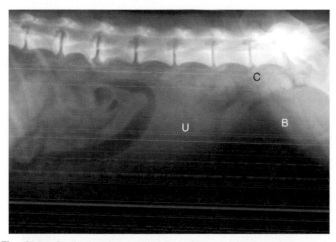

Fig. 10.38 Radiographic examination of dog with pyometra showing enlarged, fluid-filled uterus (U) in caudal ventral abdomen. Note relationship to colon (C) and bladder (B). (Radiography by Jeanne Barsanti DVM, MS, DACVIM © 2004 University of Georgia Research Foundation, Inc)

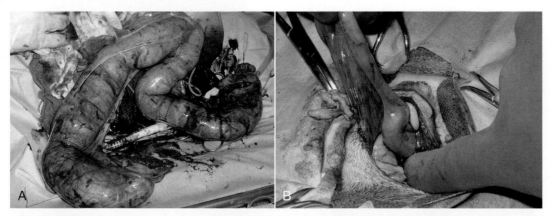

Fig. 10.39 The uterus must be carefully handled in cases of pyometra because it is often large, friable, and heavy. Compare the pyometra uterus in (A) with the normal uterus in (B). (From Bassert JM, Thomas, JA, editors: McCurnin's clinical textbook for veterinary technicians, ed 8, St Louis, 2014, Elsevier.)

anesthesia is induced. If both testicles are present, a routine castration can be performed. If only one testicle is present, the dog is considered **cryptorchid** and may require an inguinal or abdominal surgery to remove the other testicle.

For a routine castration the surgical site should be clipped from just below the tip of the prepuce to just above the scrotum. The clipped region should extend laterally into the inguinal section on both sides. The scrotum should not be clipped. The skin of the scrotum is delicate and sensitive and may be susceptible to clipper burns or tears. Irritation of the scrotum can cause the animal to lick or bite at the affected region postoperatively. The surgical site should be aseptically prepared.

Canine castration procedure. The surgeon may decide to do an open castration or closed castration. In the closed procedure, the tunics are not incised and the entire spermatic cord encased in its parietal vaginal tunic is ligated and transected. In the open procedure, the tunics are incised and the contents of the cord are ligated and transected separately.

Open castration. The surgeon selects the first testicle and applies pressure cranially to advance the testicle into the prescrotal region. The skin and subcutaneous tissues and spermatic fascia are incised (Fig. 10.40). The surgeon then incises the parietal vaginal tunic (Fig. 10.41), and the testicle is gently extruded (Fig. 10.42). A hemostat should be placed across the tunic at the attachment of the epididymis. The ligament of the tail of the epididymis is separated from the tunic. Three clamps can be placed across the spermatic cord (Fig. 10.43). The vascular cord and the ductus deferens are recognized and can be individually ligated using an absorbable suture. The surgeon may decide to ligate the vascular cord and ductus deferens together. A circumferential ligature is then placed around both the ductus deferens and the vascular cord. A hemostat is placed on the cord close to the testicle. The cord is then transected between the hemostat and ligatures (Fig. 10.44). The cord is examined for bleeding and returned within the tunic. If bleeding is noted, another ligature is placed on the spermatic cord. The second testicle can be removed in the same manner.

Closed castration. Closed castration is performed much like open castration except for the incision of the parietal vaginal tunics. Once the skin, subcutaneous tissue, and spermatic fascia are incised, the spermatic cord is exteriorized. Ligatures are placed around the entire spermatic cord and tunics, and the cord is then transected.

Closure of incision. Closure of the orchiectomy incision is usually in two layers. The subcutaneous tissues are typically closed in a simple continuous pattern with absorbable suture.

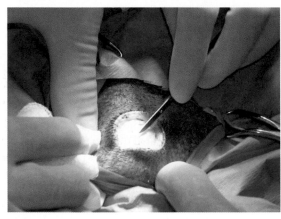

Fig. 10.40 A skin incision is made in the prescrotal region for canine castration.

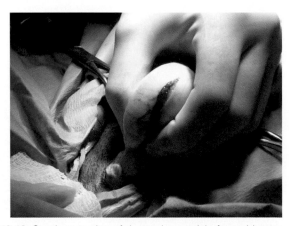

Fig. 10.42 Gentle extrusion of the canine testicle for orchiectomy.

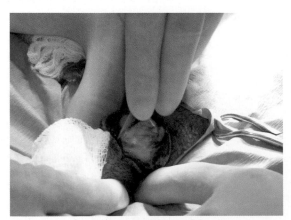

Fig. 10.41 Incision into the parietal vaginal tunic of the canine scrotum for orchiectomy.

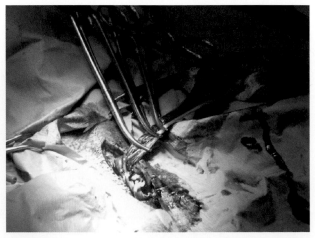

Fig. 10.43 Three hemostats are used to clamp the spermatic cord in canine castration.

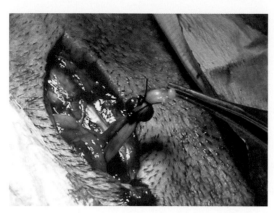

Fig. 10.44 Ligation and transection of the ductus deferens and vascular cord in canine castration. The cord is checked for hemorrhage before closing.

The skin may be closed in a simple interrupted pattern with nonabsorbable suture, or a continuous intradermal pattern can also be performed for skin closure.

Postoperative considerations and instructions. Common complications associated with canine castration include hemorrhage and scrotal hematoma. A scrotal hematoma may be the result of a hemorrhaging vessel (or vessels). Care should be taken during the surgery to provide appropriate hemostasis to avoid such complications. Cold compresses can be placed to aid in hemostasis postoperatively if hemorrhage has occurred. A complete scrotal **ablation** (removal of scrotum) may be necessary if hemostasis was unsuccessful. Other complications include self-inflicted trauma to the incision and infection or dehiscence of the incision site.

Box 10.11 shows an example of a surgery report for a canine castration.

Routine Feline Castration

Definition. Feline castration refers to the surgical removal of the testicles in the cat.

Indications. The primary indication to perform a castration is for sterilization of the male cat. Other indications include the following:

- Prevention of roaming
- Prevention of aggressive behavior or fighting
- Prevention of urine spraying or marking
- Correction of congenital abnormalities
- Treatment of scrotal neoplasia
- Treatment of scrotal abscess, infection, or trauma
- Treatment of endocrine abnormalities
- Treatment of hormone-related disease elsewhere in the body (e.g., prostatic disease, perineal hernias)

Instrumentation. No special instrumentation is required to perform a feline castration, but a 10 or 15 blade is necessary for incision into the scrotum. The surgeon may prefer to use metal clips or suture to ligate the spermatic cord.

Feline castration procedure. An examination of the testicles should be conducted before anesthesia is induced to ensure that both testicles have descended into the scrotum. The male cat should be positioned according to the surgeon's instructions (lateral or dorsal recumbency). The testicles should be prepared

| BOX 10.11 | **Surgery Report: Canine Castration** |

Animal Hospital Name
Owner: John Doe
Address: 555 Sterling Lane
Jupiter, NY 55555
Phone number: 555-5555
Animal Name: Sasha
Animal #: 65656501
Species: Canine
Breed: Labrador
DOB: 05/05/10
Date of Surgery: 01/03/2011
Primary Surgeon: Dr. Vet
Assistant: Technician Scrub
Diagnosis or Preoperative Signs: Intact male.
Surgical Procedure: Open castration.

Description of Surgical Procedure
Surgical Approach: A 3-cm ventral midline incision was made in the prescrotal region while one testicle was advanced cranially into the incision line. The incision was extended through the subcutaneous tissues.

Surgical Procedure: The right testicle was pushed up through the incision. The vaginal tunic was then incised, and the testicle pushed through. The ligament of the tail of the epididymis was bluntly dissected. The ductus deferens and the vascular cord were individually ligated with 2-0 PDS, then both were ligated together with a circumferential ligature. The testicle was then transected distal to the ligatures. The same procedure was performed on the left testicle.

Closure:
Subcutaneous tissue: 2-0 PDS in simple continuous suture pattern.
Subcuticular tissue: 3-0 Monocryl in simple continuous suture pattern.
Skin: 3-0 nylon in simple interrupted suture pattern.

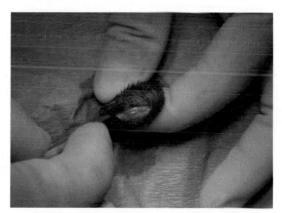

Fig. 10.45 Incision is made through the skin and parietal vaginal tunic of the feline scrotum for orchiectomy.

for surgery by either gently plucking the hair from the scrotum or by clipping the scrotal area. The scrotum should then be prepped and draped with proper aseptic technique. One testicle is held in place while the surgeon makes an incision over it (Fig. 10.45). The parietal vaginal tunic is incised, and the testicle can then be extruded from the scrotum with gentle force with the visceral vaginal tunic intact (Figs. 10.46 and 10.47).

The spermatic cord can be ligated and transected using different techniques. Once the spermatic cord is ligated, the testicle can be transected. The process is repeated on the opposite testicle.

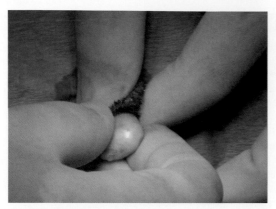

Fig. 10.46 The testicle is extruded from the feline scrotum with gentle force.

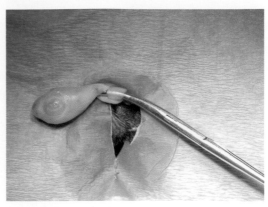

Fig. 10.48 Overhand technique for feline castration. A hemostat is placed on top of the spermatic cord, and the cord is wrapped over and around the hemostat. The cord is grabbed with the hemostat and clamped near the testicle.

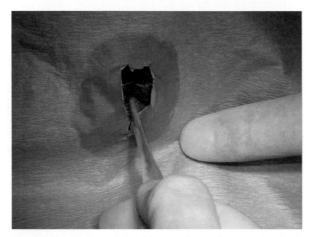

Fig. 10.47 Full extrusion of the feline testicle, allowing visualization of the spermatic cord.

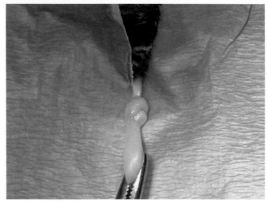

Fig. 10.49 The spermatic cord is pulled through and a knot is made with the cord in the overhand technique for feline castration.

BOX 10.12 Surgery Report: Feline Castration

Animal Hospital Name
Owner: John Doe
Address: 555 Sterling Lane
Jupiter, NY 55555
Phone number: 555-5555
Animal Name: Kitty
Animal #: 65656501
Species: Feline
Breed: Domestic shorthair
DOB: 05/05/10
Date of Surgery: 01/03/2011
Primary Surgeon: Dr. Vet
Assistant: Technician Scrub

Diagnosis or Preoperative Signs: Intact male.
Surgical Procedure: Feline castration.

Description of Surgical Procedure
Surgical Approach: A 1-cm incision was made through the skin on the left and right caudal scrotum to exteriorize each testicle.
   Surgical Pathology: None.
   Surgical Procedure: Applying pressure cranially, the right testicle was exteriorized. An incision was made over the testicle, and the spermatic fascia and parietal vaginal tunic were incised. The ligament of the tail of the epididymis was separated from the tunic using a hemostat. The ductus deferens and the vascular cord were then tied to each other and transected distal to the knot. The same procedure was repeated on the left side.
   Closure: The scrotal incisions were left open to heal by second intention.

Another type of procedure uses the reproductive anatomy to tie knots. In one such procedure the ductus deferens and the spermatic vessels are separated and used to tie square knots. Another such procedure uses an overhand technique (Figs. 10.48 and 10.49). This is done by placing a hemostat on top of the spermatic cord and wrapping the cord over and around the hemostat. The cord is then grabbed by the hemostats and clamped near the testicle. The testicle is transected and the cord pulled through to make a knot on itself.

The scrotum itself is left unsutured, allowing the incisions to heal by second intention. This helps to limit self-mutilation of the scrotum by the patient.

Postoperative considerations and instructions. Scrotal bleeding can be a common complication associated with feline castration. A cold compress can be placed on the scrotum for several minutes to aid in hemostasis. If hemorrhage continues, another surgery may be required to ligate a bleeding vessel. General discharge instructions are listed in Chapter 11. Box 10.12 shows an example of a surgery report for a feline castration.

CYSTOTOMY

Definition

Cystotomy refers to a surgical incision into the bladder to expose the lumen or interior of the urinary bladder.

Indications

A primary indication for performing a cystotomy is to remove cystic calculi. Removal of bladder stones is probably the most common bladder surgery performed in small animal surgery. Uroliths are most noted in middle-aged dogs, although they can occur at any age.

Clinical signs associated with bladder stones include hematuria, stranguria, dysuria, and pollakiuria. Stones may also become wedged in the urethra of male dogs and cause obstructions of the urethra. Radiographs should be performed on patients with suspected cystic calculi. Abdominal radiographs of animals with calculi often reveal radiopaque densities in the urinary system. It is imperative to include the urethra in the radiographs to determine if any calculi are present in the urethra, especially in male dogs. Obstruction of the urethra can lead to a buildup of urine in the bladder and can cause bladder distension. Bladder distension can lead to a rupture if left untreated. Rupture of the bladder can also result from trauma (e.g., being hit by a car) or from improper placement of a urinary catheter or forceful expression of the bladder. Most abdominal procedures require expression of the bladder before transport into surgery. *The bladder of a trauma patient should not be expressed before surgery.* The condition of the bladder may be in question, so attempts to express a traumatized bladder may lead to a bladder rupture. Clinical signs of bladder rupture can include signs of shock (tachycardia, pale mucous membranes), fever, hematuria, anuria, and abdominal pain. Urine in the abdominal cavity can cause uremia and dehydration. A bladder rupture can lead to death if identification of the rupture is delayed. Uroabdomen can be diagnosed by performing an abdominocentesis. Creatinine and urea measurements of the abdominal cavity fluid are compared with blood serum levels. If the levels of creatinine and urea in the abdominal fluid are greater than in the blood serum, a uroabdomen is diagnosed. A contrast cystourethrogram can also be performed to diagnose the exact region of the bladder leakage.

Other indications to perform cystotomy include neoplasia and congenital abnormalities. The most common neoplasia associated with the bladder in dogs and cats is transitional cell carcinoma. In the dog, bladder cancer makes up less than 1% of all canine cancers. The incidence of bladder cancer in cats is much lower.

Table 10.1 lists treatment options and preventive measures for different types of canine urolithiasis. Box 10.13 lists canine predispositions for urinary calculi.

Special Instruments

A general use soft tissue surgery pack will be sufficient for a cystotomy. A bladder spoon should be available (Fig. 10.50). Bladder spoons can aid in the retrieval of cystic calculi, especially those located in the neck of the bladder. A Balfour abdominal retractor should also be available.

Patient Preparation

The patient is placed in dorsal recumbency. The ventral abdomen is clipped and prepped, including the prepuce in a male dog, as a parapreputial incision will be performed.

Cystotomy Procedure

The patient is placed in dorsal recumbency and a ventral midline incision is performed from the umbilicus to the caudal abdomen. The bladder should be isolated and lap sponges positioned beneath the bladder to segregate it from the rest of the abdomen. Stay sutures should be placed at the apex of the bladder to assist in manipulation as well as to prevent spillage of urine into the abdomen (Fig. 10.51). The scrub technician

TABLE 10.1	Treatment and Prevention of Canine Urolithiasis	
Urolith Type	**Treatment Options**	**Preventive Measures**
Struvite	Surgical removal or dissolution Hill's s/d diet Control infection Urease inhibitor? Keep urine pH <6.5, blood urea nitrogen (BUN) <10 mg/dL, and urine specific gravity <1.020	Hill's c/d diet Monitor urine pH and urine sediment; eliminate infections quickly and appropriately
Calcium oxalate	Surgical removal	Hill's u/d diet or Hill's w/d diet plus potassium citrate
Urate	Surgical removal or dissolution Hill's u/d diet Allopurinol Control infection	Hill's u/d diet Allopurinol if necessary Correct congenital portosystemic shunts
Silicate	Surgical removal	Hill's u/d diet; prevent consumption of dirt
Cystine	Surgical removal or dissolution Hill's u/d diet d-Penicillamine N-(2-mercaptopropionyl)-glycine (MPG)	Hill's u/d diet; thiol-containing drugs if necessary

From Fossum TW, Hedlund CS, Hulse DA, et al: Small animal surgery, ed 3, St Louis, 2007, Mosby.

should grasp the stay sutures and gently lift upward to avoid spillage of urine.

A bladder spoon can be used to aid in the removal of cystic calculi, especially at the neck region of the bladder (Fig. 10.52). A red rubber catheter can be passed through the urethra, and sterile saline should be flushed through the catheter to confirm the urethral passage is clear of cystic calculi and is patent. This allows for flushing of any calculi back into the bladder, which helps avoid an additional **urethrotomy** (incision into the urethra) to remove calculi from the urethra.

Cultures of the bladder should be obtained. Some surgeons may also prefer to take a sample of the bladder for biopsy or culture. The bladder should be examined for deficiencies and closed according to the surgeon's preference. Closure of the bladder can consist of a two-layer or three-layer continuous closure or a simple interrupted suture pattern (Fig. 10.53). The stay sutures can be removed, and the abdomen may be lavaged with warm saline. The bladder can be leak tested by filling it with sterile saline through a urinary catheter and monitoring for leakage through the suture line. The abdomen should be closed routinely. Bladder stones retrieved from the bladder should be submitted for analysis so appropriate dietary therapy for calculi prevention can be instituted if necessary.

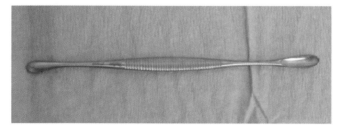

Fig. 10.50 Bladder spoon.

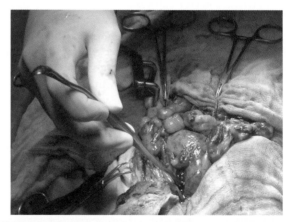

Fig. 10.52 The bladder spoon is used to remove stones from the neck of the bladder.

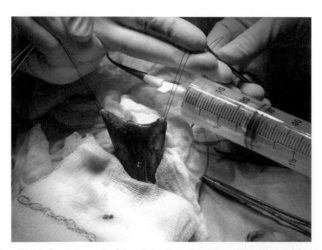

Fig. 10.51 Cystotomy incision into the ventral aspect of the bladder. Note that stay sutures are used to lift gently upward on the bladder to avoid leakage of urine. A red rubber catheter is placed to flush any stones in the urethra back into the bladder. (Modified from Fossum TW, Hedlund CS, Hulse DA, et al: Small animal surgery, ed 4, St Louis, 20013, Mosby.)

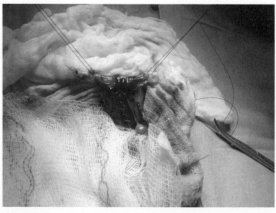

Fig. 10.53 The cystotomy incision is closed in a simple interrupted suture pattern using an absorbable suture.

Postoperative considerations and instructions. Attention must be paid to the ability of the patient to urinate. Urinary atony can occur after prolonged blockage of the bladder. Intermittent catheterization or gentle expression of the bladder may be necessary to keep the bladder from becoming overdistended, which can place stress on the bladder incision. The patient should also be monitored for signs of peritonitis (abdominal pain and fever) and urethral obstruction.

EAR PROCEDURES

Aural Hematoma Repair

Definition

Aural hematoma refers to the formation of a hematoma within the auricular cartilage on the concave surface of the ear. The hematoma forms when the cartilage in the ear pinna fractures, usually from violent head shaking or scratching at the ears secondary to otitis, foreign bodies in the ear canal, atopy, or ear mites. It is important to treat the underlying cause of the aural hematoma to prevent further injury and recurrence. Auricular hematomas occur most commonly in pendulous-eared dogs, but they also occur in cats and erect-eared dogs.

Indications

Surgical correction of an aural hematoma should be performed as soon as possible to relieve the animal's pain and to prevent a permanently scarred and thickened, cauliflower-like ear.

Instrumentation

A soft tissue surgery pack will provide the surgeon with the necessary instruments for surgical correction of an aural hematoma.

Patient Positioning

Patients are usually placed in lateral recumbency with the affected ear dorsal.

Patient Draping

A single fenestrated drape should be sufficient for the aural hematoma procedure. The drape covers the head and neck, and the affected ear is pulled through the fenestration.

Treatment Options

A variety of treatment options exist for the repair of aural hematomas. The objectives of these treatments are to eliminate the hematoma and prevent reappearance of the condition. This section describes only one common treatment option.

Incision drainage procedure. Incision drainage is probably the most widely used procedure for the treatment of aural hematomas. Its purpose is to eliminate dead space between the layers of cartilage until scar tissue can form. An incision (S-shaped or straight) is made directly over the entire hematoma. Fibrin and blood clots are removed, and the area is lavaged. Several vertical mattress sutures are placed parallel to the incision on the concave surface of the ear around the incision (Fig. 10.54). This enhances drainage of the fluid by preventing pocket formation where fluid can collect. The incision itself should remain open to allow continual drainage.

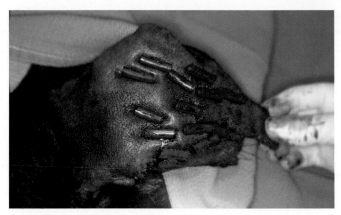

Fig. 10.54 Aural hematoma. The traditional suture technique used to treat aural hematomas is demonstrated. (From Medleau L, Hnilica K: Small Animal Dermatology, ed 2, St Louis, 2006, Elsevier.)

BOX 10.14 Surgery Report: Incision Drainage Procedure

Animal Hospital Name
Owner: John Doe
Address: 555 Sterling Lane
Jupiter, NY 55555
Phone number: 555-5555
Animal Name: Sasha
Animal #: 65656501
Species: Canine
Breed: Labrador
DOB: 05/05/10
Date of Surgery: 01/03/2011
Primary Surgeon: Dr. Vet
Assistant: Technician Scrub
Diagnosis or Preoperative Signs: Aural hematoma right ear.
Surgical Procedure: Incisional drainage of aural hematoma.

Description of Surgical Procedure
Surgical Approach: An S-shaped incision was made directly over the aural hematoma on the concave region of the pinna of the right ear. Blood and clots were evacuated.
 Surgical Pathology: Aural hematoma located on concave surface of right ear.
 Surgical Procedure: An S-shaped incision was made with a scalpel over the fluctuant part of the hematoma. Blood was drained out of the cavity, and several small clots were removed with forceps and by blotting with sponges. Numerous simple mattress sutures of 3-0 nylon were placed in a vertical orientation in a staggered pattern through the skin on the concave side of the ear and the underlying cartilage. The S-shaped incision was left open to drain, and a bandage covering the entire ear was placed.
 Closure: See above.

Box 10.14 shows an example of a surgery report for incision drainage.

Postoperative considerations and instructions. A bandage may be placed on the head, incorporating the ear. This prevents further trauma to the ear from the inevitable head shaking associated with aural hematoma repair. This also prevents trauma to the ear from the self-trauma through scratching.

Before leaving the hospital, the owner should also be instructed in the importance of keeping the bandage clean and dry. The patient will need to be scheduled for a suture removal in 10 to 14 days.

Lateral Ear Canal Resection

Definition

Resection of the lateral ear canal involves lateralization of the horizontal ear canal.

Indications

Lateral ear canal resection is indicated for animals with chronic otitis externa or neoplasia. Lateral wall resection allows drainage of the ear canal while affording ventilation of the canal. Bacteria thrive in moist and humid environments, so the extra ventilation reduces the risk of infection. Surgery improves the chronic condition in many patients, but it is not a cure. Appropriate medical management is usually required in conjunction with surgery.

Instrumentation

A soft tissue surgery pack should be sufficient for lateral ear canal resection.

Patient Positioning

The patient should be positioned in lateral recumbency with the affected ear upward and the head slightly elevated. A sandbag can be placed under the head for elevation.

Patient Draping

A four-quarter draping method should be used for lateral ear resection.

Lateral Ear Resection Procedure (Zepp procedure)

The entire ear, including both sides of the pinna and the adjacent skin, should be clipped and aseptically prepared. The ear canal should be lavaged and cleaned before the patient enters the surgery room. Once the animal is prepped and draped, the surgeon makes two parallel skin incisions from the tragus ventrally past the horizontal ear canal. The incision should extend past the region where the canal becomes horizontal. The skin flap is then excised at the proximal region. A vertical incision is made in the subcutaneous tissue over the vertical canal. The subcutaneous tissue is then reflected dorsally, exposing the auricular cartilage of the vertical canal. The cartilage of the vertical canal is then cut distally along the same incision line. The cartilage flap is reflected distally and the opening of the horizontal canal observed. The proximal two-thirds of the cartilage flap are excised, and the remaining third is reflected ventrally to form a drainboard, which is then sutured to the ventral skin incision. The drainboard technique was established by Zepp to maintain horizontal canal patency (Fig. 10.55).

Postoperative Considerations and Instructions

A bandage may be placed over the ear after the lateral ear canal resection. The owner should be made aware of possible mutilation of the surgical site by the pet. An Elizabethan collar should be sent home with the owner to avoid self-mutilation complications. Although complications are uncommon, insufficient drainage and sustained ear infections may be seen postoperatively. Most lateral ear resections still require medical management by the owner. Before leaving the hospital, the owner should also be instructed on how to clean and administer medication in the horizontal canal. Because the anatomy of the ear canal has changed, the tympanic membrane is more susceptible to damage. Analgesics should be sent home with the owner. Suture removal should be performed 10 to 14 days after surgery.

OPHTHALMIC PROCEDURES

Special Instruments

Because of the delicacy of eye procedures, specialized instruments are often required. Appropriate care and handling of the following ophthalmic instruments are important:

Half-curved tissue forceps is a smaller forceps used for handling eyelid and conjunctival tissue (Fig. 10.56). The forceps may be straight or curved with teeth structure that allows tissue to be manipulated without causing trauma.

Chalazion forceps provides tissue stabilization and hemostasis (Fig. 10.57).

The Jaeger lid plate has flat, curved ends that are placed under the eyelid to provide a firm surface when making an incision (Fig. 10.58).

Tenotomy scissors have short, blunt, narrowed tips for dividing and dissecting the muscles and tendons of the eye during recession and resection for strabismus surgery (Fig. 10.59).

Needle holders are used for handling delicate suture needles needed for placing sutures in an eye and performing neurosurgery; fine needles are held by jaws attached to spring-loaded handles that catch or release with gentle pressure (Fig. 10.60).

Patient Positioning

The patient is placed in sternal or lateral recumbency for most ophthalmic surgeries; several sandbags can be used to help position the head.

Patient Draping

Often a specialized eye drape is used for the patient undergoing ophthalmic procedures. The drape is secured with towel clamps.

Patient Preparation

Cleanliness and sterility of the surgical area are important for all patients undergoing ophthalmic procedures. Before prepping the area, a sterile lubricant, like artificial tears, should be placed in the eye to protect it. The area can then be clipped as for any surgical procedure. Then flush the eye with sterile eye wash or LRS (lactated Ringer's solution) to remove any hair or debris from the area. A very dilute (1:50) povidone-iodine (Betadine) solution can be used to aseptically prepare the area before draping. Do not use any soap-based products or alcohol because these can damage the eye.

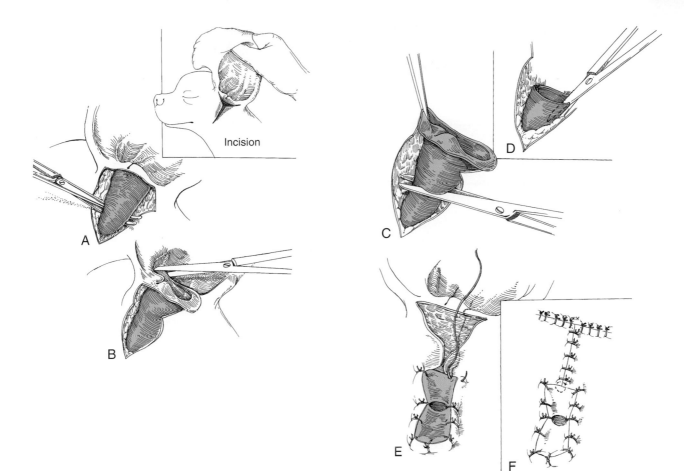

Fig. 10.55 Vertical ear canal ablation technique. Begin with T-shaped skin incision over the ear canal. A, Continue blunt dissection medially until the entire vertical canal is isolated and freed up. Dissect just underneath the cartilage to avoid damaging vascular supply to the pinna. B, Cut the auricular cartilage with heavy straight Mayo scissors, removing all affected tissue on the dorsal aspect of the medial vertical canal and pinna. This step allows complete mobilization of the vertical canal, which remains attached only at its proximal aspect. C, Remove the vertical canal approximately 1 to 2 cm distal to the annular cartilage junction. D, Incise remaining vertical canal rostrally and caudally, if necessary, to fully expose the horizontal ear canal. E, Suture the ventral flap to the skin in a fashion similar to that in lateral ear resection. F, Suture the dorsal flap to appose the cut edges of the canal and skin with simple interrupted 3-0 to 4-0 monofilament nonabsorbable material. Remaining skin is apposed to form a T-shaped closure. (From Birchard S, Sherding R: Saunders manual of small animal practice, ed 3, St Louis, 2006, Saunders.)

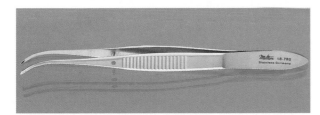

Fig. 10.56 Half-curved tissue forceps. Small forceps with fine jaws; the teeth of the forceps are structured to allow for tissue pickup without trauma. (From Sonsthagen TF: Veterinary instruments and equipment, ed 3, St Louis, Mosby, 2014.)

Entropion Repair
Definition

Entropion refers to a rolling in of the eyelid. This can mean the upper lid only, lower lid only, or both lids. Different regions of the eyelid may be involved: the medial aspect, the lateral aspect, or the entire lid.

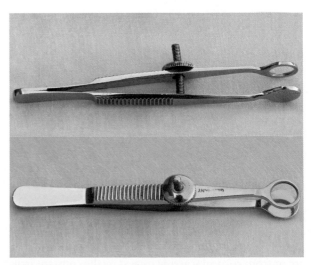

Fig. 10.57 Chalazion forceps. The ends may be circular or oval, with round, smooth edges. (From Sonsthagen TF: Veterinary instruments and equipment, ed 3, St Louis, Mosby, 2014.)

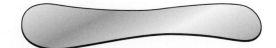

Fig. 10.58 Jaeger lid plate.

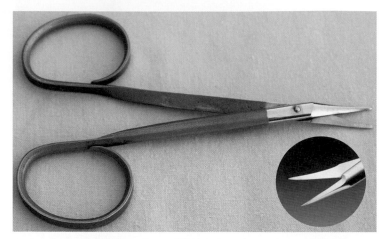

Fig. 10.59 Tenotomy scissors. (From Sonsthagen TF: Veterinary instruments and equipment, ed 3, St Louis, Mosby, 2014.)

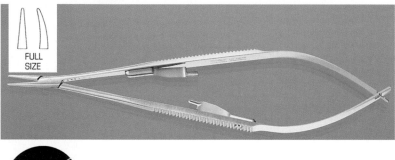

FULL SIZE

Fig. 10.60 Castroviejo needle holder with catch. (From Sonsthagen TF: Veterinary instruments and equipment, ed 3, St Louis, Mosby, 2014.)

Indications

The primary indication for an entropion surgery is to alleviate ocular irritation caused by the eyelid or by the facial hairs adjacent to it, contacting the conjunctiva and cornea.

Clinical Signs

Clinical signs of entropion may include lacrimation (tearing), blepharospasm (squinting, blinking), photophobia (sensitivity to light), enophthalmos (pulling back of the eye and a secondary, raised third eyelid), conjunctivitis (inflammation of the conjunctiva), keratitis (inflammation of the cornea) with or without corneal ulceration, and self-trauma (pawing at the eye or rubbing the eye on objects). Vision may be impaired from constant eyelid closure or from corneal scarring caused by the constant irritation.

Developmental entropion, or conformational entropion, is the most common form seen in small animals, mostly dogs. It is believed to be inherited. The most common breeds presented with developmental entropion are the Chinese Shar-Pei, chow chow, Saint Bernard, Rottweiler, Great Dane, bull mastiff, Labrador retriever, and English bulldog. Dogs with conformational entropion may have both eyes affected at the same time, but occasionally only one eye is affected.

Spastic entropion occurs secondary to ocular pain, which may result from a corneal foreign body, uveitis (intraocular inflammation), corneal ulceration, or chronic conjunctivitis. The painful eye is pulled back, causing the eyelid to roll inward. In cases of spastic entropion, the primary problem must be addressed and resolved. Application of a topical anesthetic usually temporarily resolves a spastic entropion. Dogs with developmental (conformational) entropion still have rolling in of the eyelid even after application of topical anesthetic.

Surgical Options

Eyelid tacking. Eyelid tacking is performed in young animals to roll out the eyelid temporarily (Fig. 10.61). Young puppies (usually up to 16–20 weeks) with conformational entropion are candidates for temporary placement of sutures or staples. The Chinese Shar-Pei is a breed that commonly benefits from eyelid tacking. Even though eyelid tacking is a relatively simple procedure, standard postoperative care is important. The animal should wear an Elizabethan collar until the sutures or staples are removed. In some cases, a repeat procedure may be necessary. Permanent correction is usually delayed until the animal reaches its adult conformation.

In cases of spastic entropion, temporary eyelid tacking, in addition to treatment of the underlying cause, may result in resolution of the problem.

Holtz-Celsus procedure. Several techniques are described to correct conformational entropion. The Holtz-Celsus procedure is a widely used approach that involves excision of a crescent-shaped section of skin and muscle (a "smile") from the affected portion of the eyelid. Eversion of the eyelid is accomplished by suturing the resulting skin defect.

Subcutaneous sutures are usually not necessary with the Holtz-Celsus procedure. Skin sutures are placed approximately 1 to 2 mm apart in a simple interrupted pattern. Common suture materials used are silk, gut, and polyglactin 910 (Vicryl). Small gauge sutures are preferred, usually 5-0 or 6-0, because they have a better cosmetic result.

Complications with the Holtz-Celsus procedure may result from making the initial incision too far from the eyelid margin or placing the sutures too far apart.

Postoperative Considerations and Instructions

A patient is often discharged the day the entropion is performed. Tissue swelling may occur, although it should resolve within a few days. The owner may apply warm compresses to the area to help with any swelling. Sutures are left in place for about 10 to 14 days. Nonabsorbable sutures are most often used. Absorbable sutures can also be used, especially if removing the sutures will be difficult because of an aggressive or uncooperative animal. A topical ophthalmic antibiotic is usually sent home with the owner to be used two or three times a day for 10 to 14 days after surgery.

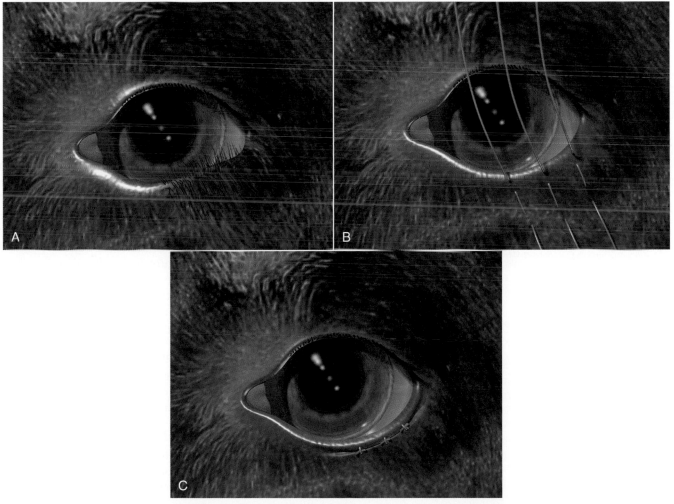

Fig. 10.61 Temporary tacking suture. A, Inferior lateral entropion. B, Vertical mattress sutures placed with first bite close to the eyelid margin and the second bite sufficient distance ventrally to create eversion when sutures were tied. C, Eversion of entropion with tacking sutures in place. (From Aquino S: Topics in Companion Animal Medicine, Vol 23, Issue 1, St Louis, 2008, Elsevier.)

The animal should wear an Elizabethan collar until the sutures are removed to prevent them from being rubbed out before healing has been completed. The awkwardness of the Elizabethan collar, especially in large dogs, often requires restriction of activity until the collar is removed.

A recheck examination is recommended 10 to 14 days after surgery or sooner if there are any problems. Box 10.15 shows an example of a surgery report for entropion repair.

Eyelid Mass (Neoplasm) Removal
Incidence and Differential Diagnosis

Eyelid masses are found in both dogs and cats. Breeds of dogs that are more predisposed to eyelid masses include poodles, Labrador retrievers, and mixed breeds. Generally, eyelid masses are seen in older dogs.

Canine eyelid masses are usually benign and may be differentiated based on their clinical appearance, but they should always be examined histologically as well.

Feline eyelid neoplasms are usually malignant and can rarely be differentiated from one another solely on their clinical appearance.

Eyelid neoplasms may be raised, alopecic (having hair loss), pigmented or nonpigmented, and may or may not become ulcerated. Cytologic examination, specifically by fine-needle aspiration (FNA) or biopsy samples of eyelid masses, may be helpful.

BOX 10.15 Surgery Report: Entropion Repair

Animal Hospital Name
Owner: John Doe
Address: 555 Sterling Lane
Jupiter, NY 55555
Phone number: 555-5555
Animal Name: Sasha
Animal #: 65656501
Species: Canine
Breed: Rottweiler
DOB: 05/05/10
Date of Surgery: 01/03/2011
Primary Surgeon: Dr. Vet
Assistant: Technician Scrub
Diagnosis or Preoperative Signs: Entropion OU.
Surgical Procedure: Holtz-Celsus entropion repair OU.

Description of Surgical Procedure
Surgical Approach: The patient was placed in sternal recumbency and the head positioned with sandbags. Each eye was clipped, prepped, and covered with a sterile eye drape. Towel clamps were used to secure the drape in place.

Surgical Procedures: Ophthalmic scissors were used to make a "smile" incision into the skin and subcutaneous tissue of the ventral eyelid approximately 5 mm from this lid margin. The incision was wider laterally and tapered medially over a distance of approximately 1 cm. Minimal bleeding was encountered and was effectively stopped with gentle pressure from a sterile cotton-tipped applicator. A simple interrupted 6-0 silk suture was first placed in the middle of this incision to appose the edges, followed by subsequent simple interrupted sutures approximately 2 mm apart to appose the skin edges.

Closure: See above.

Canine eyelid neoplasms. A *meibomian* (sebaceous) adenoma is the most common eyelid neoplasm in dogs. It arises from the meibomian gland and is found near the meibomian orifice. Other, less common benign neoplastic masses are melanomas, papillomas, and histiocytomas. Malignant neoplastic masses, which occur less often in dogs, include mast cell tumors, adenocarcinomas, basal cell carcinomas, squamous cell carcinomas, hemangiosarcomas, and fibrosarcomas.

Feline eyelid neoplasms. Squamous cell carcinoma is the most common feline eyelid tumor and is often found in cats with white or pink eyelids. Other neoplasms are basal cell carcinomas, fibrosarcomas, and mast cell tumors.

Indications for Surgery

An eyelid mass should be removed if (1) the mass becomes too large, (2) there is concern about malignancy, (3) corneal or conjunctival irritation is present, or (4) the patient is traumatizing the mass, with or without bleeding. In some cases, the owner may request removal of the mass to achieve an improved cosmetic appearance. Generally, the smaller the mass to be removed, the easier it is to reconstruct the lid, therefore preserving normal eyelid function. When the eyelid mass becomes too large (greater than one-third of the length of the eyelid), skin flaps may be necessary for eyelid reconstruction. If the eyelid mass is not completely removed, it may recur.

Surgical Options

Eyelid mass removal and subsequent eyelid repair involve careful apposition of the conjunctiva, eyelid margin, and the surrounding skin for cosmetic healing and optimal function of the eyelid. The alignment of the eyelid margin, both horizontally and vertically, is critical.

Wedge resection. A wedge resection of the eyelid mass and adjacent eyelid is a simple, common procedure. A chalazion forceps or a Jaeger lid plate may be used for stabilization. A full-thickness house-shaped incision is made with sharp dissection. The incision is closed in two layers. Subcutaneous sutures are placed in a simple interrupted pattern using 5-0 Vicryl. Skin sutures are placed using a figure-eight pattern for apposition of the eyelid margin, and a few simple interrupted sutures are placed for the remainder of the incision using 6-0 Vicryl.

The mass is routinely biopsied and submitted for histopathologic examination to confirm the diagnosis.

Postoperative Considerations and Instructions

As with other ophthalmic procedures, it is imperative that the patient wear an Elizabethan collar to prevent trauma to the incision, if it is deemed necessary by the surgeon or technician.

Prolapse of the Gland of the Third Eyelid

Prolapse, or protrusion, of the gland of the third eyelid is also known as glandular hypertrophy, glandular hyperplasia, cherry eye, and prolapse of third eyelid gland.

Third Eyelid Anatomy and Function

The third eyelid, also known as the nictitating membrane, serves as added protection for the globe. It rises up from the ventromedial aspect of the orbit and over the globe to protect it when the animal pulls its globe back into the orbit, usually as a protective mechanism. Movement of the third eyelid also aids in removal of dirt and particles from the eye. On the underside of the third eyelid is a small gland that secretes and distributes approximately 30% of the tear production. Because the gland significantly contributes to the precorneal tear film, it should not be removed. Clinical studies have confirmed extensive clinical experience that keratoconjunctivitis (KCS, dry eye) is commonly seen in animals that have their gland of the third eyelid removed, often years later. This occurs especially in breeds susceptible to prolapse of the gland, such as cocker spaniels, bull dogs, and Lhasa Apsos.

Mechanism of Prolapse

Prolapse of the third eyelid gland is the most common primary disorder of the third eyelid. A prolapse may result from a weakness in the connective tissue attachment between the ventral aspect of the third eyelid and the periorbital tissues; the result is the gland becomes everted while remaining attached to the cartilage of the third eyelid. This weakness allows the gland, which is normally found ventrally, to flip up dorsally, where it then becomes enlarged and inflamed because of chronic exposure. Abrasions and drying of the exposed gland may result in secondary inflammation and swelling. If the gland becomes severely infected, preoperative treatment with topical antibiotics is recommended.

Occasionally, in the early stages of prolapse, the gland returns to its normal position on its own or with manipulation. Unfortunately, prolapse of the gland usually recurs. Surgical intervention is the definitive treatment.

Clinical Signs

Common clinical signs of third eyelid gland prolapse include ocular discharge, conjunctivitis, and the pink, swollen mass at the medial canthus on the third eyelid seen by owners. Tear production may be affected in some patients and may be decreased.

Incidence

Protrusion of the gland of the third eyelid is usually seen in puppies and dogs younger than 2 years. It can occur in one or both eyes. Breeds predisposed to this disorder are the cocker spaniel, English bulldog, Boston terrier, Great Dane, and pug.

Surgical Options

For years, surgical removal of the third eyelid gland was the treatment of choice for third eyelid protrusion. As the role of the third eyelid gland in tear production became more apparent, however, surgical repositioning of the gland became widely recommended. As mentioned earlier, removing the third eyelid gland should be avoided, because this will likely predispose the eye to develop KCS (dry eye).

Numerous techniques are currently available for correcting prolapse of the third eyelid gland (Figs. 10.62 and 10.63), with some achieving greater success than others. The choice is usually the surgeon's preference.

Postoperative Considerations and Instructions

Inadequate positioning of the third eyelid gland may result in recurrence of the prolapse. Usually a second attempt and possibly a third attempt to secure the gland are made, typically using a different approach. Box 10.16 shows an example of a surgery report for correction of a prolapsed third eyelid gland.

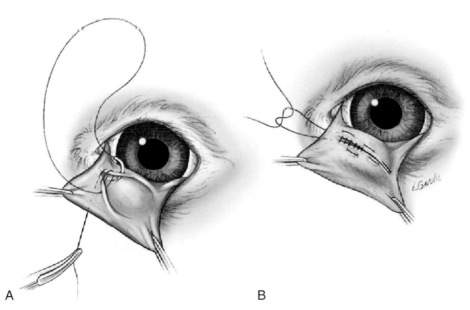

A   B

Fig. 10.62 Morgan pocket technique for repair of a prolapsed gland of the third eyelid (TE). A, This method involves securing the TE gland into a conjunctival pocket formed on the posterior surface of the TE. When the conjunctival margins are sutured, openings are left on either end to allow drainage of secretions. Suturing begins by oversewing and burying the knot (subcuticular pattern), then runs continuously through the conjunctiva from side to side, and finally is tied on the anterior ventral surface of the TE. B, This method of suturing prevents corneal irritation from the suture knots. (From Maggs D: Slatter's fundamentals of veterinary ophthalmology, ed 4, St Louis, 2008, Saunders.)

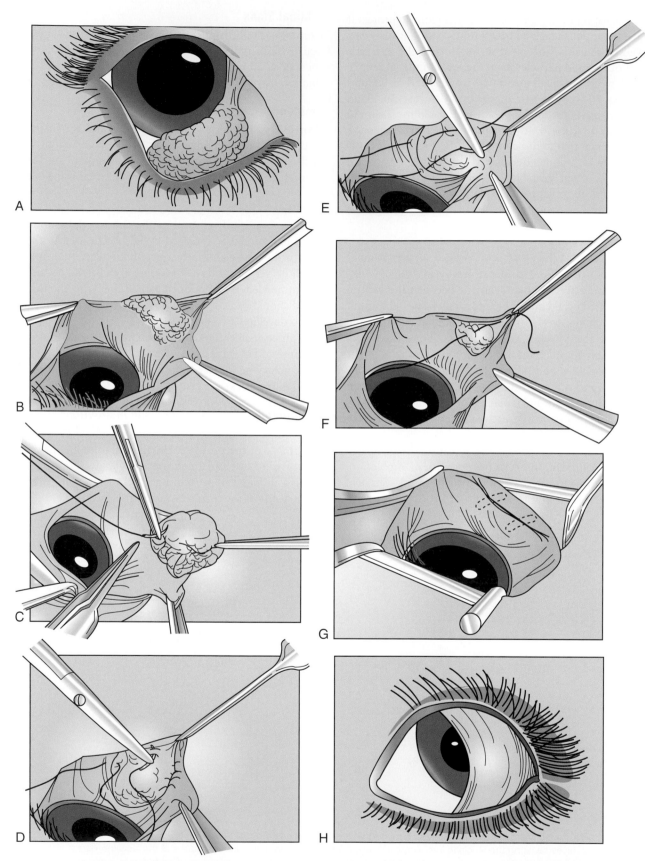

Fig. 10.63 A, Typical appearance of a prolapsed third eyelid gland. B, Elliptical incision. C, Initial anchor suture. D, Initial suture carried to the opposite side of the gland. E, Placement of a second suture. F, The initial suture is drawn together surnd tied. G, Inversion of prolapsed tissue. *Dotted lines* indicate that the suture and knots lie under the conjunctiva. H, Appearance of third eyelid immediately after surgery.

Animal Hospital Name
Owner: John Doe
Address: 555 Sterling Lane
Jupiter, NY 55555
Phone number: 555-5555
Animal Name: Fluffy
Animal #: 65656501
Species: Canine
Breed: Pug
DOB: 05/05/07
Date of Surgery: 01/03/2011
Primary Surgeon: Dr. Vet
Assistant: Technician Scrub
Diagnosis or Preoperative Signs: Prolapsed gland of the third eyelid, OD.
Surgical Procedure: Morgan pocket technique.

Description of Surgical Procedure
Surgical Approach: The patient was placed in left lateral recumbency to allow access to the right eye. The leading edge of the third eyelid was grasped with two small, noncrushing forceps and reflected away from its origin.

Surgical Procedures/Correction: With sharp dissection, two 1-cm incisions were made parallel to each other through the bulbar conjunctiva dorsal and ventral to the free margin of the gland. Blunt dissection was used to free up the conjunctiva for ease of suturing.

Closure (Technique and Suture): 6-0 Vicryl suture was used in a simple interrupted, buried pattern to appose the two incisions together, thus replacing the prolapsed gland within the third eyelid.

Surgical Samples: None

ORTHOPEDIC PROCEDURES

Definition

Orthopedic surgery is a branch of surgery dealing with the preservation and restoration of the function of the skeletal system and its articulation and association with its related structures.

Technician's Responsibilities

The purpose of this section is to familiarize the technician with the basic presentation of fractures, with fracture evaluation, and with the types of repair available for the stabilization of different fractures. Understanding fracture management and repair will make the technician an asset to any veterinary practice. The ability to triage, evaluate, and either refer or prepare the patient for orthopedic surgery are all responsibilities that may fall on the technician. Box 10.17 introduces orthopedic terms and abbreviations.

Orthopedic fracture repair is a broad and highly specialized subject; readers wanting more in-depth coverage can supplement this chapter's discussion with additional reading. Orthopedic surgery requires expensive specialized instruments and equipment along with an experienced orthopedic surgeon.

Orthopedic problems are usually not life-threatening situations. These cases can be considered life-threatening emergencies, however, if the skull or spine is involved or if the patient has lost large amounts of blood because of a long-bone fracture. Other cases that can be considered nonelective but are not

ACL: Anterior cruciate ligament.

AO: Arbeitsgemeinschaft für Osteosynthesefragen, Swiss for the Association for the Study of Internal Fixation (ASIF). These abbreviations are often seen together but separated by a slash: AO/ASIF. The AO is involved in research and development of medical devices used in orthopedic surgery. Its devices are available through a company called Synthes Holding AG (West Chester, PA).

ASIF: Association for the Study of Internal Fixation.

Articular: Pertaining to a joint.

Aseptic loosening: Breakdown of bone and loosening of prosthesis in the absence of microorganisms.

CCL: Cranial cruciate ligament.

Callus: Unorganized network of woven bone formed about ends of a broken bone, which is reabsorbed as healing is completed.

Closed reduction: Nonsurgical realignment of fracture or joint.

Delayed union: Prolonged renewal of continuity in a broken bone or between the edges of a wound.

Dislocation: Complete separation of the articular surfaces of a joint.

Elective: Referring to surgical cases that can wait for later scheduling.

HOD: Hypertrophic osteodystrophy; developmental disease that causes disruption of metaphyseal trabeculae in long bones of young, rapidly growing dogs.

Hip dysplasia: Abnormal development of coxofemoral joint characterized by subluxation or complete luxation of femoral head in younger patients and mild to severe degenerative joint disease in older patients.

IVDD: Intervertebral disk disease associated with disk degeneration and extrusion, causing spinal cord compression and nerve root entrapment.

Interfragmentary: Bone pieces of a fracture that may or may not be able to be reconstructed and stabilized.

Luxation: Complete separation of a bone from its articulation.

MPL: Medial patellar luxation.

Malunion: Faulty union and alignment of the fractured bone.

Nonunion: Failure of the fractured bone ends to unite.

Nonelective: Referring to surgical cases that cannot wait for later scheduling.

Nonreducible: Unable to be restored to the normal place or position.

OCD: Osteochondritis dissecans; inflammation of bone and cartilage that results in the splitting of cartilage pieces into the affected joint.

Open reduction: Surgical opening and exposure to realign a fracture or joint.

Reducible: Able to be restored to the normal place or relation of parts, as a fracture.

Subluxation: Partial or incomplete separation of a joint.

life threatening are open fracture or open dislocation repairs. All these cases need to be fully evaluated, and the patient should be stabilized (e.g., open airway, controlled bleeding, stable vital signs, and sufficient pain management) before further evaluation or surgery can occur. Elective orthopedic surgical cases that may present to the hospital include cranial (anterior) cruciate ligament rupture, medial or lateral patellar luxation, hip dysplasia, elbow dysplasia, or osteochondritis dissecans. These cases also need to be properly evaluated before surgery, but they are considered elective.

Patients that present with fractures can be assumed to be in significant pain and need strong analgesics. It is the technician's responsibility to see that the fracture patient receives adequate pain management as directed by the veterinarian. Any fracture noted on examination should be immobilized and bandaged accordingly. External coaptation (application of external appliance, such as a splint or cast) is important to reduce further disruption or damage to the fracture or fragments and the surrounding soft tissue and to prevent further blood loss at the fracture site. Stabilization of fractures also greatly enhances pain management and the patient's comfort level.

Types of bandages used to stabilize a fracture include the Robert Jones bandage (any long-bone fracture) (Fig. 10.64) and modified Robert Jones with metal or plastic splint (carpal, metacarpal, tarsal, metatarsal, and phalangeal fractures). A fiberglass cast with adequate padding can also be used for these same types of fractures. Fiberglass applied as a cast and not as a splint can

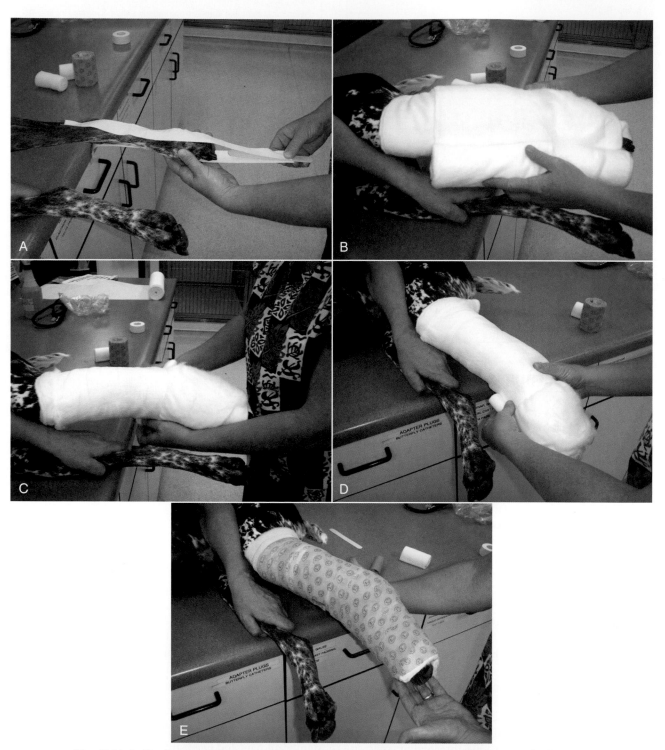

Fig. 10.64 A, Placement of stirrups. B, Wrapping the leg with large amounts of sheet cotton. C, Wrapping the cotton with roll gauze to compress the cotton. D, Wrapping the cotton with roll gauze to compress the cotton. E, Placement of Vetrap and Elastikon. (From Sirois M: Principles and practice of veterinary technology, ed 4, St Louis, 2017, Elsevier.)

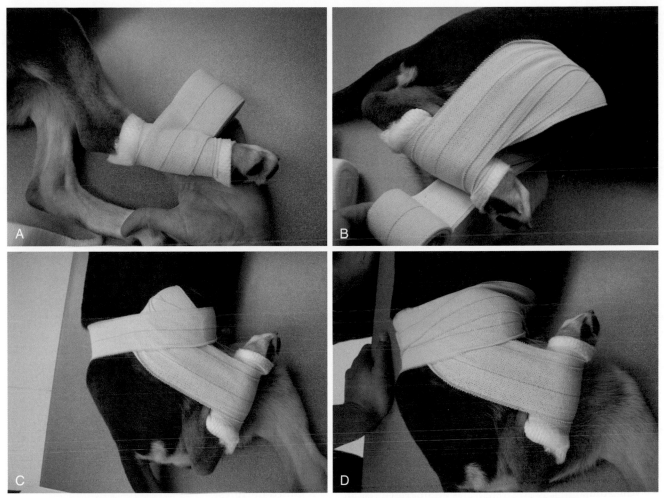

Fig. 10.65 A, Cast padding is first wrapped around the metatarsal region and then covered with Elastikon tape. B, The leg is fixed and the Elastikon is then continued around the whole leg in a figure-eight pattern. C, The wrap is extended around the abdomen and then covered with white (nonelastic) tape. D, Several layers of elastic tape are added. The finished product should then be covered with nonporous tape. (From Sirois M: Principles and practice of veterinary technology, ed 4, St Louis, 2017, Elsevier.)

make maintenance and changes technically difficult. Other bandages used for preoperative and postoperative support are the Ehmer sling (hip luxation) (Fig. 10.65), spica splint (humeral or femoral fractures) (Fig. 10.66), and Velpeau sling (scapular fractures) (Fig. 10.67). All these bandages, except for the Robert Jones, can be used as external coaptation if surgery is not an option.

Owners must always be informed of bandage and fracture complications associated with splinting or slinging. A bandage should be checked three or four times a day for signs of swelling, slippage, moisture, or soiling. If any of these scenarios occurs, the bandage should be changed.

Preoperative Considerations for Fractures

The patient history can provide pertinent information to help determine whether a patient is a good candidate for surgery and what type of fixation is best suited for a positive outcome. Patient age, temperament, health status, and activity level should be considered when recommending fixation.

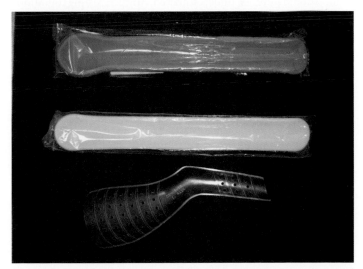

Fig. 10.66 Examples of types of splints. (From Sirois M: Principles and practice of veterinary technology, ed 4, St Louis, 2017, Elsevier.)

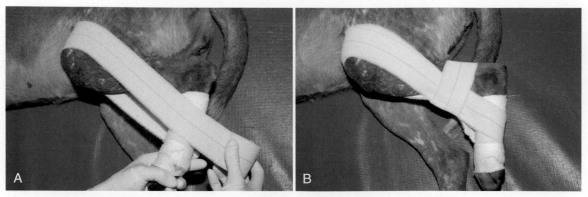

Fig. 10.67 A 90-90 flexion sling. After minimal padding has been applied to the tarsus, a sling of adhesive tape is passed along the medial aspect of the limb (see Fig. 10.64A). A, The tape is then wrapped around the hind limb with the stifle and hock held in 90-degree flexion. B, A second layer of tape is passed horizontally around the tibia to hold the previous layer in place. (From Bassert JM, Thomas, JA, editors: McCurnin's clinical textbook for veterinary technicians, ed 8, St Louis, 2014, Elsevier.)

The patient's age is significant in terms of how much more the bones need to grow and the activity level of the animal. Generally, the younger the patient, the faster is the healing time; however, there is also a greater risk of angular limb deformities if the patient's growth plates are still open and have been traumatized. Also, younger patients are more active and are more difficult to confine for long periods. Older patients tend to have slower healing time. This can contribute to an increased chance of complications because of the longer recovery time. Older patients tend to be more sedentary, which can lead to difficulty recovering normal mobility after long periods of inactivity and muscle atrophy.

The animal's size and weight can affect recovery times and success. Any animal that is overweight has an increased risk of failure for any type of orthopedic repair. Excessive force placed on any orthopedic repair too soon can cause premature loosening of the fixation and possible failure of the repair. Some large-breed dogs, as well as overweight dogs and cats, are often too weak after orthopedic surgery to lift or support their own weight and may need assistance to rise and walk.

The importance of the orthopedic surgery patient's overall health should never be underestimated. Any preexisting conditions that would increase the patient's risk during surgery, or delay healing, need to be considered and addressed preoperatively. Problems with other joints or bones, such as chronic arthritis, can contribute to poor comfort levels and increase the length of recovery.

Owner compliance is a major consideration in any orthopedic case. The animal's temperament may impact how successful owners will be at following postoperative care instructions at home. Owner compliance is probably the most underestimated component of any orthopedic patient's recovery and outcome. An animal that is aggressive, difficult to handle, or difficult for the owner to treat has a lower chance for a successful recovery than the easily handled, stoic animal. If the owners are incapable of handling and treating the patient correctly postoperatively, or cannot return for follow-up examinations, the consequences can be catastrophic.

Special Instruments

Instrumentation varies depending on the type of surgical procedure chosen for the surgical repair. Ascertaining the size of the implants (plates, screws, pins, etc.) necessary for repair, and having smaller and larger sizes available (and sterilized) in case the chosen size is not appropriate, is of the utmost importance. Communication with the surgeon prior to surgery to discuss any additional equipment is advised. Additionally, power drill equipment is also used and needs to be appropriately handled to maintain sterility.

Fracture Assessment

Fractures can be classified or described by the following factors:
1. Bone location (e.g., humerus, femur, tibia)
2. Open (compound) or closed (simple) fracture (open fractures have penetrated through the skin; the skin is intact in closed fractures)
3. Location of fracture on the bone (e.g., midshaft, articular)
4. Type of fracture (e.g., oblique, spiral, transverse, comminuted)
5. Reducible or nonreducible fracture

To assess any fracture completely, radiographs should be taken after a thorough physical examination. Some sedation is usually necessary to achieve complete relaxation and compliance of the patient for the radiographic views needed. In animals that are a sedation risk, radiographs can be taken through the bandage or splint. When radiographs are taken of any long-bone fracture, the joints above and below the fracture site should be included on the radiograph. Articular fractures should be centered on the film using the least amount of manipulation necessary. Two orthogonal views of the affected bone should be performed, usually standard cranial-caudal (craniocaudal, Cr-Ca), and mediolateral or lateromedial views are suggested for proper long-bone fracture evaluation. Radiographs should also be taken postoperatively to confirm proper alignment and repair. Preoperative radiographs also serve as a point of reference for follow-up radiographs.

Radiographs and a thorough physical examination should suffice in determining whether the fracture or fractures are open or closed. An *open or compound fracture* is a fracture in which the skin and the soft tissue covering the bone were punctured, usually by the sharp ends of the fractured bone, creating a path for external contaminants to contact the bone. The fracture is then considered to be open (no longer closed) to the external environment. If possible, open fractures should be cultured before cleaning and antibiotic therapy. Open fractures can be classified or labeled according to the mechanism of puncture and the severity of the soft tissue damage, as follows:

- Grade I open fractures have a small puncture hole in the skin around the location of the fracture. The bone broke through the skin and was exposed to external factors but is no longer visible. Soft tissue damage is minimal.
- Grade II open fractures have a larger puncture or tear in the skin around the location of the fracture, and more soft tissue damage associated with the external trauma is evident.
- Grade III open fractures have large tears and, in some cases, loss of skin at the area of impact. Soft tissue damage is extensive and usually caused by severe bone fragmentation along with the force of the external impact. Grade III open fractures can also be described as shearing injuries. The patients usually have lost so much soft tissue that the bone is exposed, and in some cases, the bone is sheared away or even missing.

Complications tend to be worse and more life threatening with open fractures than with closed fractures. Complications associated with open fractures include skin necrosis and infection leading to bone death. With both open and closed fractures, bleeding, soft tissue damage, and swelling are concerns. With any open fracture, contamination and vascular compromise are of great concern and play a large part in determining what type of repair is best suited for the condition.

A *closed or simple fracture* is a fracture that at the time of impact did not puncture or tear the skin at or around the location of the fracture. Soft tissue damage and swelling can range from mild to severe. Fig. 10.68 shows the anatomy of a long bone, and Fig. 10.69 illustrates bone planes of a femur.

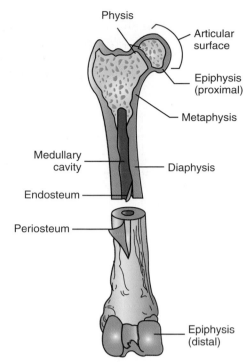

Fig. 10.68 Anatomy of a long bone (femur). *Diaphysis:* long shaft or body of bone. *Epiphysis (proximal/distal):* ends of bone, usually wider than shaft, and either entirely cartilaginous or separated from shaft by cartilaginous disk. *Metaphysis:* wider end of shaft of the bone adjacent to epiphysis. *Periosteum:* fibrous covering around bone that is not covered by articular cartilage. This layer is important for bone growth, repair, nutrition, and attachment for ligaments and tendons. *Articular surface:* smooth layer of hyaline cartilage covering epiphysis where one bone forms a joint with another bone. *Medullary cavity:* space in diaphysis containing bone marrow. *Endosteum:* fibrous tissue lining medullary cavity of bone. *Physis:* growth plate.

Types of Fractures

Five types of common fractures are shown in Fig. 10.70.

Articular and physeal fractures. Articular fractures always involve the joint. These fractures are commonly seen in young, growing animals. Physeal fractures involve the growth plate cartilage and are referred to as Salter-Harris fractures. Any fracture involving the physis or growth plate in early stages of bone development can be detrimental to development and may cause angular limb deformities. Physeal fractures can involve the physis itself or the physis and the bone above and below it. Salter-Harris fractures are identified according to the location of the fracture line and what areas of the bone are involved (Fig. 10.71).

Y fractures and T fractures are types of articular fractures that involve the distal aspect of the humerus (Fig. 10.72). The fracture lines run ventrodorsally through the humeral condyle and run in transverse (T fracture) or oblique (Y fracture) configurations through the medial and lateral epicondyles.

Surgical Options for Fracture Repair

Surgical options for fracture repair are initially basic but can become very detailed. In general, the purpose for any fracture fixation is to bring the opposing ends of the fracture and joints back into alignment. After reduction of the fracture, the bone is stabilized and supported by internal or external fixation. Once the bone has been properly immobilized, the healing process and callus formation begin. *Internal fixation* is a form of rigid fixation placed under the skin and muscle directly on or in the bone surface or medullary cavity to regain stability. Internal fixation usually involves pins or plates and screws. *External fixation* is a form of fixation applied through the exterior surface (skin and muscle) of the limb to the interior area (bone and medullary cavity) to help with stability.

Bone is the deepest tissue within the limb and therefore is afforded poor drainage in the event of infection. Bone infection (osteomyelitis) is serious and difficult to treat. Great care must be taken when preparing any patient for orthopedic surgery. A broad-spectrum antibacterial, antimicrobial, and antifungal scrub and final prep should be used before surgery, with adherence to strict sterile technique throughout the procedure to prevent contamination.

Internal Fixation

Internal fixation devices include bone plates and screws (Figs. 10.73 to 10.76), interlocking nails, intramedullary pins, Kirschner wires, and cerclage wire.

Bone plates come in a variety of shapes, sizes, and lengths. They are designed to be used with various sizes of screw. The

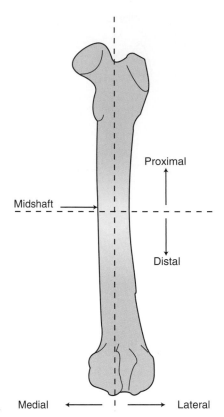

Fig. 10.69 Bone planes (femur). *Proximal:* area closest to the body or point of origin. *Distal:* area farthest from the body or point of origin. *Midshaft:* center of shaft, or toward median plane. *Lateral:* farther from medial plane. *Medial:* toward median plane (inside or middle).

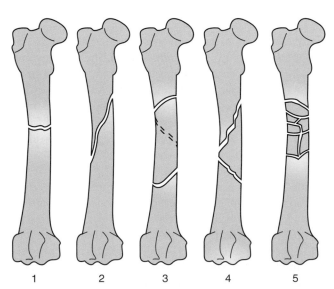

Fig. 10.70 Types of fractures. 1, *Transverse:* extending from side to side at right angle to long axis. 2, *Oblique:* being on an incline or slanting. 3, *Spiral:* curving around a center point or axis. 4, *Comminuted reducible:* broken or crushed into numerous fragments but able to be placed or aligned with opposite end of fracture. 5, *Comminuted nonreducible:* broken or crushed into numerous fragments and unable to be placed or aligned together with opposite end of fracture.

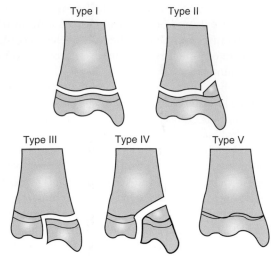

Fig. 10.71 Salter-Harris fractures. Type I fracture runs through the physis. Type II fracture runs through the metaphysis and physis. Type III fracture runs through the physis and epiphysis. Type IV fracture runs through the metaphysis, physis, and epiphysis. Type V fracture is a crushing injury to the physis; it may not always be detected initially by radiographs.

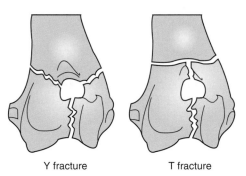

Fig. 10.72 Y and T articular fractures.

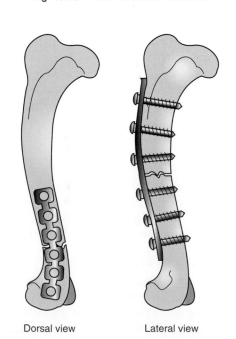

Fig. 10.73 Internal fixation (bone plate and screws).

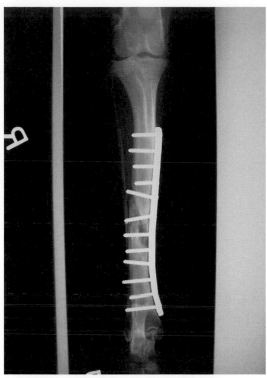

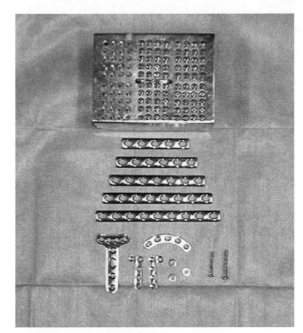

Fig. 10.76 Internal orthopedic plate and screw set.

Fig. 10.74 Radiograph (dorsal view) of a tibial fracture repair. An internal plate and screws were used for fixation.

plates are made of titanium or stainless steel and are used with screws of the same material. Soft tissue and muscle dissection is necessary to gain adequate exposure of the fracture and to afford successful reduction of the fracture.

In another type of fixation, interlocking nails are driven into the medullary cavity and secured in position by screws that engage the bone and the nail at its proximal and distal aspects. This provides stabilization without extensive soft tissue dissection and muscle manipulation to expose and reconstruct the fracture (Figs. 10.77 to 10.79).

Intramedullary (IM) pins are driven through the bone and into the medullary cavity with a Jacob's chuck. Their placement can be approached as an open surgical technique or a closed pinning technique (Figs. 10.80 and 10.81). IM pins can be used alone (single IM pin driven into medullary canal) or stacked (multiple IM pins driven into medullary canal). Intramedullary pinning is inexpensive compared with all other types of internal fixation but does not provide very rigid stability. Pins tend to migrate, and removal of the implant may become necessary.

Orthopedic wires (Kirschner or cerclage) can be used alone or combined with other fixation devices to achieve proper fixation. Cerclage wire comes in different diameters ranging from 0.4 to 1.5 mm and is used in fracture fixation for the reduction of bone fragments and the protection of fissures in bone. Cerclage wires can be applied by being passed either completely around the bone (full cerclage; Fig. 10.82) or passed through a predrilled hole in the bone (hemicerclage; Fig. 10.83).

Kirschner wires, or K-wires, are small sections of precut wire that have pointed ends (trocar) for drilling through the bone. They come in multiple diameters for stiffness and can be used in combination with cerclage wire for interfragmentary reduction.

Postoperative care. Postoperative care for internal fixation is strict confinement of the patient for 6 to 8 weeks. The patient is rechecked at suture removal, usually 10 to 14 days

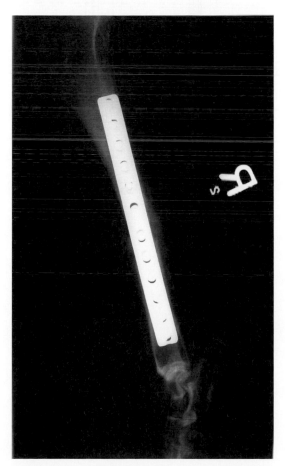

Fig. 10.75 Radiograph (lateral view) of tibial fracture repair. An internal plate and screws were used for fixation.

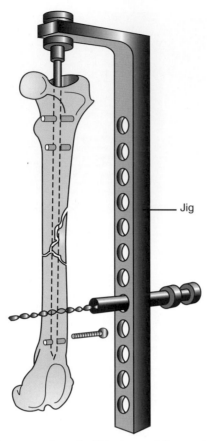

Jig

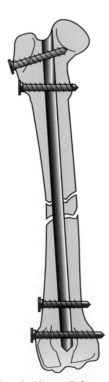

Fig. 10.77 Placement of a nail within the medullary cavity using an interlocking nail jig.

Fig. 10.78 Completed interlocking nail fracture repair. Note the two screws at proximal and distal ends of the bone used for securing the nail.

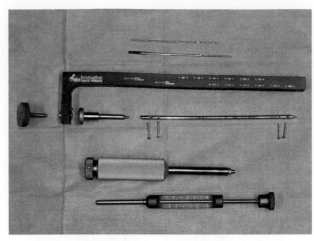

Fig. 10.79 Interlocking nail and instrument set.

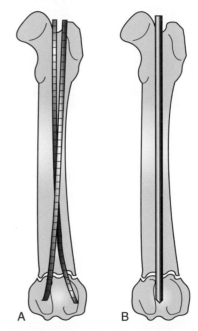

A   B

Fig. 10.80 Intramedullary pins. A, Stacked. B, Single.

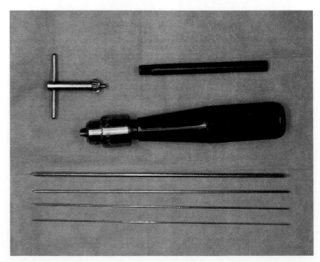

Fig. 10.81 Jacob's chuck (used to drive pins through bone) and intramedullary pins.

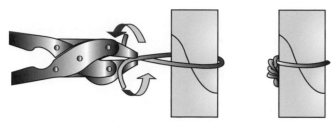

Fig. 10.82 Full-cerclage wire application for fracture stabilization.

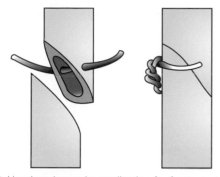

Fig. 10.83 Hemicerclage wire application for fracture stabilization.

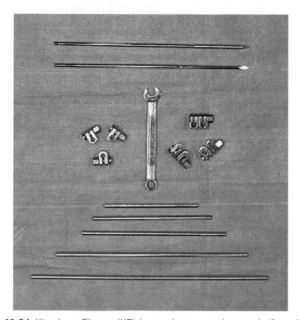

Fig. 10.84 Kirschner-Ehmer (KE) bars, clamps, and wrench (for adjustment of clamps) used for external fixation.

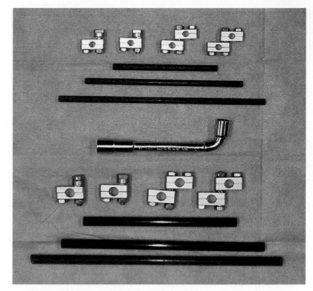

Fig. 10.85 SK rods, clamps, and wrench (for adjustment of clamps) used for external fixation.

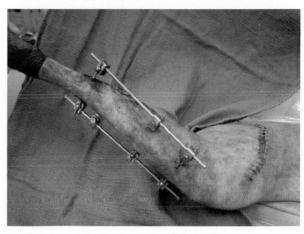

Fig. 10.86 External fixation fracture repair of tibia and fibula in a dog.

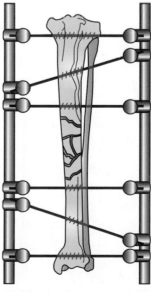

Fig. 10.87 External fixation fracture repair of tibia and fibula.

after surgery. Follow-up radiographs are taken every 4 to 6 weeks postoperatively to monitor bone healing. Young animals may need to be rechecked more frequently because of the rapid rate of bone healing and increased risk of angular complications. Internal fixation is not routinely removed unless a complication involves the implant.

External Fixation

External fixation used as primary repair includes casts, rigid splints, SK fixation, Kirschner-Ehmer (KE) fixation, and ring fixation (Figs. 10.84 to 10.87). As with internal fixation, external fixation requires specialized equipment and has many more applications beyond the scope of this chapter.

External fixation devices stabilize the bones or fracture from the exterior of the limb. These devices use threaded cross-pins that are drilled into the bone and then attached to bars with clamps, nuts and bolts, or aluminum rings to make an external tension device. This will provide rigid stability until the fracture has time to heal. Once the fracture has closed, external fixation is removed. With any external fixation device, weekly to biweekly appointments are needed for fixator adjustments, cleaning of pin tracks, and bandage changes. External fixators are an affordable treatment option for long-bone fractures or temporary joint immobilization. They are not appropriate for fractures that may involve the pelvis or pelvic joints. External fixation devices can be adjusted to best fit the fracture types and locations. The devices can be continually modified or changed throughout the healing period.

The *ring fixator,* or circular fixator, is a type of external fixator that uses different-sized rings (usually three or four) and various types of pins (Figs. 10.88 to 10.89). These pins are drilled through the bone and attached to the ring using clamps. The pin is then put under tension to pull the fracture back into alignment and is secured to the ring frame. Ring fixators have many uses in orthopedic surgery (see other texts).

Postoperative care. Postoperative care for external fixators and ring fixators includes periodic visits for cleaning of pin tracts and tightening of clamps. In most cases the external bars or rings need to be padded and wrapped to prevent trauma to the patient and to reduce the risk that the fixator will be caught on objects (e.g., bedding material, crate, furniture). Radiographs should be taken postoperatively and then every 4 weeks until the fixator is removed. Activity should be restricted for the first 4 weeks, then left to the veterinarian's discretion.

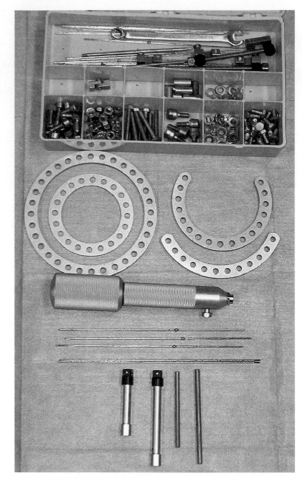

Fig. 10.89 External ring fixation set.

Complications with Fixation

The following complications may occur with internal or external fixation:

- Nonunion
- Malunion
- Delayed union
- Aseptic loosening
- Infection

Casts and Splints

Casts and splints are other external coaptation devices available for closed reduction of fractures at low cost and requiring no surgery. Anesthesia is necessary to sedate and relax the animal so that the fracture can be reduced, then splinted or cast. A radiograph is essential to ensure proper alignment before and after coaptation is applied. Splints work well on small, young, fast-healing animals. Splints are best suited for injuries that are distal to the elbow or stifle, as this allows fixation of the joints above and below the fracture site.

When fiberglass or plaster cast material is used, periodic changes can be difficult. A cast cutter or oscillating saw is needed to cut the cast, and specialized cast spreaders are required to remove the cast easily from the limb. Most patients require sedation for cast and splint changes, so they are still and

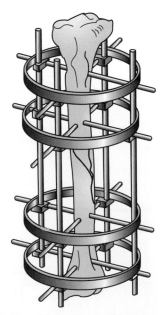

Fig. 10.88 External ring fixator of long-bone fracture.

pain free during the procedure. A sedated or anesthetized animal is also less likely to react to the loud noises associated with the oscillating saw. Most casts require additional support, such as a walking bar, to prevent normal damage to the cast from walking. Casts need to be checked at least every 1 to 2 weeks.

Splints used as primary coaptation devices are easier to manage and change than casts. As with casts, however, splints are suited only for fractures that are distal to the elbow and stifle. Any animal with a splint should have the bandage changed and the fracture rechecked once a week.

Casts and splints require similar care. They must be kept clean and dry and checked for slippage and mutilation by the animal. Any swelling in the toes or signs of malodor should also be noted. If observed, these changes need to be addressed immediately. Radiographs must be taken more often to confirm that fracture alignment and orientation have not changed. Any animal with a cast or splint must be confined to a crate or small room, with no opportunity to run, jump, play, climb stairs, or have free access to the outside until the fracture is healed.

Complications with casts and splints. The following complications may occur with casts or splints:

- Skin irritation
- Skin ulcers
- Nonunion
- Malunion
- Delayed union
- Infection

Amputation

Amputation involves the complete removal of a limb from the body. Common indications for amputation include trauma resulting in severe soft tissue damage or irreparable fractures and neurologic injuries (e.g., brachial plexus avulsion). Other indications are neoplasia, ischemic necrosis, unmanageable arthritis, and severe congenital deformities. Both hind limb and forelimb amputations are considered major surgeries and should be performed only with a thorough knowledge of the patient's physical status. Preanesthetic blood tests, including CBC, chemistry panel, electrolyte status, and blood type and crossmatch, should be obtained before surgery whenever possible. The patient's preoperative condition is extremely important because a large amount of fluid, electrolytes, and blood is lost when the limb is removed. Patients should be stabilized before surgery with appropriate fluid, electrolyte, and blood replacement therapy. A balanced electrolyte solution should also be administered throughout the procedure to help maintain hydration and blood pressure.

A variety of techniques exist for removal of the forelimb and hind limb. Forelimb amputation can be achieved by **disarticulation** of the shoulder joint or by removal of the scapula. Scapular removal is faster, easier, and allows for a more cosmetically favorable result than shoulder disarticulation. Hind limb amputation involves either midshaft femoral amputation or disarticulation of the coxofemoral joint. Midshaft amputation is considerably easier to perform than hip disarticulation. All techniques involve severing the muscles at their origins or insertions or directly through the muscle belly (Fig. 10.90).

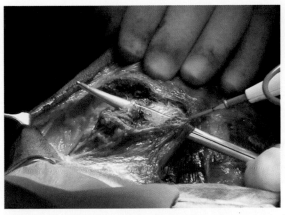

Fig. 10.90 Injection of the femoral nerve with local anesthetic before transection.

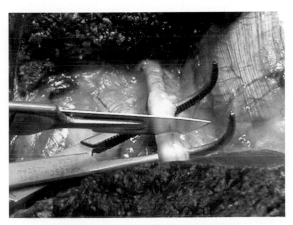

Fig. 10.91 Transection of the femoral nerve.

Major nerves are then isolated and directly injected with a local anesthetic before they are transected (Fig. 10.91). Local nerve blocks contribute significantly to postoperative pain control. Arteries and veins are isolated from surrounding tissues. Arteries are usually ligated first, thus allowing blood to drain through the venous system. In patients with neoplasia, however, veins are ligated first to limit the dissemination of tumor cells. Figs. 10.92 and 10.93 show an amputated limb and the postoperative appearance of a disarticulated coxofemoral joint.

Pain management is critical for amputation patients. A variety of analgesic protocols are currently available and are often used in combination for effective prevention of postoperative discomfort. A brachial plexus block is an excellent way to provide analgesia for a forelimb amputation. Epidural anesthesia should be performed preoperatively for a rear limb amputation and can be achieved with various drugs. Morphine is often used in forelimb amputations, and an opioid and local anesthetic are commonly used in hind limb amputations. Epidural anesthesia with both an opioid and a local anesthetic is extremely effective in controlling postoperative pain. The author refers the reader to other textbooks for more information about nerve blocks. As mentioned, intraoperative visualization of the nerves allows direct injection of local anesthetic before

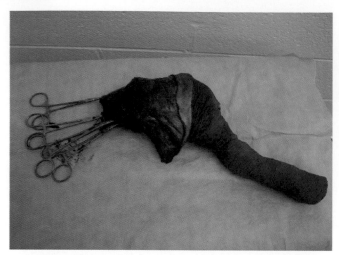

Fig. 10.92 Disarticulated amputation of the hind limb after surgery.

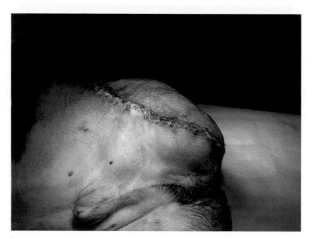

Fig. 10.93 Postoperative surgical site of hind limb amputation (disarticulated).

transection. Systemic injections of opioids and nonsteroidal antiinflammatory drugs (NSAIDs) are often administered postoperatively. Fentanyl is an opioid analgesic that can be administered for postoperative pain and will last for days. The fentanyl patch allows slow, continuous administration of fentanyl over 72 hours. The patch is applied to a clipped area of the animal's skin immediately after surgery. Transdermal fentanyl (Recuvyra®) is applied between the shoulder blades and can control pain for up to 4 days. Clients must be informed of the potential of exposure to transdermal fentanyl so appropriate caution measures can be implemented when the patient is discharged.

Postoperative Considerations and Instructions

Drain placement may be done during the procedure to inhibit seroma formation postamputation. Similarly, a bandage may be placed to limit swelling postoperatively. The drain is generally removed 24 hours postsurgery.

Clients should be educated in limiting exercise and assisting mobility with a towel or sling, especially in large- and giant-breed dogs, as the patient adjusts to the loss of the limb.

Cranial Cruciate Repair
Indications

Cranial cruciate ligament (CCL) ruptures are also referred to as anterior cruciate ligament (ACL) injury or "football player's knee" in human patients. CCL surgical repair should be performed for a partial or complete rupture of the ligament. Both the cranial and the caudal cruciate ligaments act as major stabilizing structures in the knee. The cruciate ligaments originate on either side of the femoral condyle, then course across the intercondylar fossa and attach on opposite sides of the tibia (Fig. 10.94). These ligaments function as the primary check against hyperextension of the stifle joint and limit internal rotation of the tibia. Rupture of the CCL causes instability of the stifle, which leads to degenerative changes in the joint, including synovitis, degeneration of articular cartilage, osteophyte formation, and capsular fibrosis. The medial meniscus is commonly damaged in dogs with CCL rupture. The meniscus is a fibrocartilaginous structure between the femur and tibia that functions to cushion and center the joint. CCL rupture most often causes a bucket-handle type of tear in the medial meniscus.

Rupture of the CCL is the most common cause of hind limb lameness in the dog. Ligament failure can result from both traumatic (acute) and degenerative (chronic) causes. Currently, degenerative causes are the most common reason for CCL rupture. Osteoarthritic changes act as a precursor to CCL

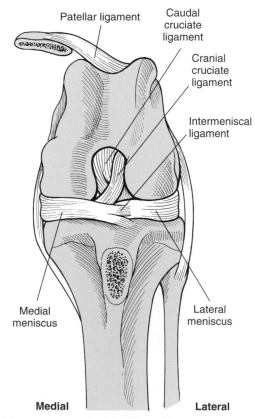

Fig. 10.94 Orientation of the cruciate ligaments and menisci. (From Fossum TW, Hedlund CS, Hulse DA, et al: Small animal surgery, ed 4, St Louis, 2013, Mosby.)

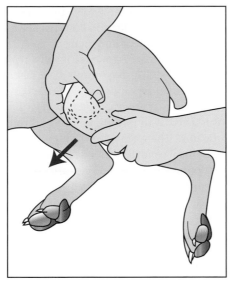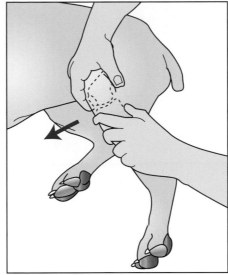

Fig. 10.95 Cranial drawer test. To examine for cruciate ligament injury, place the thumb of one hand over the lateral fabella and the index finger over the patella. Stabilize the femur with this hand. Place the thumb of the opposite hand caudal to the fibular head with the index finger on the tibial tuberosity. With the stifle flexed and then extended, attempt to move the tibia cranially and distally to the femur. (From Fossum TW, Hedlund CS, Hulse DA, et al: Small animal surgery, ed 4, St Louis, 2013, Mosby.)

weakening and rupture. Reports also indicate that 37% of dogs with a unilateral CCL tear will rupture the contralateral ligament within 2 years, indicating that degenerative processes often occur in both stifle joints.

Traumatic rupture results from hyperextension of the stifle joint or excessive internal rotation of the tibia. The CCL becomes tightly twisted, and the excessive mechanical forces cause the ligament to tear. Dogs are often presented with a history of running and catching the leg in a hole, trapping the leg in a fence or gate, or jumping to catch an object (e.g., Frisbee). Traumatic injuries account for approximately 20% of CCL ruptures.

Dogs that have sustained an acute rupture present with significant hind limb lameness. However, the degree of lameness varies widely with the increasing chronicity of the injury. The hind leg is usually carried in flexion, and the toe may touch the ground when the patient is at rest. Dogs may resist manipulation of the stifle joint because of the pain from acute inflammation. Joint effusion may also be palpable adjacent to the patellar tendon.

The major diagnostic tests for CCL injury include palpation, the tibial compression test, and the cranial drawer test (Fig. 10.95). Palpation of the affected leg often reveals muscle atrophy, pain, joint effusion, and asymmetry. Flexion and extension of the stifle joint may result in an audible click associated with displacement of the medial meniscus. Examination of the affected joint reveals a positive cranial drawer sign (cranial displacement of the tibia) and increased internal rotation of the tibia with joint flexion.

Special Instruments

A variety of retractors are typically used for CCL surgery. Hohmann retractors allow inspection of the internal surfaces of

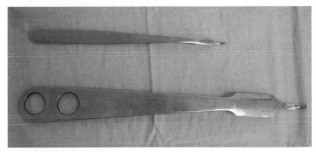

Fig. 10.96 Hohmann retractors.

the joint (Fig. 10.96). Steinmann pins and a Jacob's chuck are used to drill holes in the tibia. Many orthopedic surgeons use a high-speed drill and drill bits to drill holes. Cruciate needles allow the passage of suture through dense tendons and tissues. SECUROS currently offers a crimping system that is used for extracapsular repairs (Fig. 10.97). Both 40- and 80-lb-test nylon is available. A distractor is used to place tension on the suture loop and can be locked to check cranial drawer. Crimp tubes are then placed and crimped (with a special crimping tool) to hold the suture in place.

Patient Positioning

The patient may be placed in dorsal or lateral recumbency with the affected leg up for CCL repair. The leg should be clipped from the hip to the tarsus. An examination glove should be placed on the foot to cover the unshaven area. The leg should be suspended while it is scrubbed to ensure complete and circumferential sterility. It is important to prepare the limb in this suspended position to allow the greatest amount of manipulation during surgery (Fig. 10.98).

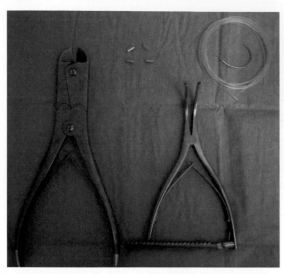

Fig. 10.97 Cruciate repair system (SECUROS, Fiskdale, MA). *Left to right,* Crimper, crimp tubes, distractor, 80-lb fishing line, and needle.

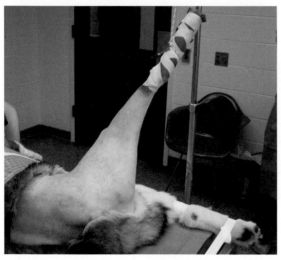

Fig. 10.98 Lateral recumbency positioning with suspended leg is usually appropriate for orthopedic surgical preparation of a limb.

Patient Draping

The surgeon should grasp the suspended leg in a sterile manner, and the foot and tarsus should be covered with an appropriately sized stockinette. The leg is held suspended, and a three-cornered draping technique is used at the hip. To improve control of postoperative infections, many orthopedic surgeons employ antimicrobial incise drapes (Ioban®; 3M, Minneapolis, MN) on the limb, instead of stockinette. This type of drape helps reduce the risk of microbes transferring into the wound because of the antimicrobial material contained in the drape adhesive. The drape is placed during patient preparation, and the incision is made directly through the drape. This drape can be left on postoperatively to control infection

Cranial Cruciate Ligament Repair

A variety of surgical techniques have been designed to restore stability to the stifle and limit secondary degenerative joint

disease. It is recommended that the joint capsule be opened with each technique to allow visualization and removal of the damaged ligament and menisci.

Intracapsular techniques involve replacement or reconstruction of the CCL using various materials, including biologic tissues (patellar tendon and fascia lata) and synthetic suture material. The joint is approached laterally (Fig. 10.99), and a graft of tissue is isolated. A tunnel is then drilled through the cranial surface of the tibia. The graft is fed through the tunnel and over the top of the lateral condyle, thereby reconstructing the CCL.

Extracapsular techniques are usually faster and easier to perform than intracapsular repairs. Extracapsular repairs involve placement of sutures outside the stifle joint and include tightrope and fascial imbrication techniques. The joint is approached laterally, and the appropriate suture (e.g., monofilament nylon, nylon fishing line) is loaded onto a properly sized cruciate needle. The needle is passed around the fabella and then through the patellar ligament. A hole is drilled through the tibial crest with a Steinmann pin, and the suture is passed through the hole (Fig. 10.100). The stifle is then flexed into a normal standing position, and the cranial drawer test is performed. Once the suture is under the appropriate tension, it is tied or crimped into place. The retinaculum should be closed with a vertical mattress pattern to provide appropriate imbrication of the joint capsule.

Both intracapsular and extracapsular reconstruction techniques rely on a recreation of the passive constraints of the stifle joint. In recent years, a technique has been developed that recreates joint stability by altering the active constraints of the joint. CCL rupture causes the tibia to slide forward and the femur to fall back, creating a shear force referred to as *cranial tibial thrust.* The tibial plateau–leveling osteotomy (TPLO) functions to change the angle of the tibia, thereby directly altering joint mechanics and creating a new plateau that eliminates cranial tibial thrust. The incision is made on the medial side of the limb. To achieve the appropriate angle of the tibia, an osteotomy of the tibial plateau is performed, the plateau is reangled, and a bone plate is placed to secure the osteotomy. Fig. 10.101 shows postoperative radiographs of a TPLO surgery. TPLO can be used in all breeds but is highly recommended for young, large- and giant- breed dogs.

Postoperative Considerations and Instructions

A soft bandage should be placed on the limb for 48 hours after CCL repair to protect the surgical site and reduce swelling. The patient should return in 14 days for a recheck and suture removal.

The most important postoperative consideration is exercise restriction. Dogs should be restricted to short leash walks for elimination only for at least 6 weeks after surgery. Activity can then be gradually increased over a 12-week period. Owners are discouraged from allowing their animals to run free, jump, climb stairs, and play rambunctiously with other animals. Failure to comply with strict exercise restriction may result in repair failure and the need for a second surgery.

Because CCL repairs are considered moderately painful, pain management is a major focus during the recovery period.

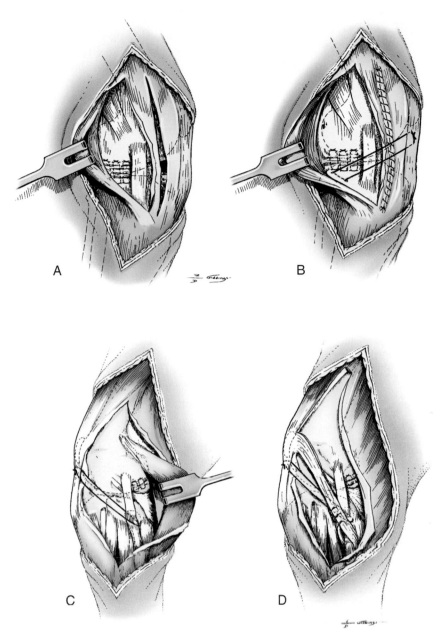

Fig. 10.99 Treatment of midsubstance rupture of the caudal cruciate ligament. The stifle has been exposed by a medial approach to the stifle joint combined with an approach to the medial collateral ligament and caudomedial compartment of the joint. A, The caudomedial joint capsule is imbricated with mattress sutures (3/0–0) placed vertically with respect to the joint, caudal to the medial collateral ligament to enhance periarticular fibrosis. B, The joint capsule is closed, and a heavy gauge suture (0–4 braided polyester, or nylon leader line) is placed from the proximal patellar ligament to a bone tunnel placed in the caudomedial corner of the proximal tibia. C, The suture is tightened with the stifle joint at a normal standing angle in a neutral position (caudal drawer is reduced). The skin is retracted to expose the lateral side of the joint, the biceps femoris fascia is incised and retracted, exposing the lateral collateral ligament and caudolateral joint capsule. The caudolateral joint capsule caudal to the lateral collateral ligament is imbricated with mattress sutures, and a heavy gauge suture is placed from the proximal patellar ligament to encircle the head of the fibula. D, The suture is similarly tightened with the stifle joint at a normal standing angle in a neutral position (caudal drawer is reduced). Further augmentation can be achieved with a strip of fascia lata that is dissected free proximally and left attached to the lateral border of the patella distally. This fascial strip is passed around the fibular head, pulled taut, and sutured to itself and the surrounding fascia lata.(From Tobias K, Johnston S: Veterinary surgery: small animal, St Louis, 2012, Saunders.)

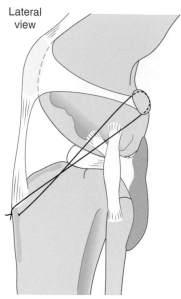

Lateral view

Fig. 10.100 Extracapsular reconstruction using a heavy, nonabsorbable suture. The suture passes through the deep fascia surrounding the fabella and through a predrilled hole in the tibial crest. Tying or crimping the suture eliminates the cranial drawer. (From Fossum TW, Hedlund CS, Hulse DA, et al: Small animal surgery, ed 4, St Louis, 2013, Mosby.)

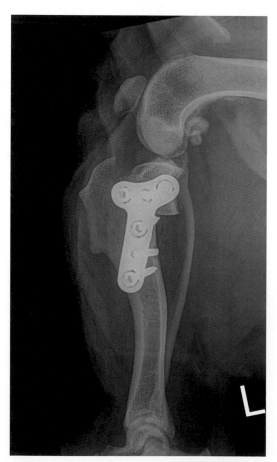

Fig. 10.101 Postoperative radiograph of an 8 year old Corgi.

Perioperative pain control involves injection of a local anesthetic directly into the joint. Preoperative epidural anesthesia greatly helps limit pain postoperatively. A new extended-release formula of bupivacaine, Nocita® (Artana Therapeutics, Leawood, KS), has been U.S. Food and Drug Administration (FDA) approved for use in CCL surgeries. Nocita is used in the closure layers and gives excellent postoperative analgesia.

Animals are often treated immediately postoperatively with a variety of injectable pain medications, including opioids and NSAIDs. Animals are then often sent home with instructions for the owner to administer an oral NSAID (e.g., carprofen) for several days after surgery. Additionally, cold packing of the incision site and stifle for 3 days postoperatively aids in controlling swelling of the joint, which can contribute to pain.

In recent years, a rigorous rehabilitation program has been advocated as part of the standard postoperative care for patients with CCL repair. Rehabilitation programs promote wound healing and decrease muscle spasm, adhesion formation, and edema while increasing muscle strength and joint range of motion (ROM). Typical programs include low-impact exercises (e.g., swimming), passive ROM exercises, heat, and whirlpool therapy.

Box 10.18 shows an example of a surgery report for a CCL repair.

Onychectomy

Definition

Onychectomy, or declawing, is the removal of the claw and its associated third phalanx and is an orthopedic procedure. The distal phalanx is surgically amputated (Fig. 10.102).

Indications

An onychectomy is an elective procedure to prevent the cat from scratching furniture of the owners. Occasionally it is a nonelective procedure required to remove neoplasia of the claw and/or phalanx or to remove an infected nail bed. Elective declaws are usually performed between 3 and 12 months of age and are typically done on the front paws only. Ideally, a declawed cat should be kept indoors, but in the event that the cat were to get outside it would still have its back claws as a means of defense. This is a painful procedure, and proper analgesia and pain management protocols need to be initiated before surgery.

Special Instruments

The procedure can be done with one of three methods: use of the Rescoe Nail Trimmer technique (Rescoe, Walled Lake, MI), with a scalpel blade, or by the CO_2 laser. Each requires its own instrumentation. A tourniquet will be required to control hemorrhage.

Patient Positioning

The cat is typically placed in lateral recumbency. The feet are not clipped unless the cat is a long-haired breed, but they are surgically scrubbed. If the laser method is used, alcohol should not be used because it will likely ignite when the laser beam hits

BOX 10.18 Surgery Report: Cranial Cruciate Ligament Repair

Animal Hospital Name

Owner: John Doe
Address: 555 Sterling Lane
Jupiter, NY 55555
Phone number: 555-5555
Animal Name: Sasha
Animal #: 65656501
Species: Canine
Breed: Labrador
DOB: 05/05/07
Date of Surgery: 12/03/2011
Primary Surgeon: Dr. Vet
Assistant: Technician Scrub

Diagnosis or Preoperative Signs: Cranial cruciate ligament rupture.
Surgical Procedure: Right stifle arthrotomy, extracapsular cranial cruciate repair.
Implants: 80-lb-test fishing line, two SECUROS clamps.

Description of Surgical Procedure

Surgical Approach: An 8- to 10-cm lateral parapatellar skin incision was made at the right stifle, and the underlying subcutaneous tissues were incised. The retinaculum and the joint capsule of the stifle were incised, and the interior of the stifle joint was visualized.

Surgical Pathology: Complete rupture of the cranial cruciate ligament.
Surgical Procedure: The remnants of the torn cranial cruciate ligament were removed, and the joint was explored. No meniscal damage was evident at this time. The joint was lavaged with sterile saline, and the joint capsule was closed with 2-0 PDS in an interrupted suture pattern. Bupivacaine (10 mL) was injected into the joint capsule. A hole was then made in the tibial tuberosity with a Steinmann pin. A wire passer was used to pass 80-lb fishing line behind the lateral femoral fabellar ligament. The fishing line was then passed (medial to lateral) through the hole in the tibial tuberosity and then under the patellar ligament. A SECUROS clamp was then placed at the end of each line. A distractor was used to tighten the lines until the joint was stable. The joint was checked for drawer as well as range of motion. A SECUROS crimper was then used to crimp each of the clamps three times. The surgical site was lavaged with sterile saline and closed routinely.

Closure:

Joint capsule: 2-0 PDS in interrupted cruciate suture pattern.
Retinaculum: 2-0 PDS in interrupted suture pattern.
Subcutaneous tissue: 3-0 Monocryl in continuous suture pattern.
Skin: 3-0 nylon in interrupted suture pattern, followed by some skin staples.

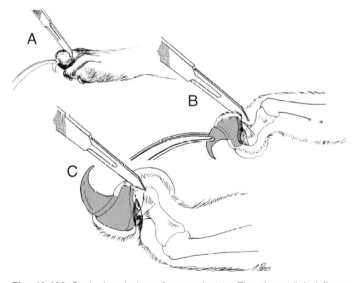

Fig. 10.102 Scalpel technique for cat declaw. The deep digital flexor tendon is filleted from its attachment to the base of P3. (From Birchard S, Sherding R: Saunders manual of small animal practice, ed 3, St Louis, 2006, Saunders.)

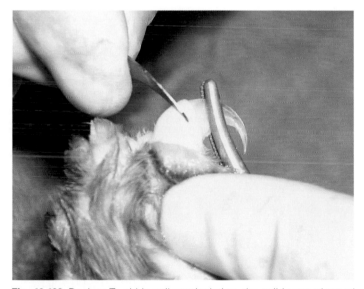

Fig. 10.103 Declaw. To aid in nail manipulation, the nail is not trimmed before surgery. (From Bassert JM, McCurnin DM, editors: McCurnin's clinical textbook for veterinary technicians, ed 7, St Louis, 2010, Elsevier.)

the prepared area. The toenails should not be clipped because their length will aid in nail manipulation during the procedure (Fig. 10.103). A tourniquet is placed on the limb, but not tightened, before aseptic preparation.

Patient Draping

A fenestrated drape should be sufficient.

Declaw Procedure

Once the foot has been scrubbed, a tourniquet should be positioned distal to the elbow and tightened. Placing the tourniquet proximal to the elbow can lead to radial nerve damage (Fig. 10.104). At this time, a nerve block may be performed (Fig. 10.105). A ring block may be administered preoperatively to limit pain during and after surgery and

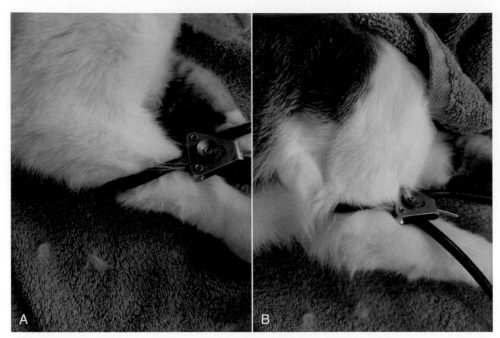

Fig. 10.104 Declaw. A tourniquet should always be placed distal to the elbow (A) rather than proximal to the elbow (B) to help prevent permanent radial nerve damage.

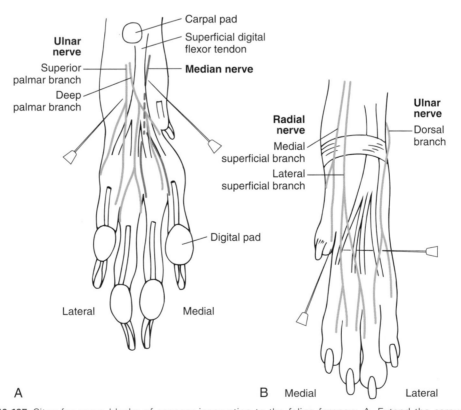

Fig. 10.105 Sites for nerve blocks of sensory innervation to the feline forepaw. A, Extend the carpus and palpate the superficial digital flexor tendon along the palmar aspect of the paw. Block the median nerve with bupivacaine just medial to the superficial digital flexor tendon. Similarly, block the palmar branches of the ulnar nerve along the lateral superficial digital flexor tendon. B, Block dorsal digital nerves II to V by inserting the needle from lateral to medial just distal to the carpus. Inject bupivacaine as the needle is withdrawn. Block dorsal digital nerve I at the articulation between metacarpal I and II with bupivacaine. (From Fossum TW, Hedlund CS, Hulse DA, et al: Small animal surgery, ed 4, St Louis, 2013, Mosby.)

helps to decrease inhalant anesthetic levels during the procedure as well.

For the Rescoe technique, the claw is extended cranially and the blade is positioned on the dorsal surface of the digit between the second and third phalanges. Care must be exercised to avoid cutting the footpad. As the cutting blade of the nail trimmer is advanced, the pad should be moved caudally and the nail should be rotated dorsally and caudally. This process is repeated for each digit.

With the blade technique, a No. 12 scalpel blade is used to excise the third phalanx. First the collateral ligaments are cut, and then the bone itself is cut away from the pad and underlying tissue.

For both the Rescoe and blade techniques, sutures or surgical glue can be placed to appose the skin edges after nail removal. If glue is used, it should not be placed on exposed bone or dropped into the wound. The wound should be closed first, and then a drop of glue added. Paws are bandaged snugly with gauze and tape. Care must be taken not to make the bandage too tight because vascular compromise and skin sloughing could occur. Once the bandage has been placed, the tourniquet can be removed.

The last technique uses a laser to disarticulate the third phalanx. A tourniquet is not necessary with this procedure because the laser provides hemostasis while cutting. Saline-soaked sponges are needed to cover the remainder of the cat's foot, all instruments, and the surgeon's fingers. The sponges prevent burning by absorbing the extra energy given off by the laser. Laser surgery is discussed in more depth later in the chapter.

The patient preparation for a laser declaw is similar to preparation for the standard declaw. Care must be taken not to use flammable liquids (alcohol) when prepping the paw skin. The surgeon will choose the wattage, mode, and tip size used for the procedure. The technician will ensure that the surgery room and its occupants are "laser safe." A hemostat can be positioned on the claw for manipulation and extension of the nail. A 360-degree circumferential incision is made through the skin and the underlying fascia between the second and third phalanges. This incision exposes the common digital extensor tendon. The laser is then used to transect the common digital extensor tendon as well as the deeper synovial layer at its insertion on the distal phalanx. Gentle distraction of the nail at this point exposes the collateral ligaments. The collateral ligaments are then incised bilaterally, and the joint between the second and third phalanges can be disarticulated. The third phalanx is further freed up by laser transection of the deep digital flexor tendon caudal to its ungual process. Care should be taken to avoid thermal damage (char) to the digital pad and other soft tissue attachments, which can be caused by misdirection of the laser beam. This procedure should be repeated on each remaining claw.

At the end of the laser procedure, each digit should be meticulously examined. Any char noted on the digit should be removed with sterile gauze. Bandages can be placed if significant hemorrhage is noted, but the laser declaw procedure is usually associated with minimal or no hemorrhage.

Postoperative Considerations and Instructions

It is imperative that multimodal pain management be used for a declaw procedure. Pain medication should be given for at least 4 to 5 days postoperatively. Consider sustained release buprenorphine injection or fentanyl patch. Robenacoxib (Onsior®; Elanco, Greenfield, IN) is an NSAID choice if the patient meets the weight and age requirements for its use. Bandages are removed within 24 hours, before the cat leaves the hospital. The owner should be advised to provide shredded paper or pelleted litter to prevent contamination of the paws with clay or clumping litter. Regular litter can be reintroduced after 10 days. The cat's activity should be restricted and excessive grooming should be discouraged until the paws have healed.

In addition to the general postoperative and discharge instructions for any declaw surgery, more specific recommendations exist for laser declaw surgery. Use of laser is purported to result in less pain and inflammation, but pain is still present. As with any procedure, appropriate analgesics should be administered postoperatively. Slight epithelial swelling is normal after surgery and may aid the redundant epithelium in covering the surgical site. Closure of the laser declaw site is usually not indicated. In most cases the patient bears weight on the paws the same day or 1 day postoperatively.

MINIMALLY INVASIVE SURGERY

Biopsy and Mass Removal

Biopsy and removal of a mass are important procedures in veterinary medicine. A biopsy is often recommended before mass removal. The biopsy sample is submitted to a lab, and histopathological examination of the sample is performed. Additionally, the histopathological report provides important information on the biologic and clinical behavior of the mass, allowing the formulation of an appropriate treatment plan and prognosis. Current biopsy techniques include fine-needle aspiration, impression smear, punch, bone, excisional, and incisional biopsies.

Fine-Needle Aspiration Biopsy

Fine-needle aspiration (FNA) represents one of the simplest methods for cytologic evaluation of a mass. The technique is easy to perform, has minimal morbidity, and usually does not require sedation; however, FNA biopsy typically has a low diagnostic yield (Box 10.19).

BOX 10.19 Fine-Needle Aspiration Technique

1. Obtain a 22-gauge or 20-gauge needle and 5-mL syringe. Place the needle into the mass.
2. Apply negative pressure by pulling back on the hub of the syringe.
3. Withdraw the needle and syringe from the mass, and then remove the needle from the syringe.
4. Fill the syringe with air, replace the needle, and gently blow the fluid and cells onto a glass slide.

This method is generally performed several times to obtain representative samples.

Impression Smears

Impression smears are as simple to perform as FNA biopsy. This technique is especially useful for ulcerated surface tumors and is often performed on freshly cut surfaces. Impression smears of excised masses can also be easily made before the samples are placed into formalin (Box 10.20).

Needle Punch Biopsy

Needle punch biopsy instruments are currently manufactured by a variety of companies. Instruments are equipped with either a cutting or a core biopsy needle and are available as manual and automatic devices (Fig. 10.106). These devices take a small piece of tissue (approximately the size of pencil lead) for histologic examination (Figs. 10.107 and 10.108). These procedures are minimally invasive and generally are performed on sedated patients. Ultrasound-guided needle punch biopsies of various internal organs, including the liver, spleen, and prostate, are also common procedures (Box 10.21).

Punch Biopsy

The punch biopsy technique is used primarily for external skin and oral masses. It has the advantage of providing a larger surface sample; however, it does not penetrate deeply into the mass (Fig. 10.109). Patients are generally placed under general anesthesia to undergo this procedure (Box 10.22).

Bone Biopsy

The most common instruments used to obtain bone biopsy samples are the Michele trephine (see Fig. 10.109) and Jamshidi bone biopsy needle (Fig. 10.110). Bone biopsies are often painful and therefore are usually performed with the patient under general anesthesia. The Jamshidi needle biopsy is less invasive but provides a smaller sample size than other methods. The Michele trephine technique removes a larger sample of bone, increasing the diagnostic yield, but it also increases the likelihood of a pathologic fracture at the biopsy site (Box 10.23).

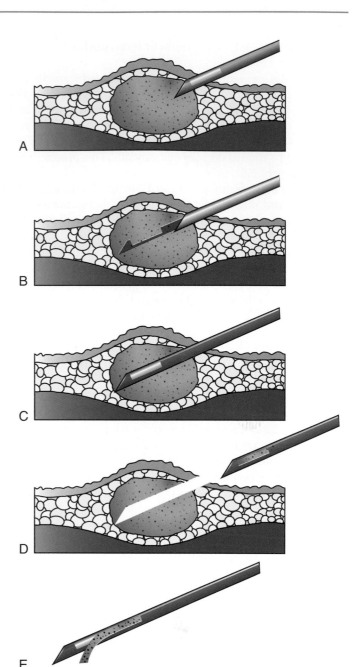

A
B
C
D
E

Fig. 10.107 Use of the manual biopsy needle requires both hands and can be awkward, resulting in more discomfort for the patient and samples of lower quality. A, The tip of needle is inserted just into the tumor. B, The inner needle is advanced without advancing the outer needle. C, Tissue from the tumor drops into the trough of the inner needle, and the outer needle is advanced to cover the inner needle, thereby cutting tissue within the trough free from the main mass. D, With the inner needle still completely within the outer needle, thus protecting the sample, the entire unit is removed. E, The inner needle is advanced beyond the end of the outer needle to allow the sample to be removed from the trough of the inner needle. (Modified from Mehler SJ, Bennet A: Surgical oncology of exotic animals. Vet Clin Exotic Anim Pract 7:783–805, 2004.)

BOX 10.20 Impression Smear Technique

1. Gently blot the surface of the mass with a paper towel to remove any excess blood and exudates.
2. Gently touch the surface of the mass to several areas of a glass slide. Take care not to twist or rub the slide against the mass, because doing so would crush cells and destroy the integrity of the sample.

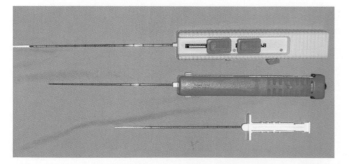

Fig. 10.106 Three varieties of needle punch biopsy instruments.

Incisional Biopsy

Incisional biopsies are generally performed only after cytology or needle core biopsies have failed to provide a diagnostic sample. A small wedge of the tumor is removed from the mass and submitted for histopathologic examination (Fig. 10.111).

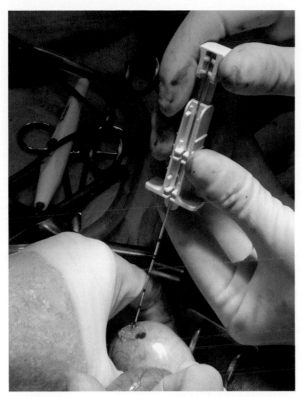

Fig. 10.108 Manual needle punch biopsy of the kidney during an exploratory laparotomy.

1. Clip and aseptically scrub the area to be sampled.
2. Block the overlying skin and muscle with a local anesthetic.
3. Hold the mass with one hand, and make a small stab incision into the overlying skin.
4. Insert the end of the needle through the stab incision (the instrument is fired, and the inner needle is advanced into the mass).
5. Withdraw the entire instrument from the mass.
6. Gently remove the sample from the sample chamber with a cotton swab or needle.

Excisional Biopsy

An excisional biopsy involves the complete removal of a mass (see Fig. 10.112). Excisional biopsies are generally performed only on benign skin tumors or when the removal of the organ is indicated.

Laser Surgery

This section discusses the role of laser surgery in veterinary medicine, laser safety, and the advantages and disadvantages of using lasers as an alternative to traditional surgery.

How Does the Laser Work?

The word *laser* is used as an acronym for "light amplification by stimulated emission of radiation." Lasers create light at distinct wavelengths and distinct delivery parameters. Laser light wavelength and frequency determine the color of the laser light and the way the laser light interacts with its target surface. When

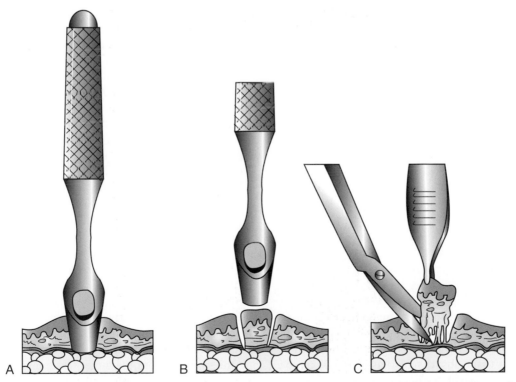

Fig. 10.109 Mechanism of punch biopsy. A, The punch is rotated back and forth over the suspect lesion until sufficient depth has been attained. B, The punch is removed or angled across the base to sever deep attachments. C, The specimen may be gently grasped with thumb forceps and cut off deeply. (From Withrow SJ, MacEwen EG: Withrow and MacEwen's small animal clinical oncology, ed 4, St Louis, 2007, Saunders.)

BOX 10.22   Punch Biopsy Technique

1. The area to be sampled is clipped and aseptically scrubbed.
2. The punch is rotated back and forth over the mass until the punch sits deeply in the lesion.
3. The punch is removed, and a scissors is used to detach the sample from its base.

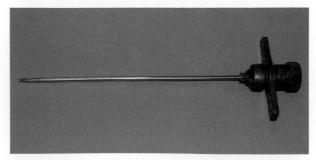

Fig. 10.111 Jamshidi bone biopsy needle.

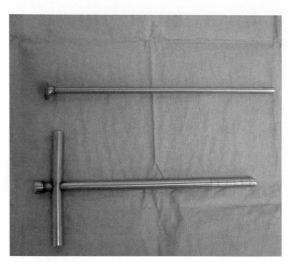

Fig. 10.110 Michele trephine bone biopsy instrument.

BOX 10.23   Bone Biopsy Technique

1. A small incision is made over the center of the lesion.
2. The trephine or needle is pushed through the soft tissues until the bony cortex is reached.
3. The stylet is removed, and the cannula or trephine is advanced through the bony cortex.
4. Once an adequate sample has been obtained, the instrument is removed and a wire is used to push the sample out of the hub of the needle. It is extremely important to avoid pushing the sample out of the tip of the needle because doing so would destroy the architecture of the sample.

laser light hits its target, it may be reflected, absorbed, scattered, or transmitted through the tissues, depending on the type of laser light being used. The types of lasers most often used in veterinary medicine are the carbon dioxide (CO_2) laser, diode laser, and neodymium:yttrium-aluminum-garnet (Nd:YAG) laser. The CO_2 and diode lasers are discussed here.

The clinical functions of the CO_2 and diode lasers consist of ablation, incision, and excision of soft tissue. Both the CO_2 and the diode lasers operate through photothermal laser–tissue interaction. This means that the laser light is absorbed and transformed into heat within the tissue. Water, hemoglobin, melanin, and some proteins absorb different wavelengths of light, causing the tissue to heat. For example, the CO_2 laser is highly absorbed by water. The diode laser is highly absorbed by melanin and hemoglobin.

Heating of the tissue at different temperatures causes certain changes in the tissue. At 42°C to 45°C, blood vessels are destroyed, resulting in necrosis of tissue. As tissue temperatures reach 50°C to 100°C, proteins denature and coagulation occurs, causing irreversible tissue damage. Once tissue temperature surpasses 100°C, solid tissue becomes gaseous vapor and smoke plume. Increased heating of tissue can cause burning, resulting in carbonization of the tissue. This carbonization is called *char*. Charring occurs when tissue absorbs heat faster than it can be released. Heating to this extent results in damage to the surrounding tissue. Carbonization of the tissue also acts as a foreign substance and can hinder wound healing as well as cause inflammation at the site.

11.2.2 CO_2 Lasers versus Diode Lasers

CO_2 lasers are available at a wavelength of 10,600 nanometers (nm) (Fig. 10.113). The CO_2 laser comes equipped with a selection of hand pieces and tips. Tips come in a variety of sizes, ranging from 0.3 mm to 1.4 mm, and specific tips are used for specific surgical procedures. The CO_2 laser is considered a class IV laser system, as are most medical lasers. Lasers are separated into classes I to IV according to the degree of possible safety hazards to patients and users. The CO_2 laser is used predominantly to create surgical incisions, to excise after incision, or for ablation of tissue. Most CO_2 lasers use a noncontact mode in which the laser tip never comes in direct contact with the tissue.

The 10,600-nm wavelength of the CO_2 laser is perfect for incising and vaporization because it is highly absorbed by water. Because most tissues have high water content, the laser energy is absorbed very close to the surface. The effect of the laser energy on tissue is determined by the laser wavelength, target tissue, spot size, power, and exposure (including exposure duration). Because laser wavelength (10,600 nm) and presumably the target tissue are known, the surgeon must choose the settings for the spot size, power, and exposure. *Spot size* refers to the diameter of the aperture. The distance of the tip from the tissue determines the exact spot size on the target tissue. Moving the tip away from the target tissue increases the spot size. Moving the tip closer to the target tissue decreases the spot size. The size of the tip also determines the spot size on the target tissue. Power settings are in watts (W), and the surgeon selects the appropriate wattage for a specific procedure. Power density

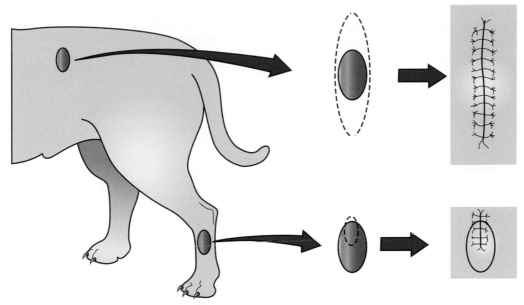

Fig. 10.112 Excisional biopsy (*top*) contrasted with incisional biopsy (*bottom*). The top tumor may be as easy to remove as to biopsy, and removal may not negatively influence other possible treatments (e.g., additional surgery, irradiation). The bottom tumor, however, requires knowledge of the tumor type before excision, because inappropriate removal could compromise a subsequent aggressive excision (short of amputation). Note that the biopsy incision is in a plane that would be included in a subsequent resection. (From Withrow SJ, MacEwen EG: Withrow and MacEwen's small animal clinical oncology, ed 4, St Louis, 2007, Saunders.)

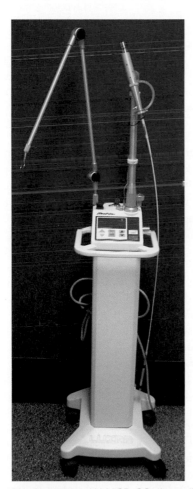

Fig. 10.113 AccuVet Novapulse LX-20SP CO_2 laser (Luxar Lumenis, Woodinville, WA).

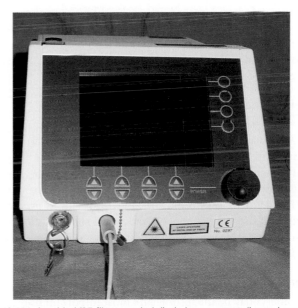

Fig. 10.114 AccuVet V25 fiber-coupled diode laser system (Luxar Lumenis).

depends on the set power, the spot size, and the distance of the tip from the tissue. The *exposure* refers to the duration of the laser beam, or how long the tissue is exposed to the laser beam. The clinician uses spot size, power, and exposure to control the interaction of the CO_2 laser beam and its effects on the tissue.

Available wavelengths for diode lasers in veterinary medicine range from 805 to 980 nm (Fig. 10.114). The diode laser is also considered a class IV laser. Diode lasers are small, compact units that emit wavelengths that are easily transmitted through small, flexible optical fibers, allowing their use with most flexible and rigid endoscopes. Diode lasers also come equipped with a variety of hand pieces and tips. The diode laser can reach its target tissue using a contact mode or a noncontact mode, whereas most CO_2 lasers use a noncontact mode of light transmission. Noncontact fibers are available in squared, cleaved, or polished tips and are more appropriate for ablation procedures. Contact fibers tend to be sculpted and are more appropriate for incisional purposes. Diode laser light has better absorption in hemoglobin and melanin, whereas the CO_2 laser light has better absorption in water. More collateral thermal damage may occur with the diode laser because of the deeper penetration, unlike the absorption of water closer to the surface with the CO_2 laser. Because of the enhanced absorption of hemoglobin, the diode laser may provide more proficient incisions and better hemostasis, especially of larger vessels.

The CO_2 and diode lasers can be used in a continuous mode or a pulse mode. The mode, tip size, and settings chosen by the clinician vary according to the type of procedure performed. When using either the CO_2 or the diode laser, the clinician should start with low power settings and a short duration of exposure until becoming familiar with the effects of the laser on the target tissue. Also, the laser energy should be delivered perpendicularly from the hand piece to the target tissue. When incising tissue, the clinician should apply lateral tension perpendicular to the incision. This maneuver helps reduce the formation of char. A record or log should be kept of each procedure performed as well as the power and duration settings. This task will most likely be the technician's responsibility. A log of procedures will help the surgeon choose settings to use for future procedures.

Laser Procedures in Veterinary Medicine

Lasers may be used for surgical procedures ranging from minor elective procedures (e.g., feline declaw, lump removal) to more extensive procedures (e.g., celiotomy, thoracotomy). Other procedures include canine and feline castration, dewclaw removal, amputation, cystotomy, soft palate resection, oncologic procedures (e.g., neoplasia removal), and ophthalmic procedures. Whether to use laser energy or traditional surgery is ultimately the surgeon's decision. (See Box 10.24 for a list of advantages and disadvantages of laser surgery.)

Laser Safety

Laser safety may be the technician's most important responsibility when assisting with laser surgery. It is imperative that precautions be taken to protect the clinical staff as well as the patient from the array of hazards associated with laser surgery. Many hospitals assign a laser safety officer, often the technician. The safety officer is responsible for following safety guidelines established by the manufacturer of the laser machine or by the American National Standards Institute (Standards ANSI Z136.3-1988 and Z136.1-1993). These guidelines give specific instructions to follow for laser safety and laser use. Most laser companies also provide user and safety training when a hospital purchases a laser machine. Laser surgery should never be performed by anyone who has not had proper training or education about laser use and

---

BOX 10.24 Advantages and Disadvantages of Laser Surgery

Advantages
- More rapid healing time of tissue
- Cauterization of blood vessels during incision
- Sterilization of tissue during incision (less risk of postoperative infection)
- Minimal risk of damage to underlying healthy tissue (CO_2 laser specifically)
- Less need for suturing
- Reduced postoperative discomfort or pain
- Reduced postoperative swelling
- Shorter surgery time in many cases

Disadvantages
- Cost
- Safety
- Need for extensive training to prevent tissue damage

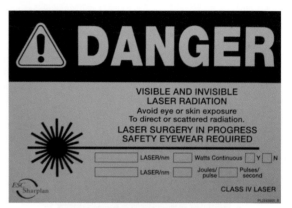

Fig. 10.115 Laser warning signs should be posted on the doors to the surgery room as well as within the surgery room.

---

safety. The ANSI standards recommend that prospective laser users become knowledgeable about policies and procedures, review clinical literature, attend courses for a certain number of hours, consult with an experienced operator of laser surgery, and receive training on specific equipment before operating laser machines.

Laser Hazards

Laser warning signs should be posted in the surgery room as well as on all doors entering it. Fig. 10.115 shows the warning sign for class IV lasers.

Dangers associated with class IV lasers include eye, skin, fire, and smoke plume hazards.

Eye hazards. Everyone in the laser surgery room must wear the eye protection goggles specific for the particular laser light (Fig. 10.116). Different lasers emit different wavelengths, and the protection worn must coincide with the laser wavelength. Scattered reflections from the laser beam can cause serious corneal or retinal damage. The eyes of the patient should also be protected from scattered laser light. When a CO_2 laser is used, moistened sponges can be placed over the eyes for protection because the CO_2 laser beam is absorbed by water. Patient eye shields are also available.

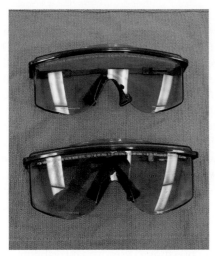

Fig. 10.116 Wavelength-specific eye protection goggles for the diode laser.

Skin hazards. Skin hazards may occur from direct or scattered laser beams. It may be in the clinician's best interest to wear gloves and a gown for added protection.

Fire hazards. Possible fire hazards include the surgical drapes, anesthetic agents, oxygen, animal's fur, alcohol products used in surgical preparation, and methane from flatulence. With the CO_2 laser, wet sponges can be placed around the surgical area for protection of drapes. Any exposed fur around the surgical region can also be moistened with water. A nonalcohol surgical prep (e.g., chlorhexidine or povidone-iodine preparation) should always be used for all laser procedures. The anesthetist should always make sure the cuff of the endotracheal (ET) tube is inflated properly to decrease the chance that gaseous vapor or oxygen will escape. Standard polyvinyl chloride (PVC) tubes may be at risk for damage and ignition during a laser procedure. Laser-safe ET tubes can be purchased for procedures within the oral cavity. Another alternative is to lay moistened sponges around the standard ET tube to prevent a possible fire hazard when CO_2 lasers are used. Because methane is considered another possible source for fire ignition, moistened sponges can be placed within the rectum of the patient during perianal surgical procedures with the CO_2 laser. Fire extinguishers should be readily available in any laser surgery room in the event of unexpected ignition.

Smoke plume hazards. The smoke plume emitted from laser contact with tissue contains toxic and carcinogenic chemicals as well as bacterial and viral particles. An evacuator is usually purchased with the laser machines. Laser procedures should never be performed without an evacuation system. The smoke evacuator should be within 1 to 2 inches of the smoke's origin. Laser surgical masks are also available. Regular surgery room masks may not filter all toxic or infectious particles.

Laparoscopy

A *laparoscopy* is a minimally invasive abdominal procedure performed for the purpose of examining the peritoneal cavity and its viscera. A type of endoscope, called a laparoscope, is placed through a small midline incision or opening into the abdominal wall for inspection of the abdominal contents. Other incisions can be made into the abdominal wall (lateral to midline) for the insertion of laparoscopic instruments through accessory ports. These specialized instruments can be used for biopsy purposes as well as to perform specific procedures (e.g., ovariohysterectomy, gastropexy) within the abdominal cavity. In many cases, laparoscopy can take the place of a full abdominal surgical procedure. In most cases, the procedure affords the patient a swift recovery with less potential for complications. Advantages of laparoscopy are listed in Box 10.25. This section describes the equipment and procedures associated with laparoscopy.

Laparoscopic Equipment

The necessary equipment to perform a laparoscopy includes the laparoscope or telescope, trocar-cannula units, fiberoptic light cable, light source, Veress insufflation needle, gas insufflator, and camera/video system (optional).

Laparoscopes. Laparoscopes for small animals range in size from 1.7 to 10 mm in diameter. The most common size tends to be the 5-mm-diameter scope for dogs and cats (Fig. 10.117). Laparoscopes are also designed with varying telescope angles. The scope with a 0-degree field of view allows the surgeon to observe the field precisely in front of the scope. Other angled scopes include the 30-degree and 45-degree fields of view. These angled telescopes enable the operator to look over the top of organs and examine small areas. Laparoscopes with an offset

---

BOX 10.25 Advantages of and Contraindications to Laparoscopic Procedures

Advantages
- Lower postoperative morbidity rate
- Lower postoperative infection rate
- Decreased postoperative pain
- Decreased hospitalization stay in most cases
- Improved patient recovery
- Smaller surgical incisions

Contraindications
- Ascites
- Abnormal clotting times
- Poor patient condition
- Obesity
- Small body size

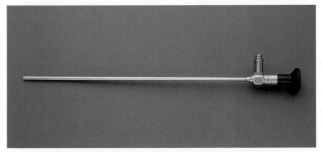

Fig. 10.117 A 5-mm laparoscope. (Courtesy Karl Storz.)

eyepiece that contains a channel for the introduction of accessory instruments are called *operating laparoscopes.* Trocar-cannula units are not needed with this type of scope.

Trocar-cannula units. Trocar-cannula units contain a trocar for puncturing through the abdominal wall and a cannula for the insertion of a telescope or laparoscopic instrument. These instruments are produced as threaded cannulas or smooth cannulas (Fig. 10.118). The threaded cannulas screw into the abdominal wall, allowing for better gripping of the cannula. Threaded cannulas are less likely to slip or fall out of the abdomen. Laparoscopic cannulas also contain a trumpet valve that thwarts the escape of gas from the abdomen.

Fiberoptic light cable and light source. A fiberoptic cable emits light from the light source to the scope (Fig. 10.119). The light from the scope illuminates the abdomen so that the operator can see the organs clearly. Light cables come in an assortment of diameters. A 4- to 5.5-mm cable is recommended for general use in dogs and cats.

Veress insufflation needle. The Veress insufflation needle is used for the original insufflation of the peritoneal cavity (Fig. 10.120), which is described later. This needle is composed of a sharp outer trocar and a blunt inner stylet. The

stylet consists of a small opening to allow gas to insufflate into the abdomen. The outer trocar functions to puncture through the abdominal wall into the abdominal cavity. The trocar is then retracted, and the inner stylet with the small opening is exposed. Gas is then insufflated through the opening.

Gas insufflator. Gas insufflators are also referred to as *laparoflators.* Tubing is connected from the gas insufflator to the Veress needle. The gas insufflator pushes gas through the tube to the needle to inflate the abdomen. This inflation lifts the abdominal wall away from the abdominal viscera, allowing the surgeon to view the abdominal organs as well as to perform biopsies or surgical procedures. Gas insufflators use CO_2, nitrous oxide, and room air. CO_2 is recommended because of its rapid rate of absorption. The laparoflators allow the operator to control the volume of gas being emitted and regulate the intraabdominal pressure. Excessive intraabdominal pressure should be avoided as it will decrease venous return to the heart and reduce the ability to ventilate. Excessive pressure can also interfere with excursions of the diaphragm. The abdominal pressures should not exceed 15 mm Hg.

Camera/video system. A camera attached to a video system and monitor is mounted on top of the laparoscope (Figs. 10.121 and 10.122). This system enables everyone in the surgery room to view the internal abdominal cavity on a monitor.

Special instruments. A general use soft tissue instrument pack should be available for laparoscopic procedures. The surgeon will require scalpel handles, blades, mosquito forceps, thumb forceps, needle holders, suture scissors, suture, and a bowl for saline. Laparoscopic instruments that should be available include biopsy instruments, cutting instruments, and palpation probe (Figs. 10.123 and 10.124). These instruments can be passed through cannulas of accessory ports to aid in biopsy

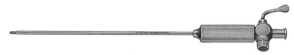

Fig. 10.120 Veress insufflation needle. (Courtesy Karl Storz.)

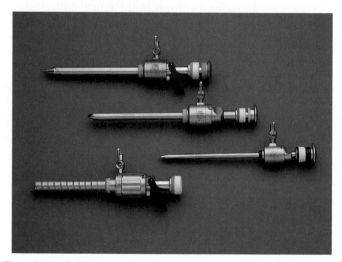

Fig. 10.118 Smooth and threaded trocar-cannula units.(Courtesy Karl Storz.)

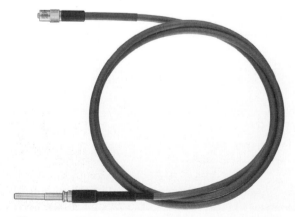

Fig. 10.119 Fiberoptic light cable. (Courtesy Karl Storz.)

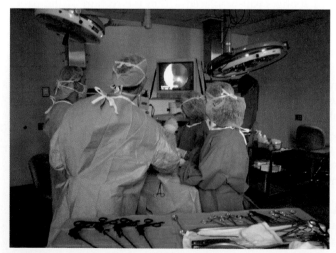

Fig. 10.121 Laparoscopic video camera is used to allow viewing of the abdominal cavity on a monitor.

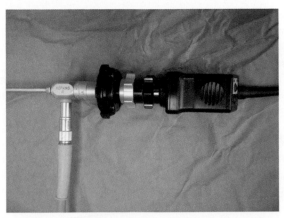

Fig. 10.122 A 5-mm laparoscope with attached light cable. The camera is attached at the eyepiece of the laparoscope.

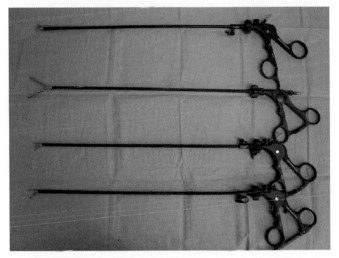

Fig. 10.123 Various laparoscopic biopsy and grasping instruments.

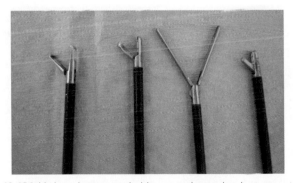

Fig. 10.124 Various laparoscopic biopsy and grasping instrument tips. *Left to right,* Atraumatic grasping forceps, biopsy forceps with teeth, bowel grasper, biopsy punch forceps.

retrieval or to perform surgical procedures. Most laparoscopic instruments are insulated so that they can be used with electro-coagulation units.

Patient Positioning

A patient undergoing a laparoscopy should be fasted for 12 hours to prevent regurgitation during anesthesia and to keep the stomach from being distended. The bladder should be expressed before the patient enters the surgery room. An increased risk of traumatic puncture by a laparoscopic instrument is present when these organs are distended. Distended organs can also make visualization of the target organs difficult. Most laparoscopic procedures are done with the patient under general anesthesia. The patient's abdomen should be clipped from the xiphoid process to the pubis as for any abdominal procedure. The clip should extend wide laterally for the placement of accessory ports. The animal may be placed in dorsal or left or right lateral recumbency. The positioning of the patient depends on the procedure. For purposes of this discussion, it is assumed that the patient has been placed in dorsal recumbency. The abdomen should be prepared routinely.

Patient Draping

A four-quarter draping method should be considered for laparoscopic procedures. Single fenestrated drapes are specifically not appropriate for this procedure.

Laparoscopic Procedure

Once the patient has been draped, the laparoscopic setup can begin. The surgeon should put on an extra pair of gloves for removing the scope and light cable from the glutaraldehyde solution in which it is stored after cleaning. A nonsterile technician pours sterile saline over the scope and light cable for rinsing purposes. The items should be rinsed thoroughly to remove all the glutaraldehyde from the cable and scope, as glutaraldehyde is toxic and irritating to tissue. The items should then be dried by a member of the sterile scrub team with a sterile towel and the extra gloves removed. Next, a sterile sleeve is used to cover the camera, and the scope is placed on the head of the camera. The camera shows the images of the abdominal contents on a monitor to allow visualization of the abdomen by everyone in the surgery room. One end of the insufflation tubing is passed to a nonsterile technician and attached to the insufflator. The other end remains sterile and will be placed on the Veress needle.

The surgeon makes a 2- to 3-mm skin incision into the abdominal skin at midline for entry of the Veress needle. Once the Veress needle is placed, a drop of saline can be introduced at the hub of the needle. This will help the surgeon know when the abdominal cavity has been penetrated, because negative pressure in the abdominal cavity will draw the saline into the needle. Proper placement of the Veress needle is important. Subcutaneous emphysema can occur if the needle is placed between the muscle and subcutaneous tissue. Once proper placement is achieved, the outer trocar of the needle is retracted, and the blunt stylet with opening is uncovered. The insufflation tubing can then be connected to the needle, and insufflation can begin. Remember: Insufflation of the abdomen should never exceed 15 mm Hg. The insufflator or laparoflator can be regulated to stop at 15 mm Hg. If pressure in the abdomen should decrease, the insufflator will automatically increase the volume of gas being released.

Once insufflation of the abdomen has been achieved, a trocar-cannula can be placed. A skin incision is made through the skin in the region of the Veress needle to reveal the abdominal wall. Next, the trocar aspect of the unit will puncture through the abdominal wall for introduction of the cannula (Fig. 10.125). When the cannula has been sufficiently placed, the trocar is removed, and the telescope (with camera) can be introduced through the cannula (Fig. 10.126). The scrub team should now be able to view the abdominal contents on the monitor. In many cases the picture appears foggy at first because of the heat from the abdomen. The scope can be removed and wiped with a warm, moistened, sterile gauze sponge. The scope can then reenter the abdominal cavity through the cannula port.

If a surgical procedure or biopsy is to be performed, the introduction of a second and a third cannula may be required for instrumentation purposes. The same technique can be used as for the telescope cannula. These cannulas will most likely be placed lateral to midline (Fig. 10.127). Placement of the cannulas will depend on the location of the organ requiring biopsy; Fig. 10.128 shows an intraoperative laparoscopic liver biopsy. Box 10.26 shows an example of a surgery report for a laparoscopic procedure.

After the abdominal procedure is completed, the instruments are removed and the incisions are closed in a routine manner.

Endoscopy

Endoscopy is the technique of examining internal body structures using specialized optical instruments. Endoscopy is generally considered a high-yield and noninvasive or minimally invasive

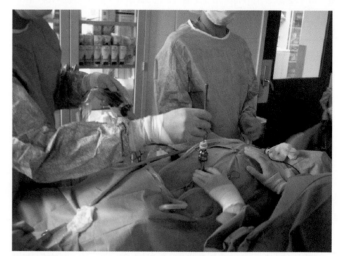

Fig. 10.127 An accessory cannula has been introduced on the right side of this dog's abdomen. A blunt probing instrument has been inserted through the cannula to allow for manipulation of the abdominal organs.

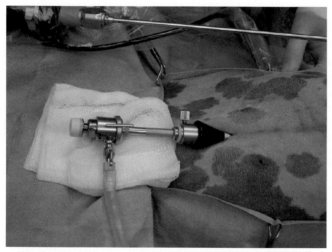

Fig. 10.125 After removal of the Veress needle, an 8-mm trocar-cannula unit is introduced at midline. The laparoscope will be introduced into the abdomen through this cannula. Note the attached tubing for insufflation of the abdomen.

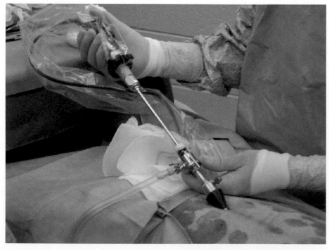

Fig. 10.126 Introduction of the laparoscope through the 8-mm cannula.

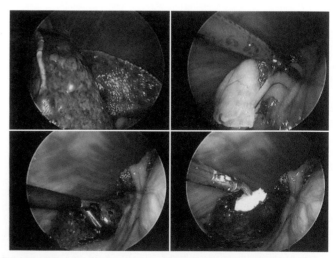

Fig. 10.128 Intraoperative laparoscopic liver biopsy. *Top left,* Laparoscopic view of diseased liver lobes. Note the many diffuse nodules throughout the liver lobes. *Top right,* A grasping instrument is placed through an accessory port to remove omentum away from the proposed biopsy site. *Bottom left,* A biopsy forceps is used to collect a piece of liver for diagnostic purposes. *Bottom right,* An absorbable gelatin sponge is placed at the biopsy site to control hemorrhage. This will stay in place and be absorbed by the body.

BOX 10.26 Surgery Report: Laparoscopic Procedure

Animal Hospital Name

Owner: John Doe

Address: 555 Sterling Lane

Jupiter, NY 55555

Phone number: 555-5555

Animal Name: Sasha

Animal #: 65656501

Species: Canine

Breed: Doberman pinscher

DOB: 05/05/07

Date of Surgery: 01/03/2011

Primary Surgeon: Dr. Vet

Assistant: Technician Scrub

Diagnosis or Preoperative Signs: Liver disease.

Surgical Procedure: Laparoscopy.

Description of Surgical Procedure

Surgical Approach and Procedure: The patient was placed in dorsal recumbency, and a Veress needle was inserted at the level of the umbilicus. The abdomen was insufflated with CO_2 through this needle until the pressure was approximately 10 mm Hg. On conclusion of insufflation, a 5-mm laparoscopic cannula was inserted into the hole created by the Veress needle. The video laparoscope was directed into the abdomen through the cannula port, and the abdominal contents were examined. A second cannula was then placed approximately 7 cm lateral to the first site for the insertion of a laparoscopic biopsy instrument. A biopsy sample was retrieved from the left medial liver lobe. The region was observed for hemorrhage. Little hemorrhage occurred.

Surgical Pathology: All liver lobes were diffusely abnormal. Small nodules (1–2 mm) were observed throughout the liver lobes.

Closure:

3-0 PDS: Closure of the small incisions in the body wall and subcutaneous tissue in a simple interrupted suture pattern.

3-0 nylon: Closure of the skin incisions in a simple interrupted suture pattern.

BOX 10.27 Common Endoscopic Procedures

Endoscopes can be used for the following noninvasive and minimally invasive procedures:

- Cystoscopy, to evaluate the bladder and lower urinary tract through the urethra
- Gastrointestinal (GI) endoscopy, including
  - Esophagoscopy, to examine the esophagus by way of the mouth
  - Gastroscopy, to examine the stomach and upper small intestine (duodenoscopy) through the mouth
  - Colonoscopy, to examine the colon by way of the anus
- Rhinoscopy, to evaluate the nasal passages through the nares
- Tracheobronchoscopy, to evaluate the trachea and bronchi by way of the mouth

Endoscopes can also be used to examine the inside of a joint (arthroscopy) or the abdominal cavity (laparoscopy), but these procedures require incision of the tissues, whereas the procedures listed above do not require incisions.

Endoscope Selection

Endoscopy equipment is now affordable for private practices and not only for referral centers and educational institutions. When purchasing endoscopy equipment, veterinarians should primarily consider (1) the probable frequency of use and the equipment's versatility, (2) the quality of the optical system, and (3) the ease of maneuvering the endoscope. Purchase price is important to many veterinarians, but purchasing a cheaper, low-quality endoscope instead of a higher quality scope can be a costly mistake; a thorough examination may be compromised by such an instrument, and a definitive diagnosis may not be achieved. High-quality endoscopes benefit hospitals because their cost can usually be recovered after 2 years; if maintained properly, these endoscopes provide many more years of service than lower quality models.

A standard flexible endoscope with a diameter of 8 to 11 mm and a working length of 100 cm is usually adequate for feline and canine upper GI examinations and colonoscopies (Fig. 10.129). An endoscope should have these features and capabilities: (1) a four-way distal tip deflection with at least 180 degrees of upward deflection (for retroflexion), (2) water flushing, (3) air

procedure. It is high yield in that it often results in diagnostic and therapeutic benefits for the patient. The body is entered ("invaded"), usually through an orifice (e.g., mouth, anus), but no incision (noninvasive) or a small incision (minimally invasive) is required to enter the body. In the diagnostic evaluation of most cases, noninvasive tests (e.g., radiography, ultrasonography, some endoscopic procedures) are performed before minimally invasive procedures (e.g., other endoscopic procedures), which are performed before invasive procedures (e.g., exploratory celiotomy) (Box 10.27).

Endoscopy allows the clinician to examine tissues directly, obtain biopsy samples, and perform therapeutic procedures, such as the removal of foreign bodies. General anesthesia and proper fasting are required for all endoscopic procedures. For each procedure that requires passing the endoscope through the mouth, the patient should be intubated with an ET tube, and a mouth speculum should be used to prevent any damage to the endoscope. The cuffed ET tube will aid in preventing aspiration of reflux or regurgitated material from the oropharynx during the procedure.

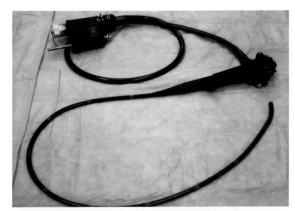

Fig. 10.129 Pentax veterinary video endoscope for small animal procedures with an insertion tube length of 100 cm and diameter of 11 mm. (PENTAX Medical Company, Montvale, NJ.) (Courtesy MJR-VHUP, Philadelphia.)

insufflation, (4) suctioning, (5) locking deflection controls, (6) an accessory channel with a diameter of 1.8 to 2.4 mm, and (7) forward-viewing optics.

Flexible Endoscopes

Because they are long and pliable, flexible endoscopes are better than rigid endoscopes for procedures that require bending or flexibility, such as examining the stomach, duodenum, and colon. Flexible endoscopes are used for noninvasive procedures and are available with either a two-way (up/down) or a four-way (up/down and left/right) distal tip deflection. The deflections are controlled by an angulation knob mounted on the control section of the endoscope. Older endoscopes have a maximum upward tip deflection of 180 degrees, whereas newer endoscopes have an upward tip deflection of 210 degrees (Fig. 10.130). Endoscopes range in length from 50 to 170 cm, with insertion tube diameters ranging from 1 to 15 mm.

There are two types of flexible endoscopes: fiberoptic (Fig. 10.131) and video (Fig. 10.132).

Fiberoptic endoscope. With a fiberoptic endoscope, a light cable carries light by fiberoptic bundles from an external light source through the control section and to the insertion tube. The control section is protected by hard plastic and contains the viewing lens, angulation control knobs, biopsy ports, white balance, and camera controls. The control section also has an eyepiece. The insertion tube houses the fiberoptic light strands and channels for air insufflation and water flushing, biopsy and retrieval instruments, and suction. When the air/water valve is compressed, water flushes and rinses the lens on the distal tip of the endoscope. When the air/water valve port is covered, insufflation occurs and can be regulated (Fig. 10.133). Insufflation aids in viewing the organs being examined.

The biopsy channel port is located at the base of the control section at the junction with the insertion tube. The insertion tube itself is protected by a waterproof sleeve. Although the endoscope has three distinct sections (light guide plug, umbilical or universal cord, and control section), it is a one-piece unit that is sealed and watertight.

The distal tip of the insertion tube can bend more easily than the rest of the endoscope because a rubber insert covers the last

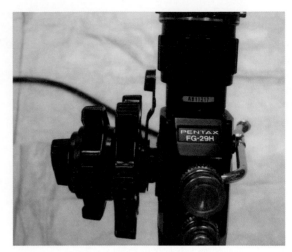

Fig. 10.131 Control section for a Pentax fiberoptic endoscope. The angulation system is on the right side of the endoscope (right side of endoscope appears on left side of figure). The large inner knob deflects up and down, and the small outer knob deflects right and left. The top valve is for suctioning, and the bottom valve is for air insufflation and flushing water to clean a dirty lens. If any images are to be taken, a camera head can be attached from the eyepiece on the endoscope to the endoscopy unit. (Courtesy MJR-VHUP, Philadelphia.)

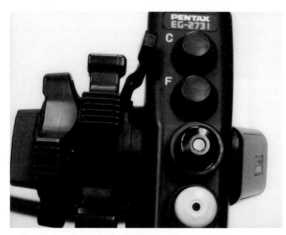

Fig. 10.132 Control section for Pentax video endoscope. The angulation knobs and valves are the same as for the fiberoptic endoscope, except that images can be directly taken from the endoscope. The F button is to freeze an image, and the C button is to capture an image so it can be printed and stored in a computer. (Courtesy MJR-VHUP, Philadelphia.)

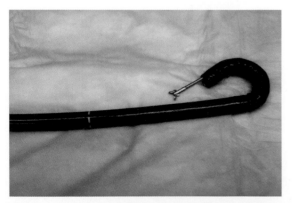

Fig. 10.130 Example of endoscope with the ability to retroflex 210 degrees. (Courtesy MJR-VHUP, Philadelphia.)

few inches. Tip deflections can be fixed in any position by using the lock mechanisms situated next to the angulation knobs. This construction allows the endoscopist to control and maneuver the endoscope with ease. The umbilical cable or universal cord connects the light guide plug to the control section of the endoscope. The light guide plug inserts into the light source. The plug has ports for the air/water and suction channels.

The fiberoptic endoscope is a direct viewing system, which means only the operator can view with this type of endoscope. Fiberoptic bundles composed of thousands of individual fibers transmit light from the light guide plug to the distal tip of the

Light guide connector section

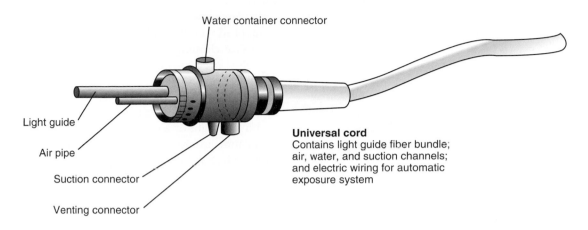

Water container connector

Light guide

Air pipe

Suction connector

Venting connector

Universal cord
Contains light guide fiber bundle;
air, water, and suction channels;
and electric wiring for automatic
exposure system

Eyepiece

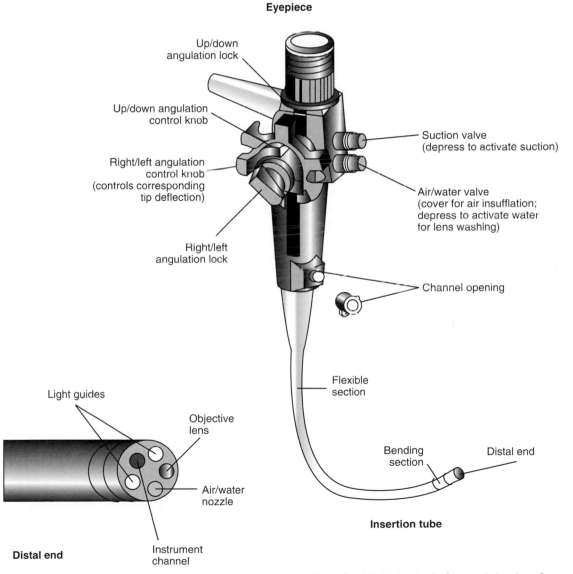

Up/down
angulation lock

Up/down angulation
control knob

Right/left angulation
control knob
(controls corresponding
tip deflection)

Right/left
angulation lock

Suction valve
(depress to activate suction)

Air/water valve
(cover for air insufflation;
depress to activate water
for lens washing)

Channel opening

Flexible
section

Light guides

Objective
lens

Air/water
nozzle

Bending
section

Distal end

Instrument
channel

Distal end

Insertion tube

Fig. 10.133 Components of a typical fiberoptic endoscope. (From Stasi K, Melendez L: Care and cleaning of the endoscope. Vet Clin North Am Small Anim Pract 31:589, 2001.)

insertion tube. The fibers' flexibility allows light to bend around corners and curves. Fiberoptic endoscopes also use a fiber bundle to transmit images from the objective lens at the distal tip, through the eyepiece, and to the endoscopist's eyes. The image guide bundles are set up so that each fiber carries a portion of the image and is in the same place at both ends of the bundle. Video cameras can be attached to the eyepiece of fiberoptic endoscopes to display images on a monitor. The final image is made up of the many small pieces of the whole image so if a fiber breaks, a black or gray dot appears on the image.

The automatic brightness system in some fiberoptic endoscopes controls the light level. Illumination decreases as the object in view draws closer, and brightness increases as the object recedes farther away. The color, texture, and reflectivity of the tissue in view all affect the intensity of brightness. The auto-brightness control compensates for these differences.

Video endoscope. Video endoscopes are similar in construction to fiberoptic endoscopes, except they do not have a direct viewing lens aided by an eyepiece. Images are seen on a video screen, which allows the entire surgical team to view the procedure. The image bundle in a fiberoptic endoscope is replaced in a video endoscope with a camera unit consisting of a lens assembly and an electronic chip known as a charged coupled device (CCD). The CCD chip is housed in the distal end of the insertion tube. The CCD chip is connected to an external video processor by approximately 16 small wires. The external video processor assembles the image and transmits it to a video monitor (Fig. 10.134).

The automatic brightness system can control the light level in all video endoscopes as in some fiberoptic endoscopes. Video endoscope systems have the capability to freeze and capture images from recording-device buttons in the control section. Other media, such as videotapes, computer files, and prints, can aid in capturing information. The light guide plug in a video endoscope is heavier than that in a fiberoptic endoscope and needs to be handled with care. The terminals in the light guide plug are not waterproof and must be covered by soaking caps (supplied with the endoscope) before being immersed in solutions for cleaning.

Rigid Endoscopes

Rigid endoscopes are better than flexible endoscopes for procedures involving a direct pathway and are more easily viewed with a straight or a direct line of sight. Such areas include the ears, nose, urinary bladder, joint spaces, and abdominal or thoracic viscera. Rigid endoscopes are used for noninvasive to moderately invasive procedures that involve tissues that lie relatively close to the body surface and can be visualized with a straight line of sight. Procedures using rigid endoscopes include otoscopy and rhinoscopy. Some procedures, such as arthroscopy, laparoscopy, and thoracoscopy, require small incisions to allow access of the object lens into the specific area to be examined. (For more information on rigid endoscopy, see Bibliography and the previous section on laparoscopy.)

Endoscopy Preparation

A technician who works with the veterinarian performing endoscopy should also have the necessary training to assist with patient preparation, equipment setup, patient monitoring, obtaining biopsy specimens, freezing/capturing and storing images, equipment breakdown, equipment cleaning, performing file backups, maintaining order of the endoscopy room, and ordering supplies.

The endoscopy technician is responsible for preparing and setting up the procedures. The endoscope of choice should be hooked up to the endoscopy machine with appropriate valves and biopsy channel covers. Before the procedure, the patient data should be ready in the computer. The machine is turned

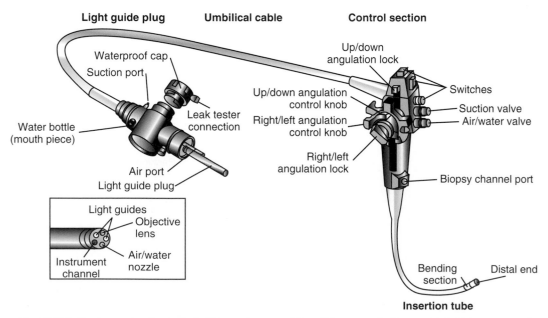

Fig. 10.134 Components of a typical video endoscope. (From Schumway R, Broussard J: Maintenance of gastrointestinal endoscopes. Clin Tech Small Anim Pract 18:254, 2003.)

on when the endoscope is attached, and the light source is checked. The endoscope should be tested while the machine is warming up. First, the technician should confirm that an adequate amount of distilled water is available for flushing; the water valve can then be depressed to confirm that water comes out of the distal end. Water flushing is done to rinse off a soiled lens on the distal tip of the endoscope. Second, the air/water valve should be gently covered and the distal end of the insertion tube submerged in a bowl of water to check for bubbles; this is a test for insufflation. Third, the tip is left submerged in a bowl of water and tested for suctioning. Any necessary accessory instruments or items, such as biopsy forceps, oral speculum, pathology request forms, water-soluble lubricant gel, gauze pads, and formalin cups or slides, should all be available and ready for use.

11.3.9 Endoscopy Work Area

The endoscopy room should be large enough to accommodate the cart or tower for the endoscopy unit (light source/suction unit, video printer/monitor, computer, keyboard), patient, anesthesia machine, and endoscopy equipment (endoscopes, accessory instruments). Additionally, a designated area to clean the endoscopy equipment, shelves and cabinets for miscellaneous storage needs, counter space, and a sink should be present in the room. Having the endoscope unit on a cart is convenient and allows portability to different areas of a hospital (Fig. 10.135).

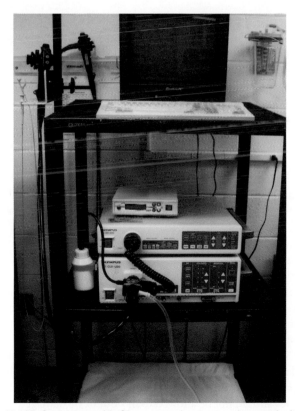

Fig. 10.135 Cart setup with Olympus endoscopy equipment (units for light source, air/suction/flushing, and brightness control), water bottle, TV monitor, biopsy forceps, and video endoscope (hanging on cart pole mount), with appropriate valves and biopsy channel cover (Olympus America, Inc., Center Valley, PA). (Courtesy MJR-VHUP, Philadelphia.)

Ideally, a well-ventilated storage cabinet will be available in the endoscopy room to protect and store the endoscopes (Fig. 10.136). If a cabinet is not available, wall mounts or cart pole mounts are acceptable (Fig. 10.137). Storing endoscopes in their original custom-padded cases is not recommended; the hanging position rather than the coiled position is strongly advised. Also, endoscopes should never be placed on a flat surface (not even temporarily) because they could fall off or be knocked onto the floor, resulting in costly repair. After cleaning, endoscopes should be hung to dry either in a

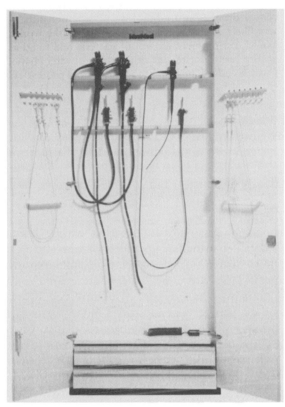

Fig. 10.136 Cabinet for storage of endoscopes and accessory instruments. (From Tams T: Small animal endoscopy, ed 2, St Louis, 1999, Mosby.)

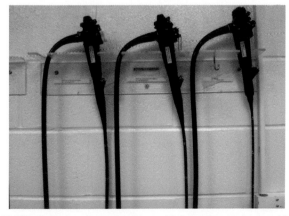

Fig. 10.137 Typical wall mount for multiple endoscopes provides appropriate hanging position, especially after cleaning and disinfecting. (Courtesy MJR-VHUP, Philadelphia.)

hanging storage cabinet or on a wall or cart pole mount, where they remain until required for another procedure. Hanging endoscopes allows any residual droplets of moisture in the insertion tube to drain. Residual moisture in the accessory channel may promote growth of bacteria and fungi and clogging of the air/water channel. Endoscopes should not be stored in their custom-padded case; if they are encased in a coiled fashion, air cannot circulate through the channels and problems are more likely to develop.

Handling the Endoscope

The control section of a flexible endoscope is the only area designed to bear its weight. During transport of an endoscope, one hand should hold the control section while the other hand holds the ends of the insertion tube and umbilical cable. The optics at the tip of the insertion tube are delicate, so extra care should be taken to protect them from damage.

There are basically two ways to hold the control section during endoscopy, described as the two-finger grip (Fig. 10.138) and the three-finger grip (Fig. 10.139). The straighter the endoscope can be maintained throughout a procedure, the more precisely it can be controlled and maneuvered. Practice and patience are required to obtain efficient and valuable endoscopic capabilities.

Biopsy Sampling

Endoscopic biopsy samples are obtained with flexible forceps. Samples obtained using forceps with a 1.8-mm cup are usually sufficient for diagnostic histopathologic examination, but cups of 2.4 mm or larger are always better because samples retrieved are substantially larger and deeper. The correct cup size is determined by the size of the endoscope's biopsy channel. Biopsy tissue samples obtained with flexible endoscopes may not always be deep enough to allow diagnosis of submucosal lesions, whereas using rigid endoscopes usually yields diagnostically sufficient amounts of tissue. It is ideal, but not always possible, to visualize the biopsy site. Depending on the difficulty in advancing the endoscope through areas of narrowing, such as the

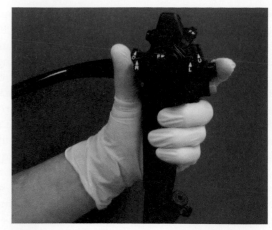

Fig. 10.139 Left-handed "three-finger" grip for holding an endoscope's control section using the third, fourth, and fifth fingers. The index finger operates the suction and air/water valves, and the thumb operates the angulation knobs. (Courtesy MJR-VHUP, Philadelphia.)

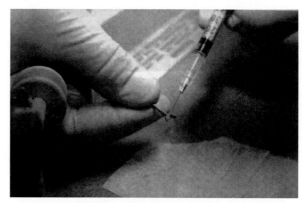

Fig. 10.140 A biopsy sample is carefully removed with a small-gauge needle. (From Tams T: Small animal endoscopy, ed 2, St Louis, 1999, Mosby.)

pyloric sphincter and ileocolic junction to obtain biopsies of the duodenum and ileum, respectively, the clinician may blindly lead the tip of the insertion tube to the site and carefully obtain blind tissue samples.

Any biopsy sample, especially an intestinal or gastric mucosa sample, must be handled carefully to minimize artifacts and distortion. If possible, tissue samples should be carefully removed from the biopsy forceps with a 25-gauge needle (Fig. 10.140). Cytology can assist in making or confirming a diagnosis, but unremarkable cytology findings do not rule out specific disorders.

It is important that tissue samples from different locations be placed in different vials of formalin and properly labeled so the pathologist can correctly identify the area sampled. Tissue samples should not be allowed to dry out or be damaged before placement in formalin.

Tissue samples that are too small and samples that have excessive artifact are common problems with endoscopy. For example, with lymphoma, neoplastic cells can be submucosal,

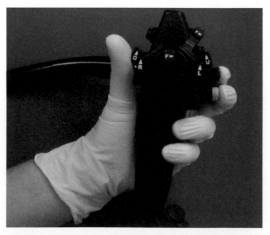

Fig. 10.138 Left-handed "two-finger" grip for holding an endoscope's control section using the fourth and fifth fingers. The index and middle fingers operate the suction and air/water valves, respectively. The thumb operates the angulation knobs. (Courtesy MJR-VHUP, Philadelphia.)

and a superficial biopsy sample may only contain reactive cells above the tumor and may miss the neoplastic cells from the tumor. This finding could be misinterpreted as a diagnosis of inflammatory bowel disease. Three to five full-thickness biopsy samples are usually sufficient, but obtaining six to eight may be more helpful, especially with both mucosal and submucosal samples. The clinician should follow up with the pathologist to determine whether the quality of the tissue samples was adequate and whether the histologic findings are consistent with the patient's clinical signs.

Even though endoscopy is considered a minimally invasive procedure, one rare but significant complication is perforation. Therefore, when biopsy samples are obtained from diseased areas, extra caution and care should be taken to avoid applying too much force against mucosal walls.

Instrumentation

Many flexible instruments are available for use with endoscopes that have an accessory channel. Both flexible and rigid endoscopes can accommodate flexible instruments. Basic instrumentation includes biopsy forceps (e.g., oval/ellipsoid cups, serrated cups, alligator cups, serrated/non-serrated bayonets), instruments for grasping foreign bodies (e.g., rat tooth forceps, wired snares, wired baskets, meshed nets, two- or three-pronged grasping forceps), cytology brushes, aspiration tubes, injection needles, and coagulating electrodes (Fig. 10.141).

Foreign bodies should not be retrieved through the accessory channel. Once the object has been visualized and firmly secured in the wired basket or forceps, the entire endoscope should be removed from the patient. Following this recommendation prevents costly damage to the accessory channel of the flexible endoscope. When removed, foreign bodies should be cleaned off as well as possible and placed in a secure bag or container for the animal's owner. Once the foreign body is removed from the instrument, the instrument can be safely removed from the endoscope.

Disposable sheathed cytology brushes are recommended for obtaining brush samples, such as a gastric or duodenal mass or intestinal mucus. One cytology brush should be used per patient because cells from one sample may be transferred to the cytologic sample of another patient if the brush is used on more than one patient. This transfer can happen because cytology brushes are difficult to clean thoroughly. Polyethylene tubing can be used to perform a duodenal wash through the endoscope to examine for evidence of giardiasis or to collect intestinal fluid for identification or quantification of bacteria.

Patient Preparation

When the esophagus, stomach, and/or duodenum are to be examined, it is important to properly prepare the patient. A 12- to 24-hour fast is recommended, and water should be withheld for 4 hours prior to the procedure.

When considering preanesthetic drugs for an endoscopy procedure that will include examination of the duodenum (duodenoscopy), it has been suggested to avoid mu opioid agonists. These drugs, such as morphine, fentanyl, and hydromorphone, may increase the tone of the pyloric sphincter, thus making entry of the endoscope into the duodenum difficult.

Esophagoscopy

Esophagoscopy is the endoscopic technique of examining the esophagus. Esophagoscopy is a useful tool in the diagnosis and treatment of esophageal disease and is indicated for the evaluation of animals with signs of esophageal disease. These signs may include (but are not limited to) regurgitation, dysphagia, odynophagia, ptyalism, change in appetite, and weight loss. Esophagoscopy is the method of choice for diagnosing disorders that affect the mucosa or alterations affecting the lumen of the esophagus (Fig. 10.142).

Esophageal foreign bodies, inflammation (esophagitis; Figs. 10.143 and 10.144), esophageal strictures, ulcers, and neoplasia are conditions affecting the esophageal mucosa or lumen that can be definitively diagnosed by esophagoscopy. However, contrast radiography is more useful than esophagoscopy in diagnosing megaesophagus, hiatal hernias, vascular

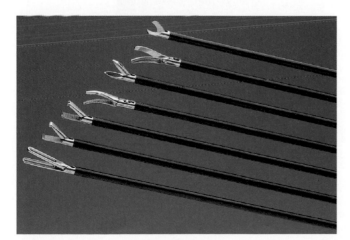

Fig. 10.141 Examples of biopsy forceps graspers and retrievers. (From Tams TR: *Small animal endoscopy*, ed 3, St Louis, 2012, Mosby.)

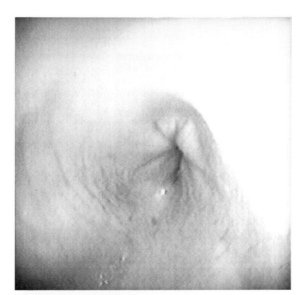

Fig. 10.142 Normal-appearing canine lower esophageal sphincter. (Courtesy MJR-VHUP, Philadelphia.)

ring anomalies, and gastroesophageal intussusception. Whenever an esophagoscopy is performed, it is important for the surgeon to advance the endoscope into the stomach. Once in the stomach, the surgeon should retroflex the scope's tip to view the gastroesophageal sphincter area to detect leiomyomas or other easily missed lesions (Box 10.28).

Canine mucosa differs from feline esophageal mucosa. A dog's esophageal mucosa is normally pale pink or grayish, and the surface is smooth and glistening. In dog breeds such as the chow chow and Shar-Pei, patches of pigmented mucosa may be observed. A cat's esophageal mucosa differs from that of a dog because of the presence of submucosal vessels and circular rings formed by circumferential mucosal folds, creating a characteristic pattern in the distal third of the cat's esophagus (Figs. 10.145 and 10.146).

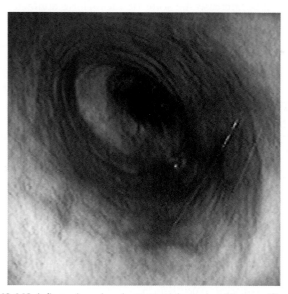

Fig. 10.143 Inflamed canine lower esophageal sphincter. (Courtesy MJR-VHUP, Philadelphia.)

Gastroscopy

Gastroscopy is the endoscopic technique of examining the stomach. Gastroscopy is indicated for the evaluation of animals with signs of gastric disease. The signs may include (but are not limited to) nausea, salivation, vomiting, hematemesis, melena, unexplained abnormal changes in breathing, and anorexia. Gastroscopy identifies abnormalities of the mucosa and reveals distortion of the stomach's normal anatomic relationship to other abdominal organs by displacement or extrinsic compression. Many consider gastroscopy to be a more valuable diagnostic tool than radiography for disorders affecting the stomach.

The following conditions can be definitively diagnosed by gastroscopy or a combination of gastroscopy and associated diagnostic tests (cytology, histology): chronic inflammation (with or without overgrowth of *Helicobacter* organisms), superficial erosions, foreign bodies, motility disorders, ulcerations, and neoplasia. Gastroscopy can also be a therapeutic intervention when used to remove foreign bodies (Figs. 10.147 to 10.149) and place feeding tubes (gastrostomy tubes and percutaneous endoscopy–guided [PEG] gastrostomy tubes).

Gastric biopsy is currently required for a diagnosis of *Helicobacter* infection. The bacteria are not uniformly distributed throughout the stomach; therefore, obtaining samples from various areas (body, fundus, antrum) is recommended. *Helicobacter* may be diagnosed by cytologic evaluation of the gastric mucosa or by examination for gastric mucosal urease activity (Box 10.29).

Duodenoscopy

Duodenoscopy is the endoscopic technique of examining the duodenum. Duodenoscopy aids in the diagnosis and treatment of small intestine disease. Clinical signs of such disease may include (but are not limited to) vomiting, hematemesis, diarrhea, melena, change in appetite, and weight loss. Duodenoscopy identifies abnormalities of the mucosa and reveals distortion of the small intestine's normal anatomic relationships by displacement or extrinsic compression.

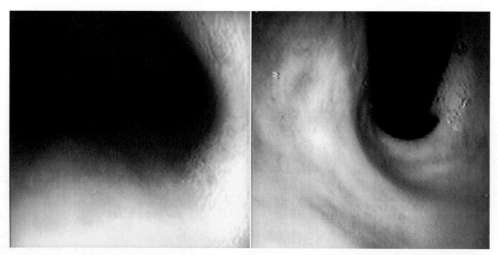

Fig. 10.144 *Left,* Mild reflux esophagitis in 10-year-old male German shepherd. *Right,* Retroflexed view of gastroesophageal sphincter and cardia. (Courtesy MJR-VHUP, Philadelphia.)

BOX 10.28 Esophagoscopy Technique

1. The anesthetized and intubated patient should be placed in left lateral recumbency with a secured oral speculum.
2. The insertion tube should be prelubricated with a water-soluble gel to aid easy passage. The endoscope is then directed centrally through the oropharynx and guided dorsal to the endotracheal tube and larynx so that the cranial esophageal sphincter (CES) comes into view.
3. The CES is the entrance to the esophagus and is normally closed; it appears as a star-shaped area of folded mucosa dorsal to the larynx. The endoscope should meet minimal or no resistance as it is being advanced within the esophagus.
4. With insufflation, the scope should advance in a slow, continuous motion, with only minor adjustments in tip deflection and torque being used to maintain a full view of the lumen and mucosal surfaces.
5. At the lumen of the thoracic esophagus, pulsations of the aorta can be seen at the level of the base of the heart.
6. When the endoscope is advanced through the gastroesophageal sphincter (GES), little or no resistance should be encountered.
7. To move the endoscope into the stomach, the tip of the insertion tube should be deflected approximately 30 degrees to the left (see note) while slight upward deflection is applied as the tip is advanced through the slit-like opening of the GES.
8. To examine the GES, the endoscope should be retroflexed. This is also known as the J maneuver. The extent of retroflexion can be 180 or 210 degrees.

NOTE: When one is referring to directional technique (i.e., left or right), the patient's orientation is the point of reference. Therefore, the instruction to turn the tip of the endoscope to the left refers to the patient's left. This principle applies to every endoscopic technique described in this chapter.

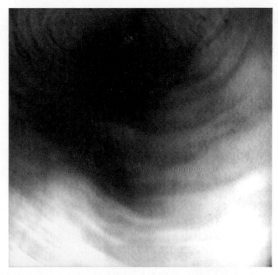

Fig. 10.146 Caudal thoracic feline esophagus with herringbone pattern not seen in canine esophagus. This esophagus is mildly inflamed. (Courtesy MJR-VHUP, Philadelphia.)

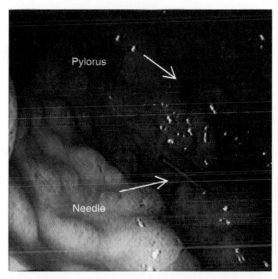

Fig. 10.147 Needle located in the pylorus of a 3 ½-year-old male Labrador; it was retrieved without complications. (Courtesy MJR-VHUP, Philadelphia.)

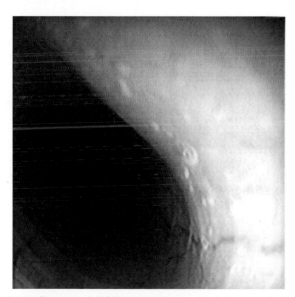

Fig. 10.145 Distal third of feline esophagus with distinctive circular ring formation (herringbone pattern). This esophagus is mildly inflamed. (Courtesy MJR-VHUP, Philadelphia.)

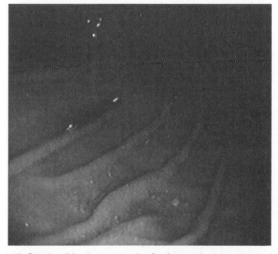

Fig. 10.148 Steel nail in the stomach of a 6-month-old male vizsla; it was retrieved without complications. (Courtesy MJR-VHUP, Philadelphia.)

The following diagnoses and conditions can be identified with the use of duodenoscopy: intestinal parasites, inflammation (inflammatory bowel disease; Figs. 10.150 to 10.152), lymphangiectasia, ulcerations, and neoplasia. Intestinal parasites (generally ascarids) are occasionally encountered on direct examination. These parasites can be easily removed, but biopsy

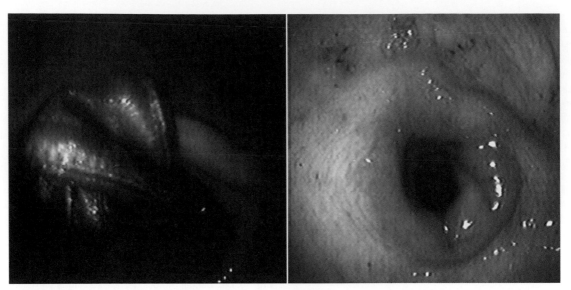

Fig. 10.149 *Left,* Article of clothing wedged in the pyloric sphincter of a 9-year-old female Alaskan malamute. *Right,* Inflammation and swelling after minor complications in retrieving object. (Courtesy MJR-VHUP, Philadelphia.)

BOX 10.29 Gastroscopy Technique

1. Fasting a patient for 12 to 24 hours and withholding water for 4 or more hours before a gastroscopy may be the key to a successful and a thorough examination.

2. The anesthetized and intubated patient should be placed in left lateral recumbency (LLR) with a secured oral speculum. With the patient in LLR, the antrum and pylorus are away from the tabletop, allowing the scope to traverse these structures more readily and the endoscopist to examine the stomach completely.

3. Because the esophagus is in a posterior plane in relation to the stomach, the tip of the insertion tube needs to be deflected in the distal esophagus before it can be advanced to the stomach.

4. The endoscope tip should be centered at the gastroesophageal (GE) orifice, and as the scope is advanced, the tip should be deflected to the left approximately 30 degrees with simultaneous slight upward deflection as the GE junction is passed. If the tip was properly directed, no resistance should be encountered as the scope advances to the stomach.

5. The endoscope tip should be positioned just through the GE junction to obtain an overview of the gastric lumen. As the tip enters the stomach, the rugal folds are seen, and the stomach is often partially or completely collapsed.

6. Gastric distension is required, so insufflation is used to the point that the rugal folds begin to separate. This step allows for spatial orientation and the identification of most gross abnormalities. In cats and small dogs, insufflation can be achieved within seconds, whereas large-breed dogs may require 30 to 120 seconds of constant insufflation for adequate distension.

7. The initial examination of the stomach should note the presence/absence of fluid or ingesta, the ease/difficulty with which the gastric walls distend with insufflation, and the gross appearance of the rugal folds and the mucosa.

8. The stomach should be empty in a properly fasted patient; however, a small pool of fluid in the fundus or at the proximal aspect of the greater curvature is considered normal. Aspiration should be performed but with great care if a large pool of fluid is present and is obscuring the rugal folds.

9. As the scope is gradually advanced through the proximal stomach, the gastric body can be evaluated if the control knobs are used to deflect the tip.

10. With the patient in LLR, the smooth lesser curvature is on the endoscopist's right and the rugal folds of the greater curvature are seen below and to the left. The endoscope is then advanced along the greater curvature until the angulus, which extends from the lesser curvature, is identified.

11. The angulus separates the body of the stomach from the antrum. The insertion tube must be maneuvered around the angulus to the antrum in order to be advanced to the pylorus through the pyloric sphincter and to enter the duodenum.

12. During a gastroscopy, the cardia and fundus can be visualized only if the insertion tube is retroflexed (J maneuver).

13. The retroflexion maneuver allows a "face view" of the angulus, cardia, and fundus. This maneuver must be initiated at a point proximal to or opposite the angulus to provide a face view of the angulus.

14. The scope is advanced along the greater curvature to the level of the distal body.

15. The tip of the insertion tube is then deflected upward as far as possible as the scope advances farther. An upward tip deflection between 180 and 210 degrees is required to visualize the cardia.

16. Panoramic examination of the proximal stomach is completed by rotation of the insertion tube. The retroflexed scope tip should be reversed gradually to allow further examination of the gastric mucosa.

NOTE: Gastroscopy should follow esophagoscopy for a thorough upper gastrointestinal examination, with the duodenum examined last and gastric biopsy specimens usually obtained after duodenal specimens.

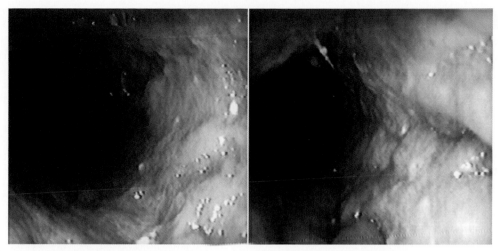

Fig. 10.150 Significant duodenal inflammation with mild ulceration from a 2-year-old female German shepherd. This dog was diagnosed with a moderate form of chronic lymphoplasmacytic and neutrophilic enteritis. (Courtesy MJR-VHUP, Philadelphia.)

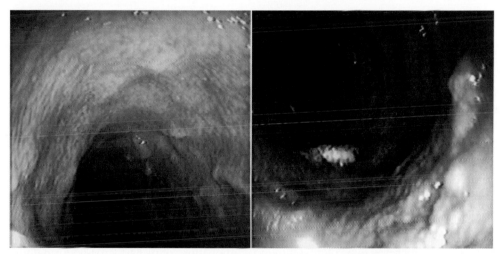

Fig. 10.151 Edematous duodenum with dilated lacteals and pinpoint ulcerations from an 8 ½-year-old bichon frise. This dog was diagnosed with chronic duodenitis. (Courtesy MJR-VHUP, Philadelphia.)

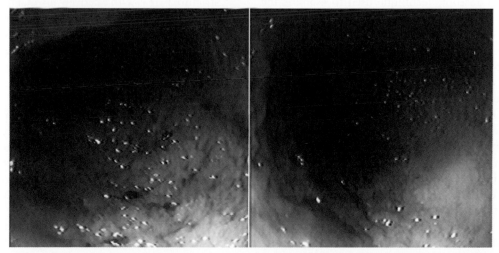

Fig. 10.152 Friable, "cobblestone" duodenum with small, ulcerated areas from a 4-year-old male domestic short-haired cat. This cat was diagnosed with severe, chronic duodenitis. (Courtesy MJR-VHUP, Philadelphia.)

BOX 10.30 **Duodenoscopy Technique**

1. Fasting a patient for 12 to 24 hours and withholding water for 4 or more hours before a duodenoscopy may be the key to a successful and thorough examination, as with gastroscopy.
2. The anesthetized and intubated patient should be placed in left lateral recumbency (LLR) with a secured oral speculum.
3. As the endoscope advances through the stomach until it reaches the pylorus, minor tip adjustments may be necessary to maintain the pyloric orifice in the center of the field of view.
4. Minimal forward pressure can be applied to advance the tip directly through the open pyloric orifice to reach the first segment of the duodenum; however, if the pyloric orifice is closed or slightly open, variable resistance may be encountered.
5. The insertion tube tip can be guided into the pyloric canal by application of leftward tip deflection alone or with slight to moderate upward tip deflection while the scope is advanced.
6. A blurred image will be seen once the insertion tube tip is in the pyloric canal, because the pyloric walls are usually pressed in around the tip of the insertion tube.
7. Turning both inner and outer control knobs on the endoscope in a clockwise direction as the scope advances provides a downward and rightward tip deflection that will aid entry into the proximal duodenum.

8. The color of the gastric mucosa is usually cream, and on entry into the duodenum, the color of the mucosa becomes pinkish red.
9. The tip of the insertion tube should then be directed into the descending duodenal lumen without the use of excessive force.
10. Because the tip of the insertion tube lies against the superior wall of the proximal duodenum, it should be angled acutely upward and sometimes also to the left. This maneuver with gentle advancement provides a tunneling view of the descending duodenum.
11. Air insufflation should be maintained to allow distension of the duodenal walls.
12. At times, minor forward or backward movements of the insertion tube may aid in freeing the endoscope tip.

NOTE: Air insufflation should be monitored carefully because excessive air may reflux into the stomach and cause unnecessary gastric distension. If this distension occurs, the endoscope should be withdrawn into the stomach and then air-suction should be applied.

---

specimens should still be obtained. If *Giardia* is suspected, a saline lavage can be performed to retrieve trophozoites. Partial-thickness specimens obtained by duodenoscopy may be preferable to full-thickness specimens obtained by abdominal exploratory surgery for patients with protein-losing enteropathy. Duodenoscopy is preferred in hypoproteinemic patients, especially if the total protein value is 3.5 g/dL or less, because surgical healing is delayed once total protein falls to that level. The most common causes of protein-losing enteropathy in dogs are inflammatory bowel disease, lymphoma, and lymphangiectasia. Lymphoma is the most common intestinal neoplasia and is believed to be more common in cats than in dogs (Box 10.30).

Colonoscopy

Colonoscopy is the endoscopic technique used to examine the rectum, large intestine, and cecum. Colonoscopy aids in the diagnosis and treatment of large bowel disease. Clinical signs may include (but are not limited to) diarrhea, hematochezia, fecal mucus, tenesmus, dyschezia, constipation, and chronic vomiting (especially in cats). Hematochezia, fecal mucus, and tenesmus are signs of diarrhea in large bowel disease, and patients with these signs usually have self-limiting disease or a disorder that can be resolved with symptomatic treatment and supportive care. Chronic vomiting is usually more common in upper GI disease, although in cats this may indicate inflammation of the ascending colon or ileum, which is why every attempt should be made to enter the ileum during colonoscopy.

Colonoscopy should be performed when clinical or laboratory findings (e.g., significant weight loss, hypoalbuminemia) suggest that a patient has a serious disorder (e.g., intussusception, histoplasmosis, adenocarcinoma) or when the clinical signs and symptoms of colonic disease do not respond to specific

therapeutic trials. However, patients who have diarrhea with large bowel disease but are otherwise healthy should be tested for parasitic disease, dietary allergy or intolerance, fiber-responsive diarrhea, and clostridial colitis before colonoscopy is considered.

The most commonly diagnosed disorders include a variety of mucosal inflammatory disorders, primarily lymphocytic-plasmacytic colitis (Figs. 10.153 and 10.154), and rectal polyps. Colonoscopy is much more accurate than contrast radiography in diagnosing large intestine disorders. Most patients with idiopathic colitis have grossly normal mucosa. It is imperative that the colon be properly prepared prior to colonoscopy (see later) to obtain high-quality biopsy samples at various levels of the colon.

Strictured areas with relatively normal mucosa usually result from a submucosal lesion. In these cases, biopsy specimen collection must be aggressive enough to ensure that submucosal tissue is obtained. Cytologic studies are sensitive in detecting histoplasmosis (*Histoplasma capsulatum* infection) and protothecosis (*Prototheca* infections) and may be useful in detecting some neoplasms and eosinophilic colitis.

Patient preparation. As mentioned previously, improper patient preparation prior to colonoscopy can affect diagnostic results. Fecal examinations for parasites and ova (e.g., whipworms, *Giardia*), cultures for pathogens (e.g., *Salmonella, Campylobacter*), fecal cytology (e.g., for *Clostridium* spores), and assays (e.g., for *Clostridium perfringens* enterotoxin) should be done before enemas or lavage solutions are administered.

The patient should be fasted for 24 to 36 hours. The colon needs to be as thoroughly cleaned as possible. Lavage solutions are best for removing food and feces from the alimentary canal. These solutions are *isosmotic* (same osmotic pressure) and

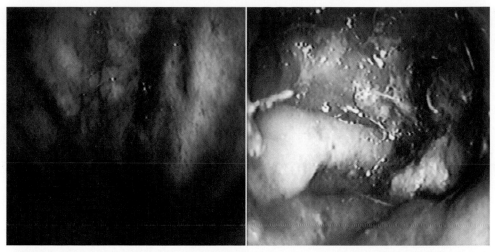

Fig. 10.153 *Left,* Moderately to severely inflamed duodenum with mild ulcerative areas. *Right,* Moderately inflamed ileocolic valve from a 2-year-old female German shepherd. This dog was diagnosed with moderate to severe lymphoplasmacytic, neutrophilic, and erosive colitis, as well as enteritis. (Courtesy MJR-VHUP, Philadelphia.)

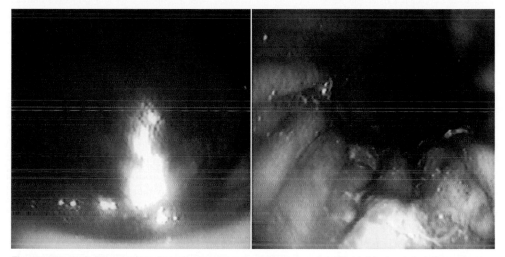

Fig. 10.154 *Left,* Rectal mass from 2-year-old male Brittany spaniel. *Right,* Moderately inflamed colon from the same patient. This dog was diagnosed with rectal papillary adenocarcinoma and moderate lymphoplasmacytic colitis. (Courtesy MJR-VHUP, Philadelphia.)

produce an osmotic diarrhea that washes particulate matter out of the colon. One example of a lavage solution is Go-LYTELY (Braintree Laboratories Inc., Braintree, MA), which is administered through a gastric or nasoesophageal tube if the patient does not consume the solution orally. GoLYTELY is a concentrated solution of polyethylene glycol and electrolytes that results in virtually no net absorption or excretions of ions or water. GoLYTELY can usually clean a bowel within 4 hours, although some patients may require more than one dosing. Large volumes can be given without causing significant changes in water or electrolyte balance. In addition to lavage solutions, an osmotic cathartic such as magnesium citrate may be used. This combination results in the best colonic preparation and minimizes artifacts induced by enema tubes.

Problems associated with lavage solutions include the following: (1) they are more expensive than enemas, (2) large volumes are needed for some patients, and (3) orogastric intubation administration can be difficult in aggressive animals.

Colonic lavages such as a warm-water enema are helpful but may need to be repeated multiple times. Improper technique can easily result in an inadequately prepared patient with possible mucosal artifacts. For this reason, it is best to fast a patient for 36 hours rather than 24 hours. When performing an enema, use a well-lubricated enema tube; the tube should not be forced if resistance is encountered because traumatic mucosal hemorrhages will likely occur and could leave an artifact that may be misinterpreted as a primary lesion during the colonoscopy. If the colon has been lavaged properly, clear water should be evacuated after the last enema. Enemas are helpful for cleaning the descending colon but are inadequate for cleaning the ascending and transverse colon and the ileocolic valve (Box 10.31).

BOX 10.31 Colonoscopy Technique

1. After the patient has been fasted properly (ideally 36 hours) and the colon adequately cleaned, the patient can be anesthetized, intubated, and placed in left lateral recumbency (LLR).
2. The flexible endoscope tip is inserted into the rectum, followed by insufflation.
3. As the tip of the scope is advanced central to the lumen, the mucosa and lumen are examined. The endoscope is advanced to its most orad (toward the mouth) limit and then slowly withdrawn so that the mucosa can be thoroughly examined.
4. The splenic flexure, the most orad part of the descending colon, is the area where the descending colon turns and becomes the transverse colon.
5. To enter the transverse colon, the distal tip of the endoscope must be diverted in the direction of the lumen, and then the tip must be carefully advanced using a blind "slide-by" technique. With this technique the distal tip usually pushes lightly against the colonic wall, and visualization is lost for 1 to 2 cm because the lens is too close to the mucosa.
6. In cats the transverse and ascending sections of the colon usually merge. It is difficult to examine the mucosa of this section because the tight bend makes it impossible for the distal tip to stay in the center of the lumen.
7. The blind slide-by technique is used from the descending colon up to the ascending colon, which leads to the cecum and ileocolic valve.
8. When the ileocolic valve is approached, careful observation is necessary, or the valve may be bypassed and the distal tip may enter the cecum.
9. If the area is adequately clean, the ileocolic valve and the cecocolic valve can both be seen. In some cases the ileocolic valve appears as another opening adjacent to the cecocolic valve. However, this area tends to be less well prepared because mucus and debris entering from the ileum may cover and hide the ileocolic valve.
10. As the distal tip reaches the ileocolic valve, minor tip adjustments may be necessary to maintain the ileocolic orifice in the center of the field of view.
11. Minimal forward pressure can be applied to advance the tip directly through the open ileocolic orifice to access the ileum; however, if the ileocolic orifice is closed or slightly open, variable resistance may be encountered.
12. If the cecum is entered and was thought to be the colon, the lumen will make additional bends that cannot be negotiated with the distal tip. No force should be applied to push the distal tip past one of these bends or the cecum may be perforated.
13. If the working length of the scope has been exhausted in the process of entering the cecum, the endoscope should be retracted slightly and air aspirated to partially collapse the lumen. This maneuver should shorten the distance to the cecocolic or ileocolic valve.
14. If rectal lesions are present, a retroflexed view is necessary. This can usually be achieved in dogs that are medium to large breeds. However, a rigid proctoscope is often the better scope for examining rectal lesions.

▮ KEY POINTS

1. To be a competent surgical assistant, the veterinary technician must have proficient knowledge of the surgical procedure, surgical instruments, and aseptic and sterile technique.
2. The intraoperative duties of the surgical assistant include retraction of tissue, bone reduction, wound sponging, suction of the surgical site, and providing hemostasis. Responsibilities also include anticipation of the surgeon's needs and performing sponge counts before surgery and before closure of the cavity.
3. Preoperative blood tests should be performed for any animal undergoing anesthesia and surgery. The surgeon will choose tests according to the patient's signalment, comorbidities, and surgery to be performed.
4. The patient's bladder should be expressed before it enters the surgery room.
5. The bladder of a traumatic injury patient should not be expressed before it enters the surgery room.
6. Patients undergoing abdominal procedures should be clipped from the xiphoid process to the pubis. This allows the surgeon to extend the incision as needed.
7. The use of Balfour retractors during abdominal surgical procedures allows for enhanced exposure to the abdominal cavity.
8. Laparotomy sponges should be used to isolate organs during hollow-organ surgery. The use of laparotomy sponges helps reduce contaminants that may enter the abdominal cavity.
9. Lap sponges can also be used to keep exteriorized tissue moist and protected during surgery.
10. Stay sutures should be placed during hollow-organ surgeries (e.g., cystotomy, gastrotomy) to allow for manipulation of the organ as well as to prevent leakage of contaminants within the abdominal cavity. The sterile surgical assistant should also take care when handling the exposed viscera; gloves or sponges used should be moistened to reduce tissue damage.
11. Abdominal lavage with warm sterile saline before closure of the abdomen helps dilute any pollutants and warm the patient.
12. A barium contrast study should never be performed if perforations of the gastrointestinal tract are suspected.
13. During an enterotomy procedure, Doyen clamps or the fingers of an assistant should be used to occlude the intestines to avoid leakage of chyme within the abdomen.
14. Abdominal incisions should be monitored daily for swelling, discharge, or malodor. Many postoperative complications are related to the incision site.
15. Patients with gastric dilation and volvulus (GDV) are considered true surgical emergencies. The immediate treatment includes decompression of the stomach, correction of fluid and electrolyte imbalances, treatment for shock, and surgery to correct the position of the stomach and gastropexy.
16. An orogastric tube should never be forced down the esophagus during placement. Gentle placement is necessary to avoid damage to the esophagus.
17. A roll of hospital tape can be placed between the upper and lower jaws of the patient receiving an orogastric tube. The tube can be placed through the hole in the roll of tape. This

will keep the jaws of the animal from biting down on the tube or the assistant's hand during placement.

18. The stomach of a dog with GDV generally rotates in a clockwise direction.

19. Animals should be spayed before their first ovarian cycle to decrease the incidence of mammary tumors. The client should discuss risk factors for their pet with the veterinarian when deciding on when to have their pet spayed.

20. The most common complication reported after an ovariohysterectomy is hemorrhage.

21. Pyometra is a potentially life-threatening condition. A complete ovariohysterectomy should be performed to remove the uterus; medical management is not recommended.

22. Care should be taken when removing an infected uterus. The organ is damaged and, in many cases, friable; purulent contents could leak out into the peritoneal cavity, leading to an increased chance of peritonitis.

23. Indications for performing a feline or canine castration include eliminating reproductive function, preventing roaming, preventing urine spraying, treating scrotal neoplasia, and treating endocrine abnormalities.

24. The client should discuss risk factors for their pet with the veterinarian when deciding on when to have their pet castrated.

25. Before placing a dog or cat under anesthesia for castration, the testicles are examined to be sure both have descended into the scrotum. If they have not, an inguinal or abdominal procedure may be necessary for testicle retrieval.

26. For cats undergoing castration, the hair of the scrotum should be gently plucked before the patient enters the surgery room.

27. Scrotal bleeding is the most common complication associated with canine and feline castration.

28. Lateral ear canal resection involves lateralization and exposure of the horizontal ear canal for drainage purposes and is generally performed in patients with chronic ear infections. Medical management is usually required even after resection.

29. *Entropion* refers to rolling in of the eyelid. Surgery is usually done to alleviate ocular irritation.

30. A meibomian (sebaceous) adenoma is the most common eyelid neoplasm in the dog.

31. Squamous cell carcinoma is the most common feline eyelid tumor and is often found in cats with white or pink eyelids.

32. A wedge resection procedure is the most common procedure performed for eyelid neoplasia.

33. Orthopedics involves injuries or diseases of the skeletal system.

34. Orthopedic injuries are usually not considered life threatening unless they involve the skull or spine or unless a long-bone fracture has resulted in a large amount of blood loss.

35. Fracture assessment should include a history, thorough physical examination, and two orthogonal radiographs.

36. When radiographs of a long-bone fracture are taken, the joint below and above the fracture site should be included in the film.

37. Open fractures are classified according to mechanism of puncture and the severity of the soft tissue damage.

38. Surgical options for fracture repair include internal fixation and external fixation. Internal fixation includes plates, screws, nails, pins, and wire. External fixation includes casts, rigid splints, and custom-made devices.

39. Casts and splints must be kept dry and clean and should be observed for slippage, self-mutilation, and toe swelling.

40. Hind limb and forelimb amputations are considered major procedures and should be performed only with a thorough knowledge of the patient's physical status.

41. Regional and local nerve blocks contribute significantly to postoperative pain control in amputation patients.

42. Cranial cruciate ligament (CCL) ruptures are also referred to as an anterior cruciate ligament (ACL) injury or "football player's knee" in humans.

43. The major diagnostic tests for CCL injury include the cranial drawer test and the tibial compression test. Palpation of the affected leg often reveals muscle atrophy, pain, joint effusion, and asymmetry.

44. Biopsy techniques for diagnostic purposes include fine-needle aspiration, impression smears, needle punch, punch, bone, incisional, and excisional.

45. Minimally invasive procedures include laparoscopy, endoscopy, and some laser surgery procedures.

46. The technician's most important role in laser surgery is laser safety. Most practices using laser surgery appoint a laser safety officer, most likely the technician.

47. Many hazards are associated with laser surgery, including eye, skin, fire, and smoke plume hazards. All safety steps should be taken to avoid potential hazards.

48. Advantages to laser surgery over traditional surgery include more rapid healing time of tissue, less risk of postoperative infection, reduced postoperative pain and swelling, and decreased surgery time.

49. Laparoscopic procedures are performed to examine and obtain biopsy specimens of the internal organs or tumors of the abdominal cavity. Laparoscopy can also be used to perform specific surgical procedures, such as a spay and gastropexy.

50. Some advantages to laparoscopic procedures include improved patient recovery, smaller surgical sites, lower postoperative infection rate, and decreased postoperative pain.

51. The patient undergoing laparoscopy should be fasted for 12 hours, and the bladder should be expressed before the patient enters the surgery room.

52. When performing endoscopy, an insertion tube should always be handled carefully. Sharp bends, tight coiling, and striking of the tube against hard surfaces should be avoided.

53. Maintaining endoscopes usually falls to the veterinary technician and involves proper cleaning and disinfection, leak testing and inspection, microbial monitoring, and storage.

54. In dogs and cats, gastric and duodenal disorders are more common than esophageal disorders. Because clinical signs

of these diseases can overlap, endoscopic examination of the esophagus should extend to the stomach and duodenum for a thorough upper gastrointestinal examination.

55. Patient preparation for colonoscopies is crucial because the whole colon needs to be visualized, and it is more difficult to clean the ileocolic valve area than the descending colon. Also, large debris cannot be aspirated as well with flexible scopes as with rigid scopes.

56. Mu opioid agonists (e.g., fentanyl, morphine, hydromorphone) should not be used for gastroduodenoscopies because they may cause pylorospasms, and entering the duodenum will be more difficult because of an increase in pyloric tone.

57. Appropriate analgesics should be administered for every surgical patient postoperatively. Multimodal analgesia is especially important for orthopedic procedures.

58. A surgical patient may need to be sent home with Elizabethan collars if the pet attempts to mutilate the incision site. Elizabethan collars should be sent home with patients that have undergone ophthalmic surgery.

REVIEW QUESTIONS

1. A circulating assistant can do which duty in the surgery suite?
   a. Opening packs
   b. Applying suction
   c. Retraction of tissues
   d. Assistance with fracture reduction

2. Balfour retractors are used to
   a. exteriorize the uterine horn during an ovariohysterectomy.
   b. hold open the abdomen for better visualization.
   c. extend an enterotomy incision to allow removal of a foreign body

3. Separation of all layers of an incision is called
   a. ileus.
   b. resection.
   c. dehiscence.

4. Evisceration puncture of the abdomen to obtain fluid is called
   a. anastomosis.
   b. intussusception.
   c. abdominocentesis.
   d. diagnostic peritoneal lavage.

5. What is a sign of intestinal viability?
   a. Vascular pulses
   b. Lack of motility
   c. Severe thinning of visceral wall
   d. Lack of bleeding on cut section of intestine

6. Which patient would be more likely to develop gastric dilation volvulus?
   a. Cairn terrier
   b. Doberman pinscher
   c. Domestic shorthair cat
   d. Cavalier King Charles spaniel

7. The primary reason for performing an ovariohysterectomy is
   a. dystocia.
   b. neoplasia.
   c. sterilization.
   d. uterine torsion.

8. What is considered the most painful part of the ovariohysterectomy procedure?
   a. Ligation of the uterine body
   b. Exteriorizing the uterine horn
   c. Plucking the suspensory ligament
   d. Transection of the ovarian pedicle

9. Which drug is used to stimulate respirations for resuscitation of newborns after a cesarean section?
   a. Atropine
   b. Naloxone
   c. Doxapram
   d. Epinephrine

10. How is the incision closed during a feline orchiectomy?
    a. The skin layer is the only layer closed.
    b. There is no closure; the incision heals by second intention.
    c. The subcutaneous layer is closed, and the skin heals by second intention.
    d. The subcutaneous tissues are closed, followed by closure of the skin.

11. What is the primary indication for a cystotomy?
    a. Neoplasia
    b. Cystic calculi
    c. Renal failure
    d. Congenital abnormalities

12. What is an indication for a patient to undergo a Zepp procedure?
    a. Dystocia
    b. Cystic calculi
    c. Urethral obstruction
    d. Chronic ear infection

13. What should be used to aseptically prepare a patient for ophthalmologic surgeries?
    a. Alcohol
    b. Chlorhexidine scrub
    c. Lactated Ringer's solution
    d. Dilute povidone-iodine solution

14. What is the medical term for the rolling in of the eyelid?
    a. Entropion
    b. Chalazion
    c. Strabismus
    d. Photophobia

15. Removal of the gland of the third eyelid can lead to
    a. entropion.
    b. cherry eye.
    c. photophobia.
    d. keratoconjunctivitis sicca.

16. Which of these procedures would be considered an elective orthopedic procedure?
    a. Skull fracture repair
    b. Open femur fracture repair
    c. Shoulder dislocation reduction
    d. Correction of medial luxating patella
17. An example of external coaptation would be placement of a/an
    a. bone plate.
    b. external fixator.
    c. intramedullary pin.
    d. modified Robert Jones bandage.
18. Salter-Harris fractures always involve the
    a. physis.
    b. diaphysis.
    c. vertebrae.
    d. humeral condyle.
19. An external fixator would be contraindicated in the treatment of a fracture of the
    a. ilium.
    b. tibia.
    c. femur.
    d. humerus.
20. Which type of fixation device can be adjusted throughout the healing period?
    a. Bone plate
    b. Cerclage wire
    c. External fixator
    d. Intramedullary pin
21. Splints should only be employed for fractures distal to the
    a. scapula.
    b. acetabulum.
    c. stifle and elbow.
    d. carpus and tarsus
22. Which of the following is a disadvantage when performing a fine needle aspirate?
    a. easy to perform.
    b. low diagnostic yield.
    c. no sedation necessary.
    d. minimal morbidity.
23. What type of minimally invasive procedure is used on cut surfaces and ulcerated surfaces of tumors?
    a. Punch biopsy
    b. Impression smear
    c. Fine-needle aspiration
    d. Needle punch biopsy
24. Which biopsy technique involves complete removal of a mass?
    a. Punch biopsy
    b. Incisional biopsy
    c. Excisional biopsy
    d. Needle punch biopsy
25. When using a laser surgical unit, exposure refers to
    a. laser wavelength.
    b. power setting of the laser.
    c. the diameter of the laser's aperture.
    d. how long the tissue is exposed to the laser.
26. The use of a specialized endoscope to perform a minimally invasive examination of the abdomen and its viscera is called
    a. endoscopy.
    b. gastroscopy.
    c. laparoscopy.
    d. abdominoscopy.
27. Endoscopic examination of the stomach is called
    a. gastroscopy.
    b. laparoscopy.
    c. duodenoscopy.
    d. esophagoscopy.
28. What is a scrotal ablation?
29. How can seroma formation be limited postamputation?
30. How can swelling be limited postamputation?
31. List two reasons to perform a gastrotomy.
32. Which type of internal fixation is less costly but may sacrifice stability?

BIBLIOGRAPHY

American National Standards Institute. *Safe use of lasers (ANSI Z136.1–1993)*. New York, 1993, ANSI.

AVMA. Elective spaying and neutering of pets, Schaumburg, 2020.

Bassert JM, Beal AD, Samples OM editors: McCurnin's clinical textbook for veterinary technicians, ed 9, St Louis, 2018, Elsevier.

Bessler M, Whelan RL, Halverson A, Treat MR, Nowygrod R: Is immune function better preserved after laparoscopic versus open colon resection? *Surg Endosc* 8:881, 1994.

Bjorab MJ, Ellison GW, Slocum B: *Current techniques in small animal surgery*, Philadelphia, 1998, Williams & Wilkins.

Blood DC, Studdert VP: *Saunders comprehensive veterinary dictionary*, ed 3, London, 2007, Saunders.

Brockman DJ, Washabau RJ, Drobatz KJ: Canine gastric dilatation/volvulus syndrome in a veterinary critical care unit: 295 cases (1986-1992). *J Am Vet Med Assoc* 207:460, 1995.

Burrows CF, Bright RM, Spencer CP: Influence of dietary composition on gastric emptying and motility in dogs: potential involvement in acute gastric dilatation. *Am J Vet Res* 46:2609, 1985.

Darvelid AW, Linde-Forsberg C: Dystocia in the bitch. *J Small Anim Pract* 35:402, 1994.

Doverspike M, Vasseur PB, Harb MF: Contralateral cranial cruciate ligament rupture: incidence in 114 dogs. *J Am Anim Hosp Assoc* 29:275, 1993.

Flanders JA, Harvey HJ: Results of tube gastrostomy as treatment for gastric torsion in the dog. *J Am Vet Med Assoc* 185:74, 1984.

Fossum TW, Cho J, Dewey C, et al Small animal surgery, ed 5, Philadelphia, 2019, Elsevier.

Gaudet DA: Retrospective study of 128 cases of canine dystocia. *J Small Anim Pract* 21:813, 1985.

Gelatt KN: *Essentials of veterinary ophthalmology*, Philadelphia, 2000, Lippincott Williams & Wilkins.

Glickman LT, Glickman NW, Schellenberg DB, et al. Multiple risk factors for the gastric dilatation-volvulus syndrome in dogs. *J Am Vet Med Assoc* 216:40, 2000.

Glickman LT, Lantz GC, Schellenberg DB, et al.: Analysis of risk factors for gastric dilatation and dilatation volvulus in dogs: a practitioner/owner case-control study. *J Am Anim Hosp Assoc* 34:253, 1997.

Gross ME, Jones BD, Bergstresser DR, et al.: Effects of abdominal insufflation with nitrous oxide on cardiorespiratory measurements in spontaneously breathing isoflurane-anesthetized dogs. *Am J Vet Res* 54:1352, 1993.

Gualtieri M: Esophagoscopy. *Vet Clin North Am Small Anim Pract* 31:605, 2001.

Harvey CE: The ear and nose. In Harvey CE, Newton CD, Schwartz A, et al.: *Small animal surgery*. Philadelphia, 1990, Lippincott.

Hitz CB: An overview of laser technology. In *Understanding laser technology: an intuitive introduction to basic and advanced laser concepts*, ed 2, Tulsa, OK, 1991, Pennwell.

Holt TL, Mann FA: Soft tissue applications of lasers. *Vet Clin North Am* 32:569, 2002.

Jacques SL: Laser-tissue interactions: photochemical, photothermal, and photomechanical. *Surg Clin North Am* 72:531, 1992.

Johanningmeier JP: TPLO repair method for CCL tears. *Vet Tech* 682.

Johnson JA, Austin C, Bruer GJ: Incidence of appendicular musculoskeletal disorders in veterinary teaching hospitals from 1980-1989. *Vet Comp Orthop Trauma* 7:56, 1994.

Johnson JM, Johnson AL: Cranial cruciate ligament rupture: pathogenesis, diagnosis and postoperative rehabilitation. *Vet Clin North Am* 23:717, 1993.

Katzir A: Medical lasers. *Lasers and optical fibers in medicine*. San Diego, 1993, Academic Press.

Katzir A: Single optical fibers. *Lasers and optical fibers in medicine*. San Diego, 1993, Academic Press.

Leib MS, Konde LJ, Wingfield WE, et al.: Circumcostal gastropexy for preventing recurrence of gastric dilatation-volvulus in the dog: an evaluation of 30 cases. *J Am Vet Med Assoc* 187:245, 1985.

Lettow E: Laparoscopic examinations in liver diseases in dogs. *Vet Med Rev* 2:159, 1972.

Lichtenbarger, M: *Gastrointinal endoscopy procedures and equipment*, Vetfolio.com, 2019

Lucroy MD, Bartels KE: Using biomedical lasers in veterinary practice., *Vet Med* 95:4, 2000.

Lumenis LX-20SP NovaPulse laser system operator's manual, Lumenis, 2002, Santa Clara, CA

Maggs D: *Fundamentals of veterinary ophthalmology*, ed 4, Philadelphia, 2008, Saunders.

Magne ML, Tams TR: Laparoscopy: instrumentation and technique. In Tams TR, editor: *Small animal endoscopy*, ed 3, St Louis, 2011, Mosby.

Marsolais GS, Dvorak G, Conzemius MG: Effects of postoperative rehabilitation on limb function after cranial cruciate ligament repair in dogs. *J Am Vet Med Assoc* 220:1325, 2002.

Matthiesen DT: Partial gastrectomy as treatment for gastric volvulus. *Vet Surg* 14:185, 1985.

Mehler SJ, Bennett A: Surgical oncology of exotic animals. *Vet Clin Exotic Anim Pract* 7:783–805, 2004.

Monnet E, Twedt DC: Laparoscopy. *Vet Clin North Am* 33:1147, 2003.

Moore CP, Constantinescu GM: Surgery of the adnexa. *Vet Clin North Am* 27:1011, 1997.

Moore KW, Read RA: Rupture of the cranial cruciate ligament in dogs. *Compend Contin Educ Pract Vet* 18:223, 1996.

Morrison WB: *Cancer in dogs and cats*, Baltimore, 1998, Williams & Wilkins.

Muir WW: Gastric dilatation-volvulus in the dog, with emphasis on cardiac arrhythmias. *J Am Vet Med Assoc* 180:739, 1982.

Nelson R, Couto C: *Small animal internal medicine*, ed 4, St Louis, 2009, Mosby.

Osborne CA, et al.: Analysis of 77,000 canine uroliths. *Vet Clin North Am Small Anim Pract* 29:1, 1999.

Palmer, R: *Understanding tibial plateau leveling osteotomies in dogs*, VeterinaryMedicine.DVM360, 2005

Pearce J, Thomsen R: Rate process analysis of thermal damage. In Welch AJ, van Gamert MJC, editors: *Optical-thermal response of laser irradiated tissue*, New York, 1995, Plenum.

Pearson H: The complications of ovariohysterectomy in the bitch., *J Small Anim Pract* 14:257, 1973.

Phillips BS: Bladder tumors in dogs and cats. *Compend Contin Educ Pract Vet* 21:540, 1999.

Piermattie DL, Flo GL, DeCam CE: *Brinker, Piermattei and Flo's handbook of small animal orthopedics and fracture repair*, ed 4, St Louis, 2006, Elsevier.

Plumb, DC: *Plumb's veterinary drug handbook*, ed 8, Ames, 2015, WileyBlackwell.

Pope, ER: Step-by-step cystotomy, *Clinician's Brief*, March 2016.

Richter KP: Laparoscopy in dogs and cats, *Vet Clin North Am* 31:707, 2001.

Robben JR, Stokhof AA, van Sluisjs FJ: Arrhythmias after surgery of gastric dilatation volvulus in dogs. *Tijdschr Diergenneeskd* 118(Suppl):67S, 1993.

Roberts SM, Severin GA, Lavach JD: Prevalence and treatment of palpebral neoplasms in the dog: 200 cases (1975-1983). ,*J Am Vet Med Assoc* 189:1355, 1986.

Rothuizen J: Laparoscopy in small animal medicine. *Vet Q* 3:225, 1985.

Sammarco JL, Conzemius MG, Perkowski SZ, Weinstein MJ, Gregor TP, Smith GK: Postoperative analgesia for stifle surgery: a comparison of intraarticular bupivacaine, morphine or saline. *Vet Surg* 25:59, 1996.

Sammarco, JL, Kahl, A: *Caesarean sections in dog: indications and techniques.* 2007.

Schneider R, Dorn CR, Taylor DO: Factors influencing canine mammary cancer development and post surgical survival. *J Natl Cancer Inst* 43:1249, 1969.

Schumway R, Broussard J: Maintenance of gastrointestinal endoscopes. *Clin Tech Small Anim Pract* 18:254, 2003.

Sirois M: *Principles and practice of veterinary technology*, ed 3, St Louis, 2011, Mosby.

Slatter D: *Textbook of small animal surgery*, ed 3, Philadelphia, 2003, Saunders.

Smeak DD: The Chinese finger trap suture technique for fastening tubes and catheters. *J Am Anim Hosp Assoc* 26:215, 1990.

Smith GK, Torg JS: Fibula head transposition for repair of cruciate-deficient stifle in the dog. *J Am Vet Med Assoc* 187:375, 1985.

Sonsthagen TF: *Veterinary instruments and equipment*, ed 3, St Louis, 2014, Mosby.

Spencer D, Daye, RM: A prospective, randomized, double-blinded, placebo-controlled clinical study on postoperative antibiotherapy in 150 arthroscopy-assisted tibial plateau leveling osteotomies in dogs, Veterinary Surgeon, 47:8, 2018.

Stasi K, Melendez L: Care and cleaning of the endoscope. *Vet Clin North Am Small Anim Pract* 31:589, 2001.

Studdert, V: *Saunders comprehensive veterinary dictionary*, ed. 4, Elsevier

Sullins KE: Diode laser and endoscopic laser surgery. *Vet Clin North Am* 32:639, 2002.

Tams T: *Handbook of small animal gastroenterology*, ed 2, St Louis, 2003, Saunders.

Tams T, editor: *Small animal endoscopy*, ed. 3, St Louis, 2011, Mosby.

Theran P: Early-age neutering of dogs and cats. *J Am Vet Med Assoc* 202:914, 1993.

3M™ Ioban™ 2 Antimicrobial Incise Drape 6661E, 2020, 3m.com, Retrieved from https://www.3m.com/3M/en_US/company-us/all-3m-products/,/3M-Ioban-2-Antimicrobial-Incise-Drape-6661EZ-50-EA-Box-4-Box-Case/?N=5002385+3294796414&rt=rud.

Tobias KM, Johnston SA: *Veterinary surgery: small animal*, St Louis, 2012, Saunders.

Troncy E, Junot S, Keroack S, et al.: Results of preemptive epidural administration of morphine with or without bupivacaine in dogs and cats undergoing surgery: 265 cases (1997-1999), *J Am Vet Med Assoc* 221:666, 2002.

Ward, E: Preanesthetic testing in private practice., *Clinician's Brief*, 1/2010

Welch AJ, van Gemert MJC: Introduction to medical applications. In Welch AJ, van Gemert MJC, editors: *Optical-thermal response of laser irradiated tissue*, New York, 1995, Plenum.

Welch AJ, van Gemert MJC, Star WM: Definitions and overview of tissue optics. In Welch AJ, van Gemert MJC, editors: *Optical-thermal response of laser irradiated tissue*, New York, 1995, Plenum.

Whittick WG: *Canine orthopedics*, ed 2, Philadelphia, 1990, Lea & Febiger.

Willard MD: *Small animal clinical diagnosis by laboratory methods*, St Louis, 2004, Saunders.

Withrow SJ, MacEwen EG: *Withrow and MacEwen*'s small animal clinical oncology, ed 4, St Louis, 2007, Saunders.

Withrow SJ, Postorino NC, Straw RC: Tumors of the gastrointestinal system. . *Clinical veterinary oncology*, Philadelphia, 1989, Lippincott.

Witney WO, Scavelli TD, Matthiesen DT, et al.: Belt-loop gastropexy: technique and surgical results in 20 dogs. *J Am Anim Hosp Assoc* 25:75, 1989.

Young WP: Feline onychectomy and elective procedures. *Vet Clin North Am* 32:601, 2002.

Zepp CP: Surgical technique to establish drainage of the external ear canal and correction of hematoma of the dog and cat. *J Am Vet Med Assoc* 115:91, 1949.

The Postoperative Patient

Ann Wortinger

LEARNING OBJECTIVES

After completion of this chapter, the reader will be able to:

- Monitor the patient during the anesthesia recovery period.
- Identify the proper time to extubate the patient.
- Safely extubate the patient.
- Recognize and administer prescribed treatments for prevention of postanesthesia complications, such as hypothermia, emergence delirium, and prolonged recovery.
- Recognize and administer prescribed treatments for postsurgical complications, such as hemorrhage, seroma, dehiscence, self-trauma, and infection.
- Thoroughly and properly cleanse wounds, understanding the principles of lavage and débridement.
- Maintain and monitor bandages, casts, splints, and slings.

- Maintain and monitor surgical drains.
- Maintain and monitor indwelling venous and urinary catheters.
- Provide nutritional support for postoperative patients through the techniques of force feeding and tube feeding.
- Understand the basic forms of physical therapy.
- Provide effective postoperative analgesia.
- Understand the importance of preemptive, preoperative analgesia on the success of postoperative analgesia.
- Safely combine different classes of analgesics to provide effective postoperative pain management (multimodal analgesia).

KEY TERMS

Active drains	Emergence delirium	Passive drains
Autotransfusion	Fenestrated	Pétrissage
Brachycephalic	Hypoglycemia	Semiocclusive wound dressing
Cryotherapy	Hypothermia	Seroma
Débridement	Lavage	Thermoregulatory
Dehiscence	Normothermic	Wind-up
Dissociative anesthetic	Occlusive wound dressing	

The work of the veterinary technician is still far from complete even when the last suture is placed and the surgeon leaves the surgical suite. The patient still needs to recover from the anesthesia, and postoperative pain needs to be recognized and controlled. The surgical wounds need to heal. The surgical procedure has yet to be proved successful. The patient and the owner need help and guidance during the recuperation period. Careful patient monitoring and owner mentoring are important responsibilities of the veterinary technician.

Compassion, caring, and concern are the hallmarks of an excellent technician. All hospitalized patients need an advocate. The observant and trained technician who advocates for the patient's needs and points out changes in the patient's physical status to the attending veterinarian is an invaluable asset to both the patient and the veterinarian.

RECOVERY FROM ANESTHESIA AND EXTUBATION

Shepherding the patient from the surgical plane of anesthesia back to consciousness is the first step in the recovery process. The recovery period starts with the cessation of anesthesia and continues until the patient's vital signs and level of consciousness have returned to normal. The length of this period depends on many factors that include the length of the anesthetic period, the condition of the patient, the type of anesthetic agent used and the route of administration, the patient's body temperature, and the breed of the patient.

First, the patient must be safely extubated. The steps in the process of extubation are outlined in Box 11.1. It is important to remember that the inhaled gas is not metabolized by the patient, and will be exhaled into the room environment after disconnection from the anesthetic machine. To help prevent personal and environmental contamination, it is recommended to not put your face near the mouth of a recovering animal, to maintain the patient on oxygen for as long as possible to prevent environmental contamination, and to limit the number of recovering animals based on the size of the area and capability of the ventilation system in the area.

Brachycephalic breeds of dogs, such as English bulldogs, pugs, and Pekingese, are prone to developing complications while recovering from anesthesia. These short-headed dogs often have stenotic nares and elongated soft palates and are predisposed to laryngeal obstruction during sedation. An elongated soft palate can occlude the larynx and prevent the passage of air through the mouth. The stenotic nares do not allow sufficient air

---

BOX 11.1 Sequence of Events for Endotracheal Extubation

1. Turn off the anesthetic vaporizer and leave the patient on oxygen for 5 minutes if possible.
2. Find an empty syringe with the plunger depressed completely. Attach a syringe to the cuff if using a silicone tube with a spring valve in the pilot tube (non–red rubber tube), and deflate the cuff. Leaving the cuff inflated without having it securely fastened can lead to tracheal trauma, necrosis, or tearing. It is imperative to monitor the patient for any signs of vomiting or regurgitation once the cuff is deflated to prevent aspiration.*
3. Untie the endotracheal (ET) tube attachment from the patient's head or muzzle.*
4. Check the patient's reflexes. Not every patient will stay under for the full 5 minutes. The anesthetist must know whether or not the patient is close to jumping off the table.
5. Untie the patient from the table, detach all monitoring devices, and decrease fluid administration to a maintenance rate. Remove the V-trough or sandbags and place the patient in lateral recumbency. When rotating the patient into lateral recumbency, guard the tube and do not let it rotate in the patient's trachea. It is important to prevent twisting injury to the trachea. Small patients are especially prone to this injury.
6. Take the immediate postoperative temperature at this point. Continue anesthetic monitoring of the vital signs every 5 minutes until the patient is sufficiently recovered to be returned to the cage.
7. Once the 5 minutes of oxygen administration are completed, disconnect the patient from the anesthesia machine while the oxygen is flowing. This will ensure that the patient always has a source of oxygen in case of an emergency. Place a hand over the end of the Y-piece and squeeze the reservoir bag. This will empty the circuit of most of the gas through the exhaust system.
8. Now shut of the oxygen at the flowmeter.
9. Recheck the reflexes and determine the patient's stage of anesthesia. If the patient is still "asleep," stimulate the patient by rubbing its thorax, stroking the neck, and gently pulling the tongue or ears. It may also help to gently rotate the animal from side to side.
10. Once the patient has swallowed two or three times, gently pull the ET tube down and out of the mouth. (See exception for brachycephalic breeds noted on page 214.)*
11. Check the end of the ET tube for blood, regurgitated stomach contents, and food. If the animal has regurgitated material in the mouth, hang the head down off the surgical table to allow the material to drip out of the mouth. Quickly determine whether the patient needs to be reintubated or the pharynx needs to be suctioned. Carefully rinsing the mouth gently with water may suffice, provided that it does not cause the patient to gag and choke from the rinsing process.
12. Take the patient to the recovery cage.
13. Place the patient in the recovery cage, so that the animal can be easily monitored for mucous membrane color and respiratory rate.
14. Continue to monitor the patient every 5 to 10 minutes to ensure that recovery is a safe and smooth event until complete. At this point, give postoperative pain medications as instructed. Generally, if the patient's temperature is less than 98° F postoperatively, opioid drugs will not be given. Hypothermia concerns are discussed later.

Alternative Steps

If the ET tube cuff is not deflated before being untied, extreme care must be taken to ensure tracheal trauma does not occur; the following alternative steps should be used:

*2. Untie the ET tube attachment from the patient's head or muzzle.
*3. Find an empty syringe with the plunger depressed completely. Attach the syringe to the cuff if using a silicone tube with a spring valve in the pilot tube (non–red rubber tube). Do not deflate the ET tube cuff yet.
*10. Once the patient swallows two or three times, deflate the cuff and gently pull the ET tube down and out of the mouth. (See exception for brachycephalic breeds noted on page 214.) The ET tube cuff should never be deflated before the patient regains the ability to swallow. A patient that cannot swallow is vulnerable to aspiration of material that has pooled in the pharynx. A properly inflated ET tube cuff prevents such aspiration.

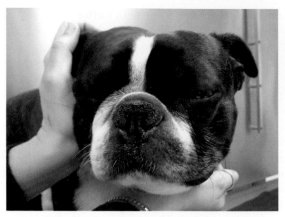

Fig. 11.1 Brachycephalic breeds of dogs and cats often have nasal openings that are extremely small. Breathing through the nose is difficult. This condition is known as stenotic nares.

to pass through the nasal passages (Fig. 11.1). When managing a brachycephalic dog under anesthesia, the best course of action is to delay extubation as long as possible. Many anesthetists will extubate brachycephalic dogs only after they can lift their heads by themselves. Allow these patients to recover as fully as possible before pulling the endotracheal (ET) tube. Once the ET tube is out, closely monitor the patient for any signs of dyspnea and cyanosis (blue mucous membranes). Optimizing tissue perfusion and maintaining adequate oxygen delivery are the main goals of anesthetic recovery.

POSTOPERATIVE MONITORING

Close monitoring and documentation of vital signs are usually discontinued after the patient is extubated and placed in the recovery cage. Although the recovery period technically begins when the animal is disconnected from anesthesia, the patient is not completely recovered until all physiologic parameters, including neurologic responses, are normal. This period can last for hours and can be dependent on the patient and the anesthetic used. Potential complications include airway obstruction, hypotension, thermoregulatory problems (primarily hypothermia), and cardiac arrhythmia. Although patient monitoring

may not need to be as frequent, regular monitoring should continue.

The recovery area should be a separate and quiet area in the animal hospital dedicated to recovery from anesthesia. The recovery area should be constantly staffed with one or more technicians. The area should be fully stocked with drugs and equipment necessary to handle any emergency. In small hospitals with limited personnel, recovering patients should be placed in a staffed area where they will be observed frequently. Patients should never be left unattended, because many accidents and complications can occur during this time.

At-risk patients should be monitored closely while recovering. A charting system should be used to help the recovery technicians identify trends and initiate appropriate treatments. The vital signs may be plotted on a graph similar to the anesthesia form, or the vital sign readings may be written in a chart (Fig. 11.2). To minimize problems during recovery, the patient should be positioned in the recovery cage so that mucous membranes and respiration can be easily observed. This usually means the animal's head is towards the front of the cage and uncovered to aid observation. Do not tightly curl their bodies, with their noses in a back corner of the cage.

COMPLICATIONS RELATED TO ANESTHESIA

Hypothermia

Thermoregulation occurs when temperature variations are detected by thermal receptors in peripheral tissues (e.g., skin, extremities, and subcutaneous) and core zone regions (e.g., brain, heart, and great vessels) and transmitted to the posterior hypothalamus by way of the spinal cord. Thermal homeostasis is achieved by modulating the flow of blood to organs, viscera, and skin via vasoconstriction or vasodilation.

Heat loss occurs in two stages: In stage one, heat is transferred from the core to the skin. Stage two occurs when heat is ultimately lost to the environment by conduction, convection, radiation, and evaporation of moisture from the skin and respiratory tract. Prevention of heat loss requires that these four ways of loss are controlled or moderated.

Time				
Temperature				
Pulse				
Respiration				
Blood tests				
PVC/TS				
Electrolytes				
Blood gases				
Other				
Blood pressure				

Fig. 11.2 Postanesthesia monitoring form. Vital signs and *PCV/TS*, Packed cell volume/total solids.

Most patients lose body heat while they are anesthetized. Mild hypothermia, or body temperature no lower than 97° F (about 36° C), is expected and is usually well tolerated by the patient. A body temperature below 93° F (about 34° C) is worrisome and can affect the patient's recovery adversely. Small patients are at the greatest risk of hypothermia because of their small body surface–to–mass ratio. Most heat loss (Fig. 11.3) occurs within the first 20 minutes of general anesthesia. As the body temperature decreases, the amount of anesthetic required decreases. For every 1.8° F (1° C) decrease in body temperature there is a 5% decrease in minimum alveolar concentration (MAC) requirements.

The metabolism of the body cells functions best at normal body temperature. As the body temperature drops, normal metabolism slows down, adversely affecting the functioning of all organs of the body. The brain and heart are particularly sensitive to hypothermia. Almost every major organ and system is adversely affected by hypothermia. Hypothermia can cause decreased cardiac output, increased risk of arrhythmias, hypoxia, and reduced tissue perfusion. Decreased hepatic metabolism results in delayed drug clearance and intestinal hypomotility and can prolong anesthetic recoveries. Suppressed immune function can lead to increased infection rates and delayed wound healing. The net effect of hypothermia is increased morbidity and mortality.

For a normal animal, when vasoconstrictive efforts by the body fail to mitigate heat loss and maintain core temperature, heat production is augmented via increasing muscle tone and shivering. Shivering is very effective in restoring body temperature but is uncomfortable for the animal and can be associated with a significant increase in metabolic oxygen demand (40%–200% or more). As the body cools, the anesthetized animal cannot compensate by shivering or seeking a warmer environment. Muscular activity involved with shivering increases body heat. The anesthetized patient is lying still, so body heat production from muscular activity is absent. Because most anesthetized animals have been fasted, the heat produced during digestion is also not available.

Rewarming should be considered when hypothermic patients have a temperature less than 97.6° F. There are three techniques for rewarming patients: passive external rewarming, active external rewarming, and active core rewarming.

During rewarming, an after-drop occurs because of a large temperature gradient created by colder peripheral blood being transferred to the relatively warmer core, resulting in a further reduction in the core body temperature. Therefore, warming the torso region while the (cooler) extremities remain vasoconstricted can be advantageous. Decrease rewarming efforts as the patient's temperature approaches normal to avoid rebound hyperthermia, especially in cats and small dogs. Once the temperature has reached 100°F (37.7°C), rewarming efforts can be discontinued.

Monitor the temperature of hypothermic patients every 30 minutes. Hypothermia results when body heat loss exceeds heat production. Causes of hypothermia are related to the effects of anesthesia and the consequences of surgery such as removing the hair coat during surgical prep, opening the abdomen during surgery, and prolonged inactivity and the inability to shiver. Preanesthetic and analgesic drugs can alter the thermoregulatory center in the brain, thus interfering with the maintenance of a constant, optimum body temperature. All animals undergoing a surgical procedure are at risk for development of hypothermia. Neonates, very lean animals (Body Condition Score < 2/5 or 4/9), and geriatric animals are at greatest risk for hypothermia. Numerous procedures are performed on the surgical patient that increase the loss of body heat (Box 11.2).

Various means to prevent hypothermia during surgery are discussed in Chapter 5. Treatment of hypothermia is discussed here. Many of the treatment measures are similar to the measures used to prevent hypothermia. The hypothermic patient needs to be monitored closely and frequently. Placing pads or blankets with circulating warm water or air under, over, and around the patient is a first step (Fig. 11.4). SnuggleSafe Microwave Heat Pad (SnuggleSafe, Lenric C21 Ltd., Littlehampton, West Sussex, UK), Hot Dog warmer (Augustine Temperature Management, Eden Prairie MN) (Fig. 11.5), sacks of rice or lentils heated in a microwave oven, and warm water bottles or bags can supplement other measures. The patient, including its head, can be placed under a tent made by blankets and warming objects. The air under the blankets is warmer than the room air; breathing in the warmed air helps warm the body. Fluids administered subcutaneously or intravenously should be warmed to approximately 98° to 99° F. The fluid temperature can be

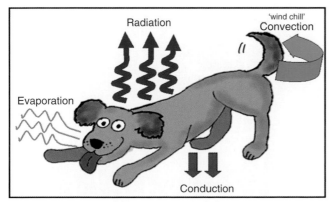

Fig. 11.3 Heat loss methods. (Image courtesy Heidi Reuss-Lamky LVT, VTS [Surgery, Anesthesia].)

BOX 11.2 Procedures That Lead to Body Heat Loss

The surgical site is shaved.

The surgical site is cleaned with surgical scrub and water followed by alcohol. The evaporation of these cleansing agents quickly cools the skin.

The patient may be maintained on gas anesthesia carried by cold oxygen. The source of the oxygen is a compressed oxygen tank. Any gas stored under pressure is cold. The cold gases entering the lungs cool the body.

Room-temperature fluids administered intravenously will lower body temperature.

A body cavity may be opened, exposing the internal organs to room-temperature air.

The patient may be laying on a metal or grate surface that quickly wicks heat away from the body.

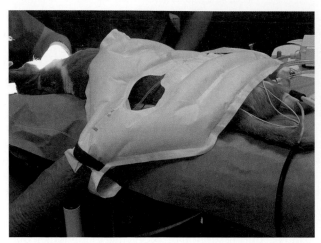

Fig. 11.4 Gaymar convection-air patient-warming system blanket is placed over cat recovering from anesthesia. The warm air diffuses around the patient, providing a warm microenvironment.

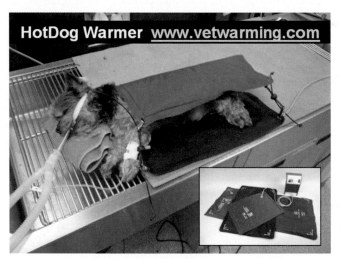

Fig. 11.5 Hot Dog warming system provides warming of both the top and bottom of the patient. (Image courtesy Augustine Biomedical & Design.)

tested on the technician's wrist, as in testing for the proper temperature of baby formula before feeding. Warming devices for intravenous (IV) fluids are also available.

Water-filled balloons or latex gloves can be used instead of bottles. Expired fluid bags can be heated in a microwave oven and are effective in warming the patient. These are softer than bottles and mold to the contours of the patient's body. Towels or blankets can be warmed in the dryer and then wrapped around the patient with an outer blanket to help trap the heat. While this method is convenient, there is significant risk of thermal burns when the bags are heated too much, and they lose heat quickly and must be monitored and reheated often.

Uncooked rice or lentils can substitute for the water in bottles, balloons, or gloves. The rice-filled containers are placed in a microwave oven for several minutes. The time required depends on the power level used, the oven's wattage, and the size of the bottle or bag. The technician must experiment beforehand to determine the proper heating time needed. These containers

tend to remain warmer for a longer time than water bottles. Care must be taken not to leave plastic containers in the microwave too long; overheating could melt the plastic. The technician must ensure that none of these warming devices is in direct contact with the skin, which might cause thermal burns. Either the patient or the warming device should be wrapped in at least a single layer of cloth to protect the skin. The patient is unable to move away from these heat sources if they are too warm or if damage to the skin is occurring; this can result in significant thermal burns, especially in areas where the protective fur layer has been removed for the surgical procedure. As the warm water bottle cools and its temperature falls below the temperature of the hypothermic patient, the bottle that was warming the patient will now be cooling the patient. The water bottles should be re-warmed frequently. Also, leaking of the warm water on to the patient is a concern. A wet patient is at risk of becoming a colder patient. All homemade warmers tend to lose heat quickly and must be monitored often to ensure they do not cause thermal burns by being too hot or further exacerbate hypothermia by being too cool.

Electric heating pads should not be used. They can become too hot for the recumbent patient, and severe thermal burns of the skin may occur. Such burns usually do not become evident until several days later. Large areas of skin that were in contact with the electric heating pad may be affected. Significant skin sloughing can be a serious complication. The electric heating pad can also prove to be a source of electrocution if the patient decides to chew on the cord or pad.

Emergence Delirium

Occasionally when recovering from general anesthesia, the animal exhibits signs of excitement, possibly with exaggerated and uncontrollable movements. The patient may thrash around in the cage, cry out, or paddle all four legs. This phenomenon is called **emergence delirium** (Fig. 11.6).

Emergence delirium occurs for several reasons. During the recovery process the animal travels back through the stages of anesthesia. Stage II is the "excitement" stage of anesthesia. In

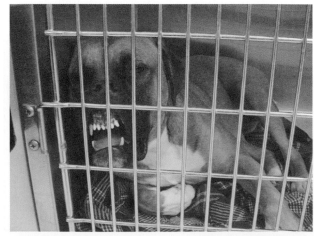

Fig. 11.6 Dog exhibiting emergence delirium. Between periods of thrashing in the cage, the dog presses its nose against the cage door.

some cases, the patient passes slowly through stage II and spends several minutes exhibiting signs of excitement. Analgesic and anesthetic side effects contribute to the development of emergence delirium. Opioids are given for their analgesic effects, but these drugs can sensitize the patient to loud auditory stimuli and bright visual stimuli. When stimulated, these patients may be aroused and may exhibit erratic behavior. Dissociative anesthetic agents, such as ketamine, are known to cause hallucinations in humans, so animals also may undergo hallucinations when given these agents.

If the patient thrashes violently in the cage, problems may arise. The surgical site may undergo severe trauma and possibly dehiscence. The animal may smash its head against the hard side of the cage, causing bruising, scraped skin, and even fractured teeth. Toes can become wedged into the bars of the cage, causing skin damage or even broken bones. The patient that is wildly thrashing in the cage may also become hyperthermic, so a body temperature reading should be taken as soon as possible. Howling and screeching may become loud and may disturb other patients, hospital personnel, and clients.

The animal undergoing emergence delirium needs to be approached carefully. This animal is capable of hurting itself as well as the staff. Nevertheless, this patient needs to be calmed; in some cases, "tincture of time" and holding the animal are sufficient. Some animals benefit from administration of a tranquilizer. The technician should notify the veterinarian in charge of the case for a consultation if the animal has injured or may injure itself or if the delirium lasts several minutes.

Prolonged Recovery

Some animals may take an unexpectedly long time to recover from the anesthesia. Most animals are able to maintain sternal recumbency and lift their head within several minutes after extubation. The patient that is unable to raise its head or to be aroused while recovering in its cage is a concern for the recovery room nurse. There are many reasons why a patient may have a prolonged recovery from anesthesia.

Anesthesia-Related Causes

Excessive depth of anesthesia. If the patient was maintained for a long time under anesthesia (>1 hour) and the depth of anesthesia was maintained at a deep level (stage III, plane 3), the patient will have a high concentration of the anesthetic in the body tissues. Gas anesthetics must pass out of the body tissues into the bloodstream and be eliminated by the lungs. A small percentage of a gas anesthetic is metabolized by the liver.

Breed predisposition. Sight hounds are sensitive to barbiturate anesthetics. In most dogs, barbiturates are redistributed from the vessel-rich tissues of the brain and muscles to the fat stores. Once in the fat stores, the barbiturate slowly reenters the bloodstream and is eventually metabolized in the liver. Sight hounds do not typically have as much fat on their bodies as most other breeds. Therefore, when the muscles become saturated, the barbiturate has no place for storage and is recirculated back to the brain, thus prolonging anesthesia recovery. Of all of the barbiturates previously available, only pentobarbital

sodium is still regularly used for induction of general anesthesia. This is only used in laboratory animals by intraperitoneal injection and is not commonly seen in general practice.

Patient-Related Causes

Hypotension, poor perfusion, or shock. *Hypotension* is defined as a systolic pressure less than 80 mm Hg or a mean arterial pressure (MAP) less than 60 mm Hg. The patient that is in shock or has hypotension is not effectively perfusing the organs and tissues. This is especially important for the kidneys and brain. The anesthetic is therefore not being delivered effectively to the organs that will utilize and eliminate it. Blood pressure can be measured using a couple of methods. The most accurate is the direct measure in which an arterial catheter is placed in the animal, and blood pressure is measured directly from this site. This practice is more technically difficult than venous catheter placement and, if placed when the animal is awake, is very uncomfortable. More commonly, indirect means of measurement are used in practice. These include Doppler and oscillometric measurements. Both of these means are noninvasive and require the use of an occlusive cuff. Doppler readings are believed to be more accurate in cats but do require more "hands-on" use. Oscillometric measurement requires the use of a specialized machine that automatically inflates and deflates the cuff, detecting oscillations in the flow through the artery. Oscillometric measurements may not be accurate if cardiac arrhythmias, slow pulse rates, or low blood pressure are present.

Liver or kidney disease. Many anesthetics are metabolized and eliminated through the liver or kidneys. Patients with compromised liver or kidney function eliminate these anesthetic agents more slowly than patients with healthy organs. Preanesthetic blood tests help identify such patients. The dose of anesthetic should then be reduced for these patients, or an alternative anesthetic agent should be used.

Intracranial disease. Patients with an altered level of consciousness (LOC) caused by central nervous system (CNS) disease are especially sensitive to the side effects of certain anesthetics. Some anesthetics increase intracranial pressure. Patients with a history of head trauma or seizures may not be able to tolerate anesthetic agents that lower the seizure threshold. In these patients a different anesthetic protocol should be used.

Hypoglycemia. Neonatal patients are extremely susceptible to development of hypoglycemia. Glucose is stored in the form of glycogen in the liver and muscle for use between periods of eating. Because of their small size and immature livers, these animals tend to not have as much stored glycogen as older animals and may become hypoglycemic much sooner than one would expect. These patients should not be fasted, or fasted for only 1 to 2 hours, before anesthesia. Hypoglycemia adversely affects the patient's recovery from anesthesia and predisposes the patient to seizures. If the blood glucose becomes lower than 50 mg/dL, seizures can be seen. Food should also be offered as soon after anesthesia recovery as possible. Once they are swallowing, are normothermic, and have had their pain managed, the patients can be offered food. There is no reason to wait until the next day to offer food after an anesthetic event. A veterinary recovery diet is usually a good option to offer during this recovery period. These diets are higher in protein and fats and lower in carbohydrates than typical maintenance diets. This allows for a more gradual increase in blood glucose and helps to prevent another decrease later in the day. Small meals offered frequently are preferred over a single large meal. Palatability of recovery diets also tends to be higher, allowing easier feeding.

Hypothermia. The cells of the body function best at a normal body temperature. The cellular enzymes involved in metabolizing anesthetic drugs are less active when the body temperature falls. Bradycardia and subsequent perfusion abnormalities are other consequences associated with hypothermia. If perfusion and circulation are adversely affected, the anesthetic cannot be redistributed to the organs that will eliminate it.

Therapeutic Measures

The patient recovering slowly from anesthesia needs to be assessed by the veterinarian, who may order laboratory tests to be run. Additional nursing care measures may be instituted as well. Close monitoring is important because this is a fragile patient in which a life-threatening complication could develop. Several methods can be used to hasten the patient's recovery from anesthesia.

Physical stimulation. Physical stimulation by rubbing, massaging, and turning from side to side are simple ways to increase the patient's level of consciousness. Talking to or whistling to the animal can help speed up the recovery.

Ventilation. The patient that is still intubated can be manually ventilated with pure oxygen. Gas anesthetic agents are mainly eliminated through the lungs. Ventilating the patient with pure oxygen and increasing the frequency of respirations raises the rate at which the gas anesthetic leaves the body. Normal oxygen saturation should be greater than 95% using a peripheral pulse oximeter. A pulse oximetry reading of less than 90% requires an immediate response by the technician. Care must be taken not to overventilate the patient and cause apnea. The pure oxygen in the system triggers the respiratory center to decrease respirations, causing a decrease or cessation of respirations. If the system is not scavenged for waste anesthetic gases (WAGs), care needs to be taken by the staff during this period because the residual waste anesthetic gas is exhaled by the patient into the recovery room environment, increasing secondary exposure by the staff to the gas.

Fluid therapy. A bolus of IV fluids can help increase the blood pressure of the hypotensive patient and improve perfusion of internal organs such as the lungs, liver, and kidneys. Warmed fluids can help raise the core body temperature. Blood pressure should be monitored using either Doppler or oscillometric devices to assess response to fluid resuscitation efforts.

Reversal agents. Some injectable anesthetic agents have reversal agents. The technician should consult with the veterinarian before administering a reversal agent. Giving an opioid antagonist, such as naloxone, reverses all the effects of the opioid, including its analgesic effects. The loss of analgesic effects could be detrimental to the patient. Dexmedetomidine is reversed by atipamezole. It works by simply displacing the dexmedetomidine from the alpha$_2$ receptors allowing nerve function to return to normal. Doxapram is a respiratory

stimulant that helps to arouse the deeply anesthetized patient; it is not a specific reversal agent.

Warming measures. The hypothermic patient recovers slowly from anesthesia and will benefit from warming measures (see earlier discussion).

Dextrose. Hypoglycemia may be documented through a blood test or may be suspected from the patient's symptoms and risk factors. Clinically, patients with hypoglycemia may appear disoriented, may gaze blankly off into space, may be slow to respond to noxious stimuli, and may have either a prolonged recovery from anesthesia or seizures.

Dextrose solution administered intravenously is the preferred treatment. Due to the high osmolality of the original 50% dextrose solution, for IV administration, dilute 1:1 with sterile water or 0.9% saline. The solution should be administered slowly to patients with marked hypoglycemia. The desired effect includes increased awareness and consciousness. A constant-rate infusion (CRI) of 2.5% to 5% dextrose solution may be required to maintain blood glucose levels high enough to eliminate signs of hypoglycemia.

Dextrose should not be given orally. Oral administration may lead to aspiration if the gag reflex is diminished or absent. Due to the high osmolality of the original solution, dextrose should also not be given by intramuscular or subcutaneous (SC) injection, as it will result in significant tissue irritation. The dextrose solution is hypertonic and will draw fluid into the SC space from the cellular space, causing cellular dehydration and cell death. Dextrose will not be efficiently absorbed from the SC space into the bloodstream because of poor peripheral perfusion.

The most important monitoring technique for a patient is clinical assessment by the technician's own senses. Catastrophic consequences can occur when too much attention is placed on information provided by the monitoring equipment and not enough attention is focused on the patient's physical exam.

COMPLICATIONS RELATED TO SURGERY

Hemorrhage

The surgical incision should be routinely inspected during postoperative monitoring. Any bleeding at the surgical site should be attended to (Fig. 11.7). If direct pressure applied to the site for 5 to 10 minutes does not stop the bleeding, a bandage should be applied if possible and the surgeon notified. Excessive bleeding at the surgical site that does not stop may indicate that bleeding is also occurring internally or that a coagulopathy has developed.

Internal bleeding can manifest as the following clinical signs: pale mucous membranes, slowed capillary refill time (>2 seconds), rapid respiratory rate, abdominal bloating, swelling at or around the surgical site, and hypotension, ultimately culminating in hypovolemic shock. An abdominocentesis (abdominal tap, "belly tap") can be performed using a 22-gauge needle and syringe. Collecting frank blood from the abdominocentesis is a positive diagnosis for internal bleeding into the peritoneal cavity. A thoracocentesis (chest tap) is performed if internal bleeding is suspected after thoracic surgery. The blood collected from these taps will not typically clot because it is already defibrinated. This means that it has

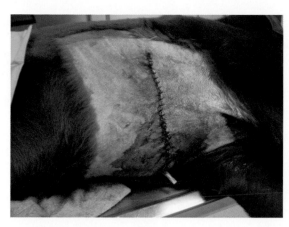

Fig. 11.7 Bleeding at the surgical site is often seen when drains are placed. It is important to clean the blood from the surgical site or cover the site with a bandage temporarily. Dogs and cats otherwise are driven to lick at the surgical site covered with blood.

already clotted once, using up all the fibrin, and even though it looks like fresh peripheral blood, it is actually older blood that has already begun breaking down its fibrin clots. If clots are found, this indicates active, fresh bleeding.

Excessive postoperative bleeding occurs for several reasons. The patient may have a coagulation disorder. A surgical ligature around a major vessel may have dislodged. Smaller arteries that were not bleeding intraoperatively because of hypotension may begin to bleed as the patient regains normal blood pressure and the effects of anesthesia wear off.

Coagulation disorders may predispose the patient to hemorrhage. Certain breeds, such as Doberman pinschers, may have a genetic disorder called von Willebrand disease, which manifests as a primary coagulation problem caused by decrease or lack of von Willebrand factor. Animals with chronic liver disease may have secondary coagulation problems caused by a clotting factor deficiency. Intrinsic clotting factors are produced primarily in the liver, and when it is not functioning properly, these may not be synthesized normally or in sufficient amounts to allow formation of a stable blood clot. Preanesthetic assessment of animals with chronic liver disease should include a coagulation profile. This usually consists of a complete platelet count, prothrombin time (PT), and an activated partial thromboplastin time (aPTT). Certain toxins, such as rodenticides, can cause coagulation disorders. Platelet decreases caused by immune-mediated disease (e.g., immune-mediated thrombocytopenia) or infectious disease (e.g., Rocky Mountain spotted fever) can predispose the patient to hemorrhage.

In some cases, the surgeon may decide to reanesthetize the patient and go back in. The patient may need to be surgically explored to find the bleeding vessel or vessels. This patient is at high risk for additional anesthetic complications. Fluid therapy should be maintained, and colloid fluids may replace the crystalloid fluids. Colloid fluids, because of their larger molecule size, will remain within the vessels for a longer period of time than will crystalloids, allowing for better maintenance of peripheral blood pressure. It is important to be prepared for emergency situations and to work efficiently. An additional venous access site may be needed for administering a blood transfusion or blood component therapy. In general, a blood transfusion refers to administering whole blood (fresh or stored) from one patient to another. Depending on how recently the whole blood was collected from the donor and when it is administered to the recipient, it may contain red blood cells (RBCs), white blood cells (WBCs), platelets, plasma proteins, and functional coagulation factors. Blood component therapy involves separating out the parts of whole blood and administering only those parts that the patient needs (e.g., plasma, packed RBCs, platelet-rich plasma), which will extend the usefulness of the blood collected from the donor (Table 11.1).

The blood pooling in the abdomen or thorax can be aseptically collected, passed through a blood transfusion micropore filter, and readministered to the patient. This procedure is called an autotransfusion. If an exogenous source of blood is needed, ideally crossmatched units of blood are administered. Whole blood increases the colloid pressure and oxygen delivery to the tissues. If stored blood is used, the RBCs can take up to 24 hours before they become fully functional again. Administering blood rich in clotting factors improves coagulation. Some practices have blood products such as fresh plasma, fresh frozen plasma, and platelet-rich plasma available for administration.

Another manifestation of excessive bleeding is the formation of a hematoma at the surgical site, such as in the scrotal sac after a castration procedure (Fig. 11.8). The surgical site may be traumatized if the patient has a difficult recovery (e.g., emergence delirium). Clots covering the cut ends of small subcutaneous blood vessels can become dislodged, allowing blood to pool under the skin at the suture site. Initially, a soft, fluctuant swelling is observed. Aspirating the lump with a 22-gauge needle and syringe shows the lump to be filled with blood. The presence of the hematoma impedes the healing process by separating the layers of tissue.

The surgeon may order application of warm, moist compresses to the area multiple times daily. This helps speed up the flow of blood into the area, allowing quicker reabsorption of the hematoma. The surgeon may choose to suction the blood with a needle and syringe, followed by application of a pressure bandage. Alternatively, a Penrose drain can be surgically placed for continuous drainage.

Seroma

A seroma is a collection of tissue fluid (serum) in a pocket under the skin that forms at an area of excessive movement. A seroma may develop at the surgical site in a patient that is overactive postoperatively. The irritation from the scraping of rough sutures can cause inflammation. When tissues are inflamed, serum leaks from the capillaries. The serum collects in the potential space between the skin and muscle layers (Fig. 11.9). This seroma interferes with the normal healing process. If the serum leaks through the skin suture line, bacteria from the skin may contaminate the serum in the pocket and an abscess may form.

Seromas appear as lumps at the surgical site. An abscess, hematoma, or hernia can also resemble a seroma. Aseptically aspirating the mass with a 22-gauge needle and syringe allows a differential diagnosis. A straw-colored or light-red fluid is seen if the mass is a seroma. Hematomas are filled with blood. Purulent fluid fills the syringe when the swelling is caused by an abscess. The syringe

TABLE 11.1 Blood and Fluid Products: Indications for Use and Doses

Product	Indications	Infusion Rate
Isotonic crystalloid solutions*	Shock Dehydration Maintenance	Dogs: Up to 90 mL/kg (to effect) Cats: Up to 60 mL/kg (to effect) Maintenance rate is approximately 66 mL/kg/day for a 10-kg dog; larger dogs need less (e.g., 44 mL/kg/day for a 40-kg dog), whereas smaller dogs need more (e.g., 81 mL/kg/day for a 5-kg dog)
Hetastarch	Shock Hypoalbuminemia	Dogs: 10–20 mL/kg/hr (shock) Cats: 10–15 mL/kg/hr over 10–15 min (shock) 5–10 mL/kg (can repeat) or constant-rate infusion (1–2 mL/kg/hr) up to 20 mL/kg/day (hypoalbuminemia)
Dextran 70	Shock Hypoalbuminemia	Dogs: 10–20 mL/kg/hr (shock) Cats: 10–15 mL/kg/hr (shock) 5–10 mL/kg (can repeat) or constant-rate infusion (1–2 mL/kg/hr) up to 20 mL/kg/day (hypoalbuminemia)
25% Human serum albumin	Shock Hypoalbuminemia	5–25 mL/kg; maximal volume 2–4 mL/kg (bolus or slow push) 0.1–1.7 mL/kg/hr as a constant-rate infusion‡
7% Hypertonic saline†	Shock Hypoalbuminemia	4 mL/kg over 5 min, then isotonic crystalloids (10–20 mL/kg/hr) to effect
Fresh whole blood	Anemia Hemorrhage Coagulopathy Shock	10–22 mL/kg; in general, 2 mL/kg will raise the PCV by 1% For shock: 22 mL/kg/hr maximum
Stored whole blood	Anemia Hemorrhage	10–22 mL/kg; in general, 2 mL/kg will raise the PCV by 1%
Packed red blood cells	Anemia Hemorrhage	6–10 mL/kg and then reassess the patient's PCV to determine whether more is necessary; in general, 1 mL/kg will raise the PCV by 1%
Platelet-rich plasma	Thrombocytopenia Coagulopathy	1 unit/3–10 kg
Fresh frozen plasma	Coagulopathy Hypoproteinemia Disseminated intravascular coagulation	10–20 mL/kg; then reassess serum albumin or antithrombin III concentration to determine whether more is necessary
Cryoprecipitate	Von Willebrand disease Hemophilia	1 unit/5–15 kg
Oxyglobin	Anemia Shock	Dogs: 15–30 mL/kg at a maximum rate of 10 mL/kg/hr Cats: 5–10 mL/kg at a maximum rate of 5 mL/kg/hr

PCV, Packed cell volume.

*Monitor central venous pressure to prevent fluid overload.

† To prolong the effect of hypertonic saline, hetastarch or other colloid may be administered simultaneously. Do not exceed the maximum rate for either fluid.

‡ Data from Mathews KA, Barry M: The use of 25% human serum albumin: outcome and efficacy in raising serum albumin and systemic blood pressure in critically ill dogs and cats. J Vet Emerg Crit Care 15:110, 2005.

Modified from Fossum TW, Hedlund CS, Hulse DA, et al: *Small animal surgery*, ed 3, St Louis, 2007, Mosby.

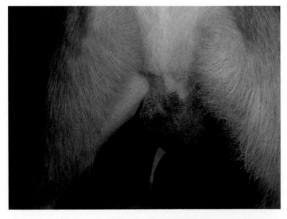

Fig. 11.8 Postoperative scrotal hematoma. Bleeding into the scrotal sac has occurred. This picture was taken 18 hours after the castration surgery.

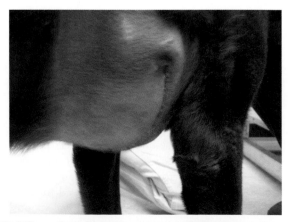

Fig. 11.9 Formation of large seroma around the surgical site caused when the dog scratched at the site over a 24-hour period.

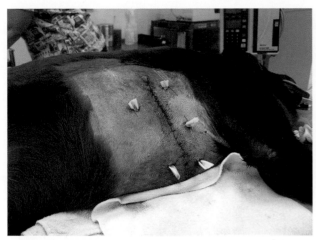

Fig. 11.10 Postoperative seroma drainage. Penrose drains were placed on each side of the surgical incision to allow drainage of the seroma fluid.

appears empty or has a small drop of liquefied fat if the lump results from herniation of omentum. When in doubt, make a smear of the fluid, stain with Diff-Quik–type stain, and look at the fluid under a microscope. Serum is absent of any cells but may have a purple hazy background consistent with protein. Hematomas and abscesses will have RBCs and WBCs, respectively.

Seromas are treated much like hematomas. Small seromas can be managed by warm, moist compresses applied multiple times during the day. The pocket can be drained using a syringe and needle, followed by a pressure bandage. Large seromas need to be drained surgically (Fig. 11.10). Surgical drainage also allows the surgeon to explore the surgical site to ensure that all the muscle-layer sutures are intact.

DEHISCENCE

Postoperative dehiscence is the premature loss of sutures that allows the surgical site to open. Dehiscence exposes underlying tissues to contamination. Any or all layers of the surgical closure may undergo dehiscence. If a thoracic surgical site dehisces, pneumothorax can follow. Dehiscence can have serious and even fatal consequences.

The animal can cause dehiscence by excessively licking or chewing at the surgical site, which can weaken or remove the sutures. Infection of the site can also weaken the tissues, and the suture can tear through the skin and muscles. Blunt trauma to the surgical site can cause sutures to rip through healthy tissue. Active playing with other dogs or falls while climbing steps postoperatively can create blunt trauma extensive enough to lead to dehiscence.

Self-Trauma

Self-trauma may be a problem in the postoperative patient. Excessive licking, scratching, or rubbing of the surgical site slows the healing process and can lead to dehiscence.

Animals instinctually lick their wounds. Sutures are at risk of being removed by the animal before healing is complete. When licking occurs, bacteria from the mouth can be deposited deep into the surgical incision. The surgical site becomes contaminated, and the animal runs the risk of infection.

Preventive Measures

Prevention of self-trauma is essential. The strategy for keeping the postoperative patient free of self-trauma requires two tactics: (1) preventing the animal from reaching the surgical site and (2) preventing the animal from wanting to reach the surgical site.

Block access to surgical site

Elizabethan collar. The flat, plastic Elizabethan collar, or E-collar, is placed around the neck. It is attached to the animal's collar, or a gauze strip is threaded through the collar stays. The plastic shield blocks the patient from licking surgical sites caudal to the neck (Fig. 11.11). The animal can still scratch or rub the site. The pet is awkward and has no peripheral vision while wearing the collar. The pet should never be loose outside while wearing an E-collar. The pet will probably knock things over and collide with door frames. It is also imperative to ensure that the animal can still eat and drink with the E-collar in place. In some instances, the E-collar makes contact with the floor around the bowl, preventing the animal's mouth or tongue from reaching the bowl.

BiteNot collar. While fitted with the BiteNot Collar (BiteNot Products, Inc., San Francisco), the patient is unable to bend its neck to reach any part of its body and lick. As with an E-collar, the pet wearing the BiteNot Collar can still scratch or rub at the site (Fig. 11.12).

Bandaging the area. A bandage may be enough to block the patient from licking the area (Fig. 11.13). Surgical sites are not always in areas that can be easily bandaged. A pet may find a way to remove the bandage or may even eat the bandage. Thus, it is essential that the bandage be monitored closely for signs of slipping or wetness and for tooth marks. Placing a shirt over a thoracic surgical site can also act as a barrier for the animal. Ensure that it fits properly and is kept clean and dry.

Basket muzzle. A dog can be fitted with a basket muzzle, which prevents the patient from chewing at the site. The dog may rub the site with the muzzle and may also be able to lick. However, this type of muzzle may act as an effective psychological barrier.

Hobbles. Taping the hind legs together can prevent the patient from scratching at the surgical site (Fig. 11.14).

Block desire to reach surgical site

Foul-tasting product applied around the site. Bitter-apple liquid and Yuk2e or YukForte ointments (Vet Planet LLC,

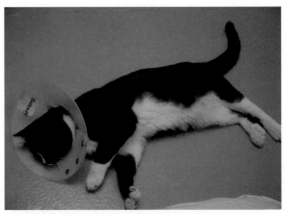

Fig. 11.11 Elizabethan collar is applied to prevent licking and chewing on a drain.

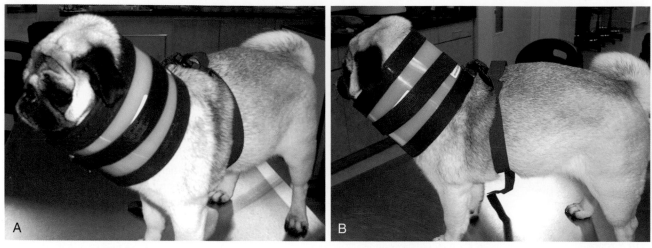

Fig. 11.12 A and B, The BiteNot Collar (BiteNot Products, Inc., San Francisco) properly placed.

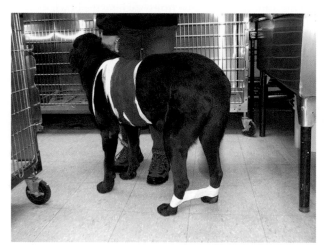

Fig. 11.13 This pet had a bandage that encircled the chest. The bandage covered Penrose drains that had been placed to drain a seroma. The bandage also helped to keep the dog clean during the first 12 hours postoperatively. The hind legs are taped together ("hobbled") to prevent scratching at the chest area with the rear paws.

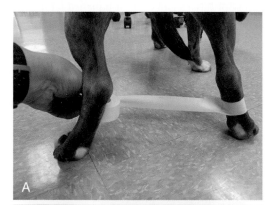

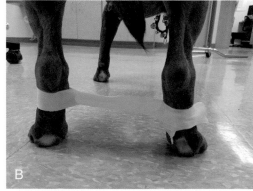

Fig. 11.14 Hobbles. A, Adhesive tape wide enough to cover half of the metatarsal region is placed loosely around the metatarsal region. B, The tape is then adhered together between the legs and placed around the opposite metatarsus. The hind limbs are positioned apart at a distance equal to the width of the pelvis.

Boyds, MD) are examples of bitter-tasting applications that can be placed on the skin around the surgical site. The foul taste may deter the patient from licking the area.

Sedation. Chemical restraint can be very effective. Chronic tranquilization during the recuperative period may be necessary to prevent licking as well as overactivity.

Stainless steel suture or staples. The surgeon may anticipate a problem with licking and elect to place staples in the skin rather than to close with sutures. Stainless steel sutures prick the tongue when licked. Staples can withstand more licking than sutures or tissue adhesive (skin glue).

Adequate pain management. For many animals, licking is a self-soothing behavior elicited by pain at the surgical site. When this pain is adequately management, the licking behavior will stop. Ensure that the pain associated with the surgery has been managed for the entire time required for healing, not just for the first 24 hours.

INFECTION

When the surgical site becomes infected, healing is delayed. The patient is in pain and may have a fever. The surgical site is swollen, red, and draining, and the sutures are at risk of falling out.

Surgical débridement and resuturing may be necessary. Some animals may have an allergic reaction to the absorbable sutures that has the appearance of an infected wound. In either instance, the surgeon will cut away the dead tissue and suture healthy tissue together using less reactive suture material. The patient will most likely receive systemic antibiotic therapy. Warm, moist compresses and cleaning of the site with dilute antiseptic solution also may be prescribed.

POSTOPERATIVE NURSING CARE

Wound Management

A wound occurs whenever there is an interruption in the normal integrity of the tissue. Wounds can be purposeful, such as a surgical incision, or incidental, such as a traumatic injury. Wound healing begins directly after the injury occurs and is a dynamic process, with more than one phase of wound healing occurring at the same time (Box 11.3).

Wound healing can be influenced by many factors, including host factors, wound characteristics, and external factors (Box 11.4). Successful management of the wound requires accurate assessment and planning.

Wound Classification

Wounds are classified by several means. One method of classification is by etiology, or cause. In this scheme a surgical wound is called an incisional wound, because the soft tissue damage (or wound) is caused by the surgeon's scalpel. Another method of classification is based on the duration and degree of wound contamination. Class 1 wounds are 0 to 6 hours old with minimal contamination; most surgical wounds fall into this class. Class 2 wounds are 6 to 12 hours old with significant contamination. Class 3 wounds are more than 12 hours old with profound (gross) contamination. However, this system fails to address the contaminated wounds that are new or a few hours old, such as traumatic wounds sustained in animal fights or automobile accidents.

A more useful classification scheme is based only on the degree of contamination. Age of the wound is not part of this

---

BOX 11.3 Phases of Wound Healing

Inflammatory
Begins immediately after injury; characterized by formation of blood clot; platelets stimulate other stages by release of growth factors.

Débridement
Part of inflammatory phase; characterized by influx of white blood cells (macrophages, monocytes) into wound; occurs approximately 6 hours after injury; wound healing is sustained by release of growth factors from multiple cell types.

Repair (Fibroblastic)
Begins 3 to 5 days after wounding; characterized by invasion of fibroblasts and development of granulation tissue; wound strength increases exponentially.

Maturation
Characterized by remodeling of the collagen of the scar and slow gain in wound strength; begins approximately 3 weeks after injury and may take weeks to years to complete.

From Bassert JM, McCurnin DM, editors: *McCurnin's clinical textbook for veterinary technicians*, ed 7, St Louis, 2010, Saunders.

BOX 11.4 Factors Affecting Wound Healing

Host Factors
- Geriatric patients: Debilitated state decreases wound healing.
- Malnourishment: Decreased protein levels delay wound healing.
- Hepatic disease: Clotting factor deficiency.
- Underlying disease: Hyperadrenocorticism or diabetes mellitus.

Wound Characteristics
- Foreign material: Drains, implants, sutures, and so on can cause inflammatory responses that interfere with healing, and soil, gravel, or plant material can introduce infection-causing agents.
- Type of incision: Electroscalpel or electrocoagulation causes more necrosis than a conventional scalpel.
- Infection of any kind.

External Factors
- Drugs: Corticosteroids depress wound healing and increase the chance of infection. Chemotherapeutic agents and radiation therapy can also delay wound healing.

BOX 11.5 Wound Contamination Classifications with Examples

Clean
Created under sterile conditions. Does not enter into the gastrointestinal tract, respiratory tract, or the urogenital or oropharyngeal areas.
Examples: Surgical wound.

Clean-Contaminated
Minimal contamination; the level of contamination can be removed or reduced.
Examples: Surgical incision into the gastrointestinal tract, respiratory tract, urogenital or oropharyngeal areas.

Contaminated
Heavy contamination present.
Examples: Leakage of intestinal contents into the peritoneum during an enterotomy. Traumatic wounds that are presented shortly after they occur (e.g., road rash after animal is hit by a motor vehicle).

Dirty
Old traumatic wound; active infection with purulent exudate.
Examples: Laceration that was left unattended and became infected.

---

system. Using degree of contamination to classify wounds guides the veterinarian in making decisions regarding wound management. There are four classes: clean, clean-contaminated, contaminated, and infected (Box 11.5).

Clean Wound

Surgical wounds made under aseptic conditions are considered clean. Surgical sites of castration or ovariohysterectomy are considered examples of clean wounds (see Fig. 11.15).

Clean-Contaminated Wound

Surgical wounds that are contaminated with contents from the gastrointestinal (GI), respiratory, or urinary tract are considered clean-contaminated wounds. The contamination is minimal and easy to remove. Traumatic wounds can be considered clean-contaminated wounds after lavage and débridement (Fig. 11.16).

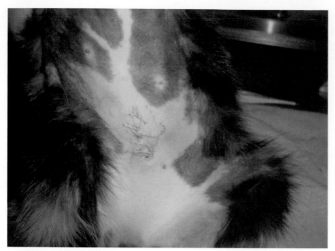

Fig. 11.15 Surgical wound 24 hours after completion of procedure; clean wound.

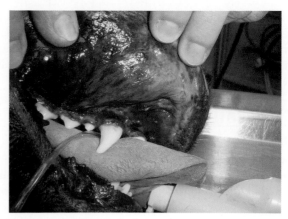

Fig. 11.17 The wound in this dog's mouth was caused by a spider bite. Dark red tissue is necrotic. The wound was flushed with sterile saline, and the dog received a regimen of broad-spectrum antibiotics. Because the wound was located in a contaminated area, in this case the mouth, the wound was initially classified as a contaminated wound.

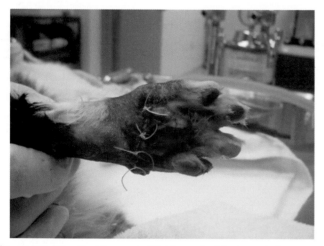

Fig. 11.16 After flushing and débridement, this lacerated paw was sutured closed; clean contaminated wound.

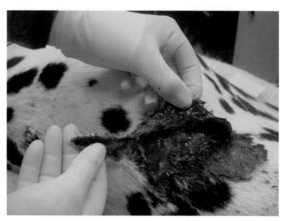

Fig. 11.18 This open, infected wound was covered with a thick layer of dried, purulent fluid, blood, and fur.

Contaminated Wound

These types of wounds have heavy contamination. Foreign material (e.g., grass, asphalt) and compromised tissue are incorporated in the wound. The wound can become contaminated when there is major spillage from the GI tract. Wounds sustained in fights with another animal can be examples of contaminated wounds. Wounds located within the mouth cavity are immediately contaminated by oral cavity flora (Fig. 11.17).

Infected Wound

Infected wounds are inflamed, contaminated with many bacterial organisms (by definition more than 100,000/gram of tissue), purulent discharge (pus), and varying amounts of necrotic (dead) tissue. Traumatic or surgical wounds can progress to become infected if treatment is inadequate or nonexistent (Fig. 11.18).

Wound Cleansing

Regardless of the wound classification, it must be managed properly in order to facilitate healing. Box 11.6 lists the fundamentals

---

BOX 11.6   Fundamentals of Wound Management

1. Temporarily cover the wound to prevent further trauma and contamination.
2. Assess the traumatized animal and stabilize its condition.
3. Clip and aseptically prepare the area around the wound.
4. Culture the wound.
5. Debride dead tissue and remove foreign debris from the wound.
6. Lavage the wound thoroughly.
7. Provide wound drainage.
8. Promote healing by stabilizing and protecting the cleaned wound.
9. Perform appropriate wound closure.

From Fossum TW, Hedlund CS, Hulse DA, et al: *Small animal surgery*, ed 3, St. Louis, 2007, Mosby.

---

of wound management. Surgical site preparation, sterile gloving, sterile draping, use of sterile instruments, and adherence to aseptic technique all minimize initial contamination of the surgical wound. Circumstances such as immunosuppressed patient status, self-mutilation, or unavoidable intraoperative contamination can render the surgical wound contaminated. Cleansing of contaminated wounds facilitates healing. Whether caused by surgery or trauma, contaminated wounds are cleansed of debris and protected from microorganisms through numerous means, including lavage, débridement, dressings, and antimicrobial agents.

Lavage

Lavage is the procedure of forceful rinsing of a wound (Fig. 11.19). Anesthesia may be necessary if the patient is in pain and struggles. Thorough lavage flushes out foreign debris, purulent fluid, and microorganisms from a wound. The goal of a successful lavage is to reduce the number of microorganisms in the wound to a level that the immune system can handle. As the criticalists say, "the solution to pollution is dilution."

Solutions used to lavage external wounds include tap water, sterile saline, lactated Ringer's solution, diluted chlorhexidine, and diluted povidone-iodine. Although tap water is not sterile,

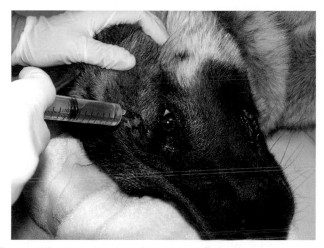

Fig. 11.19 Lavage procedure. Syringe with dilute chlorhexidine solution (1:40 dilution) is flushed around the wound to rinse debris and blood from the area.

it is still a safe and effective lavage agent for external wounds that do not penetrate a body cavity (thorax or abdomen) or joint. Two percent chlorhexidine solution is diluted 1:40 with water to make a 0.05% concentrated solution for lavage. Povidone-iodine (10% stock solution) is diluted 1:10. These diluted solutions should be prepared fresh daily; their potency diminishes with time. When adding dilute antiseptics to lavage fluids, the cytotoxic potential must be kept in mind. (See Table 11.2 for a list of lavage solutions with their advantages and disadvantages.)

Débridement

Débridement is the removal of adhered debris and dead tissue from the wound. Surgical débridement is the cutting away of dead tissue from the living tissue until fresh bleeding edges are exposed. Dead tissue or foreign material left in a wound will delay healing as the body must still get rid of this material, usually though phagocytosis. After the area is debrided, the fresh skin edges are sutured together. Usually, surgical débridement is performed with the patient under anesthesia. General anesthesia is used if the animal is stable and the involved area is large. Local anesthesia is often administered for debilitated animals and smaller wounds (see anesthesia texts for specific techniques).

During the early phase of wound healing, débridement may need to occur. The primary layer of bandage material can provide a means of débridement. Dry mesh gauze directly applied to an open wound with embedded foreign material or necrotic tissue is called a *dry-to-dry bandage.* Removal of the dry-to-dry bandage can be painful because the adhered wound material is removed with the bandage material.

Mechanical débridement can also be accomplished on a daily basis through the use of wet-to-dry bandaging techniques. The *wet-to-dry bandage* is used with open wounds that have embedded foreign material, devitalized tissue, and viscous exudates. A primary layer of sterile, saline-soaked gauze sponges is applied directly to the wound. A secondary layer of dry gauze

TABLE 11.2 Lavage Solutions

Cleanser	Advantage	Disadvantage
Tap water	Availability Inexpensive Ease of application	Hypotonic Cytotoxic trace elements Not antimicrobial
Balanced electrolyte solution: Lactated Ringer's solution (LRS); Normosol	Isotonic Least cytotoxic	Not antimicrobial
Normal (0.9%) solution	Isotonic	Slightly more acidic than LRS Not antimicrobial
0.05% Chlorhexidine (1 part stock solution to 40 parts sterile water or LRS) or (≈25 mL stock solution per liter)	Wide antimicrobial spectrum Good residual activity Not inactivated by organic matter	Precipitates in electrolyte solutions More concentrated solutions are cytotoxic and may slow granulation tissue formation *Proteus, Pseudomonas,* and *Candida* are resistant Corneal toxicity
0.1% Povidone-iodine (1 part stock to 100 parts LRS) or (≈10 mL stock to 100 mL LRS)	Wide antimicrobial spectrum	Inactivated by organic matter Limited residual activity Cytotoxic at concentrations greater than 1% Contact hypersensitivity Thyroid disorders if absorbed

Modified from Fossum TW, Hedlund CS, Hulse DA, et al: *Small animal surgery,* ed 3, St Louis, 2007, Mosby.

sponges and rolled-cotton batting is layered onto the primary layer and then secured to the animal with rolled gauze and tape. The dressing is changed two or three times daily. When the primary layer is removed, the foreign matter and necrotic debris that have dried to the gauze are pulled off the wound. As with dry-to-dry bandaging, the patient may need to be sedated for bandage changes because this procedure tends to be painful.

Wet-to-dry and dry-to-dry bandages have the disadvantage of possible bacterial growth in the bandage. A moist environment at the wound surface dilutes the viscous exudates, allowing the secondary layer to absorb the fluid more readily.

Enzymatic preparations of trypsin or chymotrypsin can be applied to wounds to digest and remove necrotic tissue. These are both naturally occurring pancreatic enzymes that assist with protein digestion. This technique is indicated when (1) further surgical débridement may damage important nerves and blood vessels, (2) deeper fistulas exist, or (3) the patient is a poor anesthesia risk.

Wound Dressings

Wound dressings are categorized as two types, semiocclusive and occlusive. Wound dressings are the contact, or primary, layer of a bandage. Semiocclusive dressings include the wet-to-dry bandages used to debride wounds mechanically. Cotton and polyester gauze pads, petroleum jelly–coated gauze pads, antibiotic ointment–coated polyethylene glycol sponges, and polyurethane foam sponges are examples of nonadherent, semiocclusive dressings. Semiocclusive dressings allow excess fluid to be absorbed by the secondary layer.

Occlusive dressings are impermeable to air and produce a moist environment that facilitates wound healing. These dressings are used in the later stages of wound healing, when the bandage needs less frequent changing. Examples of occlusive dressings are natural cellulose and gelatin, as well as polyethylene polymers attached to a synthetic film. These occlusive dressings do not adhere to the wound.

Antimicrobial Agents

Antimicrobial agents may be applied topically to superficial wounds. However, the use of antimicrobial agents is not a substitute for appropriate and careful débridement and lavage.

Large multiuse tubs or tubes of antimicrobial agents may be a source of patient-to-patient contamination through introduction of bacteria unless strict aseptic technique is used to retrieve the contents. Just because the product contains an antibiotic does not ensure that there is no bacterial growth in the tub. A better option is the use of single-dose packets of antibiotic ointment. Topical treatment can be discontinued once granulation tissue appears in the wound. If single-use products are not an option, using a clean tongue depressor to remove a volume of ointment and transfer to a sterile gauze before use can help to maintain product sterility.

Drains

A *drain* is a surgically placed implant that is temporarily affixed in the wound. The drain provides a channel through which unwanted fluid or gas may leave the wound. When surgery or other trauma to the skin disrupts the hypodermis, the skin may no longer adhere to the underlying fascia. This creates a potential space that the body will try to fill with tissue fluid; this results in the formation of a seroma. Healing occurs most rapidly if the fluid is evacuated. Drawing the fluid out through a needle is only effective temporarily. Continuous drainage needs to be provided.

The two basic categories of drains are passive and active. Passive drains use gravity and overflow gradients to evacuate the fluid or gas. Active drains create negative-pressure gradients to the area and suck the fluid and gas from the wound.

Passive drains are typically made of soft, pliable latex tubing. Red rubber tubes and silicone tubes are stiff, less compliant, and potentially more irritating. Teat cannulas, originally made to drain purulent fluid from infected mammary glands in cows, are also used to drain aural hematomas in dogs. Teat cannulas are made of polyethylene plastic and are quite hard (Fig. 11.20).

The passive drain exits the skin at the most ventral (gravity-dependent) spot possible. The drain does not exit from the primary surgical incision. A small stab incision is made through the skin adjacent to the surgical incision. The drain is secured to the skin by one or two sutures. The opposite end of the drain may remain buried below the skin or may exit at the opposite end of the wound. Whether the end of the drain is buried or exits to the surface, a suture secures the end of the drain (Fig. 11.21).

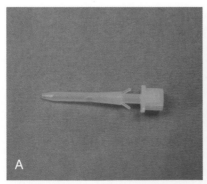
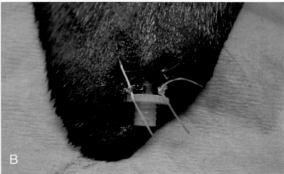

Fig. 11.20 Plastic teat cannulas are also used to drain aural hematomas in dogs. A, Teat cannula has two small prongs that help keep it in place. B, Cannula is sutured into place at the most dependent aspect of the hematoma pocket to allow gravity to assist in drainage.

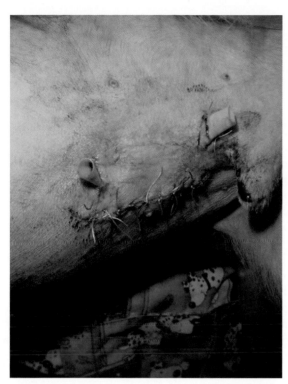

Fig. 11.21 Each end of the drain is sutured to the skin to keep it in place.

An *active drain* is usually made out of polymeric silicone (Silastic), red rubber, polyethylene, or polypropylene plastic. The drain is **fenestrated** (has holes) in multiple places. The fenestrated section of the drain is placed in the area that requires draining. Many commercial suction devices are available. Attaching a syringe to the tube can make a simple, homemade suction device. The plunger of the syringe is pulled back and secured by a pin placed through a predrilled hole in the plunger's shaft to hold the plunger in place.

All drains must be kept clean. Dried fluid accumulates around the drain where it exits the skin. Placing a warm, moist cloth over the drain loosens the dried material. The cloth is soaked in a bowl of water or dilute solution of an antiseptic such as chlorhexidine (1:40 dilution). This procedure may need to be repeated several times daily. The skin surrounding the drain may become raw and irritated from contact with the serous or purulent fluid; this is termed serum scald. Petrolatum-based ointments applied to the skin can facilitate cleaning and protect the skin from further damage.

The veterinary surgeon determines the best time to remove the drain. Usually, the drain is removed 3 to 5 days after surgery. Any dried fluid is cleaned out, and all sutures securing the drain are cut. The drain is firmly grasped and pulled out with one swift motion. If the proximal end of the drain is not buried, one end is freed and pulled as much as possible from the incision and then cut. The other end is then freed, and the remainder of the drain is removed.

If the patient has removed the drain prematurely, the owner should be asked to bring the drain in for inspection. It is important to determine that the pet has removed the entire drain. A piece of drain left under the skin will fester. The immune system will treat the piece of drain as a foreign invader, surrounding it with fluid and inflammatory cells. This drain piece will have to be surgically removed.

WOUND CLOSURE

The choice of wound closure will be based on the nature of the wound. It may be closed immediately (primary closure), several days after the injury (delayed primary closure), after the formation of granulation tissue (secondary closure), or it may not be surgically closed (secondary intention or contraction or epithelialization) (Box 11.7).

Wounds heal quickest when sutured closed. Depending on the level of contamination, however, the wound may not be sutured closed immediately. If a wound is sutured closed immediately, it has received *primary closure*. If a wound is left open for a few days, protected with dressings, and sutured closed later, *delayed primary closure* has been performed. Leaving the wound open for a longer period (5–7 days) and then suturing it closed is known as *secondary closure*. It is important to appose healthy skin edges that have an adequate blood supply with sutures or staples. Apposing necrotic skin edges or compromised skin edges (rather than healthy skin edges) together will result in dehiscence (sutures pull apart) because there is inadequate blood supply to begin healing.

Some wounds may be left to heal closed without suturing. This method is known as *second-intention healing* (Fig. 11.22). This is most commonly seen with shallow injuries or holes as with tube removals. Scarring is most likely to occur in second intention healing.

Bandages, Splints, Casts, and Slings

Bandages, splints, casts, and slings are frequently applied after surgical procedures or trauma to a limb. The purposes of these applications are to protect wounds, speed the healing process, and immobilize the extremities. Immobilization helps the patient by decreasing pain and facilitates healing by securing bone fragments and soft tissue pieces closer together to allow healing.

Bandages have three basic layers: primary (contact) layer, secondary (padded) layer, and tertiary (outer) layer (Table 11.3). The primary layer is in contact with the wound. This contact

---

BOX 11.7 Methods of Wound Closure

Primary Closure
Closed immediately. Used for clean, new wounds with little to no contamination.

Delayed Primary Closure
Closed within 1 to 5 days after the injury occurs. Used for moderately contaminated or traumatized wounds. The wound should be free of infection, and granulation tissue has not formed.

Secondary Closure
Closed after 5 days. Granulation tissue has formed. Used for severely contaminated or traumatized wounds that require extended wound management.

Secondary Intention
Wound is not closed. It is allowed to heal by contraction and epithelialization.

layer may adhere to the open wound or may be nonadherent. Adherent materials such as cotton gauze are usually applied early in the healing process and allow débridement when the bandage is changed because dried tissue and cells will be removed along with the bandage material. Nonadherent dressings are used later in the healing process or to cover wounds closed by sutures. These do not stick to the wound and allow a stable granulation bed to form and close the wound.

The secondary layer secures the contact layer to the wound and provides an absorptive layer for blood, serum, and purulent fluid. This padded layer also provides support to the extremity. It applies pressure to the wound, thus compressing any dead space and preventing seroma formation and hemorrhage. Rolled cotton, synthetic polyester batting, multilayer absorbent pads, or cast padding may be used. Rolled gauze is used to hold the layer in place, with pressure applied to compress the padding underneath. It is important not to use too much pressure and occlude the blood supply to the extremity. Mastering the technique of applying the proper pressure and placing a comfortable, supporting bandage on a patient requires practice. An experienced technician or veterinarian should supervise the first few bandage wrappings attempted by newer personnel to ensure the technique and pressure used are appropriate.

When a bandage, cast, or sling is applied immediately after trauma to an extremity, swelling of the limb is expected. When the limb is confined by such a stabilizing measure, swelling may result in cessation of blood flow to the extremity. Toes can be left exposed at the distal end of the bandage or cast to monitor

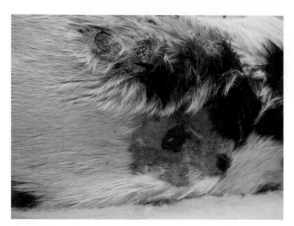

Fig. 11.22 These wounds were left unsutured. They healed as open wounds.

TABLE 11.3   Characteristics of Primary, Secondary, and Tertiary Bandage Layers

Type	Indication and Purpose	Example
Primary		
Adherent	No longer indicated in wound care	Dry gauze (dry-to-dry) Wet gauze (wet-to-dry)
Hypertonic	Contaminated and infected wounds; hypertonicity is antimicrobial and draws fluid and tissue debris from wound	Hypertonic sodium chloride dressing (20%) (e.g., CURASALT*)
Nonadherent semiocclusive	Moderately or copiously exudative wounds; keeps wound surface moist, draws fluid and tissue debris from wound	Transparent polyurethane film—Polyskin II* With hydrophilic properties: hydrogel (e.g., Curagel*), absorptive foam (e.g., Hydrasorb*) Hydrocolloid (e.g., Ultec Hydrocolloid Dressing*)
Nonadherent occlusive	Minimally exudative wounds; partial-thickness wounds (abrasions); keeps wound surface moist and promotes epithelialization; protects new epithelium	Without hydrophilic properties: OpSite,* Tegaderm Transparent Dressing,* BIOCLUSIVE Transparent Dressing† With hydrophilic properties: hydrogel (e.g., NU-GEL†), hydrocolloid (e.g., Hydrocol Dressing†)
Nonadherent without occlusive properties	Intact wound surface (e.g., surgical wound, recently epithelialized wound)	Petrolatum-impregnated gauze (e.g., Adaptic†); rayon or Teflon pads (e.g., Telfa pads†)
Secondary		
Padding	Absorbs exudate, pads and supports the wound	Cast padding—Specialist Cast Padding‡ Roll cotton
Tertiary		
Conforming gauze	Conforming and holding layer	Conforming gauze (e.g., Kling,*)
Nonocclusive elastic adhesive tape	Holding and protective layer, permeable to moisture	Elastikon,*
Nonocclusive elastic bandage	Holding and protective layer, permeable to moisture	Vetrap§
Occlusive tape	Contraindicated	Waterproof tape
Occlusive wrap	Contraindicated	Plastic wrap

*Tyco Healthcare/Kendall, Mansfield, MA.
†Johnson & Johnson Medical, Arlington, TX.
‡Johnson & Johnson Orthopedics, Raynham, MA.
§3M Animal Products, St. Paul.
From Bassert JM, McCurnin DM, editors: *McCurnin's clinical textbook for veterinary technicians*, ed 7, St Louis, 2010, Saunders.

the amount of swelling under the bandage. The nails of the two middle toes should be only a few millimeters apart. If the nails are farther apart, the toes are swollen. If the toes look swollen, the bandage should be removed immediately. If the nail beds appear blue or maroon, there should be concern about blood flow to the extremities. The bandage may be too tight to allow proper blood flow and will need to be replaced immediately.

The tertiary layer of the bandage is made of porous adhesive tape or elasticized tape, such as Vetrap (3M, St Paul, MN) or Elastikon (Tyco Healthcare/Kendall, Mansfield, MA). This layer provides protection to the secondary layer. If this outer layer becomes wet, either from moisture on the outside (e.g., soiled by rainwater or urine) or seepage from the inside as with wound drainage, the entire bandage must be changed immediately.

It is important to keep these bandages intact, secure (no slipping down the leg), and dry. Stirrups are used to help stabilize the bandage and prevent slippage off the leg. The stirrups are applied before the primary layer, typically to the side of the extremities but away from any injury. Animals may try to remove the wrappings by gnawing, violently shaking the extremity, or prying off the bandage. It is important to use Elizabethan collars to prevent damage to the bandage. After several days, stretching of the outer layer and compression of the inner padding will loosen the bandage, which may slip or shift position. Also, the skin adjacent to the edges of the bandage, sling, splint, or cast may become abraded. Wetness, staining, and odor may also be noted. If any of these problems occur, the bandage, cast, or splint should be removed, the area investigated, and the bandage replaced.

INTRAVENOUS CATHETER MAINTENANCE

IV catheters are placed and maintained for extended periods in some surgical patients. Common veins used for peripheral catheter placement include the left and right cephalic, left and right lateral saphenous (dogs), and left and right medial saphenous (cats). The left and right jugular veins are generally used for central catheters. Central catheters (central lines) allow the technician to measure central venous pressures, collect blood samples for frequent blood checks without a separate venipuncture for each sample collected, administer multiple medications or solutions when utilizing multiport catheters, and administer hypertonic solutions such as total parenteral nutrition (TPN).

All IV catheters provide direct access to the patient's vascular system, and therefore all catheters should be placed using aseptic technique. All connections among the catheter, connector sets, and IV lines need to be left untaped but secure. Access to these connections must be available at all times without having to untape the connections. The patient often attempts to pull or chew out the catheter. Sufficient taping and restraint devices (e.g., E-collar) can prevent many problems. Fig. 11.23 shows a cage that was occupied by a cat that pulled off the catheter cap (catheter remained intact).

Previously, the recommendation was that peripheral IV catheters were replaced every 3 days, regardless of condition. It is now recognized that as long as the appropriate catheter

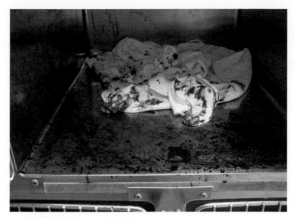

Fig. 11.23 Consequence of a lost catheter cap.

monitoring and maintenance has occurred, many catheters can be left in place for well over the 72 hours without additional complications. A catheter placed into a central vein may remain in place for as long as there is no indication of phlebitis and the catheter remains patent. The old catheter is removed only after the new catheter is secured in place. If no continuous infusion is being administered through the catheter, the catheter is flushed with 1 to 5 mL of saline every 6 to 8 hours. Research has consistently shown no benefit to the use of heparinized saline compared to straight 0.9% saline in ensuring catheter patency. It is the act of flushing that keeps the catheters patent, rather than the additional of heparin. This procedure helps ensure that the catheter remains patent the entire time it is in place. Bandages securing catheters in place should be changed if they become soiled with vomitus or other contaminants.

Each time the catheter is flushed, the insertion site and all connections should be checked. If the tape is soiled, it should be retaped. If swelling is noted in the paw, the tape may be wrapped too tightly, and it should be replaced. If swelling is noted proximal to the catheter, the catheter may be perivascular (not in the vein). If the catheter bandage is soaked, the entire catheter should be replaced at a different site. The old catheter site is covered for a few minutes with a piece of gauze. A spot of antibiotic ointment can be applied to the gauze, which is secured by adhesive tape.

When administering medication through the catheter, the technician should check for patency using a 0.9% saline flush before drug administration. After the medication is administered, the catheter is flushed again with saline. Blood samples are often collected through the IV catheter, but the clinician must keep in mind that residues from medications administered through the catheter could interfere with test results. A three-syringe technique can be used to help decrease the incidence of contaminants in a blood sample collected from an IV catheter. A 3-mL syringe is half filled with heparinized saline (to help prevent the blood pulled into the syringe from clotting), and blood is withdrawn into the syringe from the catheter. This helps clean any contaminants from the catheter. Then the second syringe is used to withdraw the appropriate sample and place it in the desired collection tubes. Lastly, the original syringe is used to replace the withdrawn blood and flush the catheter with the remaining heparinized saline.

URINARY CATHETER MAINTENANCE

Patients recovering from back surgery, urinary tract surgery, and orthopedic procedures may have a urinary catheter placed. The urinary catheter helps ensure urethral patency, allows for quantification of urine production, and helps keep the patient clean.

The catheter is placed aseptically. The distal end is secured to the patient with tape and sutures. An empty, sterile IV fluid bag and administration set are connected to the distal end of the catheter. The bag is suspended below the level of the bladder for urine flow by gravity.

It is important to check the patency of the urine collection system regularly. The tubing may become kinked. As the patient turns in the cage, the collection tubing may become twisted and cause the tube's lumen to collapse. The collection tube can be pinched in the cage door as it is closed. Blood clots can be passed and form obstructions in the tubing. The catheter and tubing should be checked for leaks. Often the patient attempts to pull out the catheter, and tooth marks may be detected. Leaking systems are replaced, and the patient is fitted with an Elizabethan collar to prevent further problems. Replacement of the entire collection system every 24 hours is recommended to decrease the incidence of opportunistic bacterial infections. If long-term use is required, the catheter itself should be replaced every 3 to 5 days.

NUTRITIONAL SUPPORT

All animals need to maintain appropriate levels of nutrient intake, but this need is especially important in patients recuperating from surgery and serious illness. Inadequate nutrition can negatively affect the animal through decreased wound healing, suppression of the immune system, decreased cardiac and respiratory function, and increased bacterial translocation from the gut. Voluntary oral intake is the preferred route for food administration but may be insufficient to meet the animal's energy requirements. The animal needs to be able to consume at least 85% of the calculated resting energy requirements (RER) to be able to feed orally. Feeding a calorically dense, highly palatable food may help increase voluntary oral intake (Fig. 11.24). If needed, oral intake can be supplemented with the use of assisted feeding techniques, pharmacologic appetite stimulants, and tube feedings.

Assisted feeding is best accomplished with pureed or liquid diets and a catheter-tip syringe. The food needs to be of a consistency that can be easily administered through the syringe. If necessary, small amounts of water can be added to commercial gruel diets to increase their ease of passage through the syringe and catheter. The food may be smeared on the animal's lips to initiate licking and cleaning. A lump of food may be applied to the roof of the mouth. A liquid diet may be squirted through a syringe into the cheek pouch. Assisted feeding is a labor-intensive and time-consuming

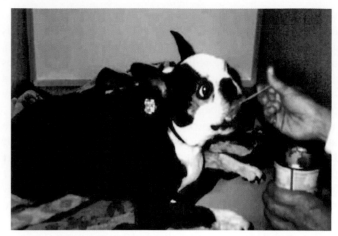

Fig. 11.24 Hand-feeding a highly palatable food.

process and often falls short of the required caloric goal. Additionally, calculating the actual amount of food that the animal consumed can be very tricky. The animal often fights the feedings and may become stressed. Aspiration of the food into the lungs from the mouth during the struggle is a major concern. No patient should be allowed to have a decreased nutrient intake for longer than 3 days, which includes the time prior to surgery/hospitalization. Metabolic changes begin within this time that can have a significantly negative impact on recovery.

Animals should be offered food as soon after anesthesia recovery as possible. They need to be able to protect their airway, to be normothermic, and to be able to swallow before being fed. There is no nutritional reason to delay postoperative feeding and numerous reasons why the animals should be fed. Delayed wound healing has been demonstrated in animals from which food has been withheld in the first 24 hours postoperatively. With small and neonatal animals, feeding is even more important because their functional reserves of carbohydrates in the form of glycogen and fats are significantly less than older, larger animals.

Several pharmacologic agents are thought to increase the appetite of dogs and cats. The benzodiazepine tranquilizer diazepam has been found to stimulate the appetite of cats. An IV injection generally induces the cat immediately to eat any palatable food within reach. The food should be in place and warmed to body temperature before the cat is returned to the cage after the injection. Cyproheptadine is a serotonin antagonist that stimulates the appetite of both dogs and cats. It is typically given orally. It is not unusual for a cat or dog to pout through any appetite stimulation. Corticosteroids and progestational steroids (e.g., megestrol) work well in humans but are seldom used in dogs and cats because of potential adverse side effects, such as diabetes mellitus, immunosuppression, and delayed healing. When these medications are given as treatment for a disease, increased appetite may be a beneficial side effect of treatment. Mirtazapine is a new class of drugs used for appetite stimulation. It is a noradrenergic and specific serotonergic antidepressant (NaSSA) used in people to manage anxiety and depression. It is useful for long-term appetite stimulation and has the advantage of not requiring daily administration. Capromorelin (Entyce, Aratana) is currently the only U.S. Food and Drug Administration (FDA)-approved appetite stimulant for dogs. It works by stimulating the dog's natural "hunger hormone" to trigger a feeling of hunger, hopefully causing the animal to eat. Acupuncture also may stimulate a surgical patient's appetite postoperatively, in addition to providing some pain relief. A veterinary acupuncturist should be consulted for these cases.

Effective pain management is also important; many animals have suppressed appetite secondary to unrecognized or untreated pain. Nausea caused by therapeutic medications such as narcotics and antibiotics can also suppress appetite. If nausea occurs, a decision to change medications may need to be made, if possible, to allow increased food intake.

The initial amount of food that the patient will need per day is calculated in the following way.

For those who do not have calculators that do logarithms, the following formula can also be used. This formula is most accurate for patients weighing more than 2 kg and less than 30 kg:

$$\text{Dogs weighing 2 to 50 kg: (wt [kg]} \times 30) + 70 = \text{RER}$$

$$\text{Cats: wt [kg]} \times 40 = \text{RER}$$

$$\text{Estimated food intake} = \text{Resting energy requirement}$$

Calculate food intake by finding RER and then determine the caloric density of the food being used. Divide the caloric density by the RER to determine the quantity that should be fed every 24 hours. If the animal has not eaten in more than 3 days, start the initial food intake at 30% to 50% of RER for the first 24 hours. Small, frequent meals also help to decrease food-related discomfort as well as nausea.

Enteral tube feeding may be necessary to meet nutritional needs. Neonatal animals adapt well to repeated orogastric tubing. Juvenile and adult animals deal better with the placement of a semi-permanent, indwelling feeding tube. The feeding tube may be placed through the nose (nasoesophageal or nasogastric), esophagus (esophagostomy), or stomach (gastrostomy). A tube placed through the abdominal wall into the stomach, known as a gastric tube or percutaneous endoscopic gastrostomy (PEG) tube, is the easiest of all feeding tubes to maintain but does require more anesthesia and equipment than some of the other types of tubes for placement.

Using an indwelling feeding tube is convenient, less time consuming, and less stressful to the patient than force feeding or syringe feeding, but indwelling tubes are not without problems. A nasoesophageal or esophagostomy tube (Fig. 11.25) that passes down the esophagus may irritate the esophagus or, if passed through the cardiac sphincter into the stomach, can irritate the stomach wall, cause gastroesophageal reflux, and may initiate vomiting. The tube can be vomited up, displacing it from the esophagus so that it instead comes out of the mouth, and the patient may then chew through it. A nasogastric tube must be very small in diameter to pass through the nasal turbinates and therefore can easily become obstructed when food is administered through it. The nasogastric tube

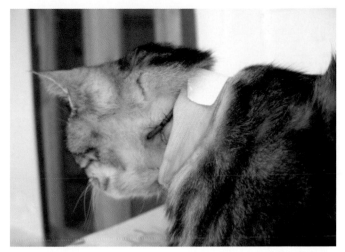

Fig. 11.25 Esophagostomy tube.

can cause nosebleeds, sneezing, and inflammation of the nasal passage with mucus discharge. Premature removal of the tube by the patient is a complication inherent in all types of feeding tubes.

The gruel or liquid diet may be homemade or commercially purchased. The benefit of commercially prepared recovery diets is that their nutrient content and caloric density are known, making food administration calculations easier. Any food that can be blenderized can be fed through a feeding tube of a large enough diameter (typically at minimum a 12-14 French tube). Feeding of a raw or uncooked diet through a feeding tube is not recommended because of the possibility of bacterial contamination of the food. When the tube feedings are initiated, the amounts should be small (2–10 mL, depending on animal's size) and administered frequently (about every 2 hours). The desired amount to be fed is based on the RER. For the first day, 50% of the RER is divided up into multiple equal sized feedings administered every 2 to 4 hours. Use of a gastrostomy tube should be delayed for 12 hours after it is placed to allow a temporary stoma to form internally between the visceral peritoneum and the parietal peritoneum (Fig. 11.26).

Vomiting of food occurs most commonly in the first or second day. Once the feedings are tolerated, larger amounts and less frequent feedings can be done. After the first day, 75% to 100% of RER can be given divided up into four to six equal feedings throughout the day. The food is slowly administered over 10 to 20 minutes through the feeding tube with either an infusion pump or a catheter-tipped syringe to allow the stomach to accommodate gradually to the presence of the food. After the food is injected, 10 to 15 mL of water is slowly administered through the catheter to rinse the inside of the tube and remove any food that may have remained in the tube. This step helps prevent tube obstruction. The tube is closed with a Luer-Slip adapter plug. How the tube is managed externally depends on which type of feeding tube is placed, the condition of the animal, and the desires of the veterinarian. Some tubes are not secured at all to the animal, and others are glued or sutured in place.

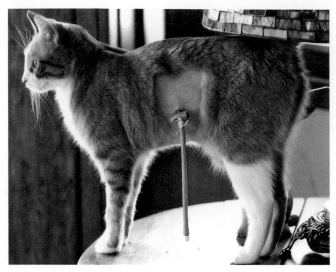

Fig. 11.26 Gastrostomy (percutaneous endoscopic gastrostomy [PEG]) tube.

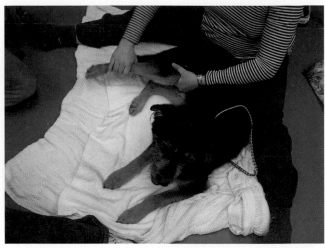

Fig. 11.27 Physical therapist demonstrating passive range-of-motion movements.

Depending on the type selected, the feeding tube may remain in place for a period of 3 to 5 days (nasoesophageal) to the remainder of the animal's life (gastrostomy/PEG). Tube removal also depends on which tube is selected.

Physical Therapy

Physical therapy techniques can benefit most patients. Immobility resulting from sickness, trauma, or surgical procedures can complicate recuperation. Physical therapy techniques enhance patient comfort, prevent complications from disuse, and hasten healing. The success of many orthopedic procedures rests on the rehabilitation of the patient. Veterinarians, veterinary technicians, and owners can perform many physical rehabilitation techniques to improve surgical outcomes and ensure client satisfaction. Some states have limited the practice of physical therapy on animals to licensed physical therapists. Therefore, many veterinarians prefer to use the term *physical rehabilitation* when referring to the following techniques.

Massage, application of heat or cold, bandaging, range-of-motion (ROM) exercises, and physical exercise are all therapeutic techniques that may be prescribed. Under the supervision of the attending veterinarian, the veterinary technician or owner may perform the techniques with the patient. Detailed descriptions of these techniques are found in other texts and articles; this section briefly describes the various types of physical therapy that may be used postoperatively.

In the first 72 hours after surgery, opioid analgesics, antiinflammatory drugs, passive ROM exercises, and cryotherapy are used to decrease pain, prevent edema formation, and gradually improve range of motion. Pain management is discussed later. Cryotherapy is the application of cold, such as ice packs wrapped in a towel, to the affected limb. The packs can be affixed to the limb with elastic wraps. The cold packs are applied for up to 30 minutes two to four times a day. The cold causes vasoconstriction, which decreases blood flow and limits edema

formation. The cold temperature of the tissue also reduces nerve conduction, producing analgesia.

Passive ROM exercises are exercises that support a joint while moving it to the extent of its limitations (Fig. 11.27). The best time to perform passive ROM exercises is shortly after administration of analgesic drugs. This procedure should be performed slowly with the muscles relaxed, as follows: While supporting the limb, slowly and gently flex and extend each joint one at a time, taking care to keep all the joints in the working extremity in their normal anatomic alignment throughout the exercise. Flex and extend each joint only to the extent that the joint just begins to resist the degree of flexion or extension applied to it. Passive ROM helps prevent contracture, improve blood and lymph flow, maintain normal range of joint movement, and stimulate sensory awareness. Ten to fifteen repetitions should be performed two or three times daily. Treat every joint of the affected limb, starting with the joint distal to the injury or surgical site.

Between 3 and 5 days after surgery, other physical therapy procedures may be added. Cryotherapy is replaced with *thermotherapy*. Warm, moist heat is applied to the injured area. The heat causes vasodilation, increases local circulation, and provides mild pain relief. Thermotherapy should be applied for 10 to 20 minutes before passive ROM, massage, or exercise. Massage therapy relaxes muscles, breaks down adhesions, improves blood and lymph flow, and relieves pain. The massage session starts with gentle running of the hands over the surface of the animal's skin (effleurage, frottage). The stroking movements should start distally and move proximally. The second massage method kneads the muscles in small circles with the pads of the fingers (not the fingertips) or the heel of the hand with a gradual increase in pressure (**pétrissage**). The massage session lasts about 20 minutes and is done every 24 to 48 hours (Fig. 11.28).

Exercise that elevates the heart rate and increases muscle tone can be initiated about 2 weeks after surgery. Initial exercise

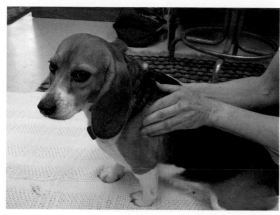

Fig. 11.28 Massage can relax the pet as well as increase blood and lymph flow, relieve pain, and break down adhesions.

is assisted by slings and harnesses. Swimming is also a good initial exercise; the buoyancy of the water helps support the patient. This low-impact exercise is replaced in a few weeks with unassisted exercise, such as leash walks. As the patient's stamina increases, the length of time spent exercising also increases.

Although physical therapy has many benefits, contraindications to it do exist. Massage should not be performed over open wounds, infected areas, or malignant tumors. Animals with thromboembolic disease and those receiving anticoagulants should not be massaged. Cryotherapy is avoided in patients with ischemic injury, diabetes mellitus, vasculitis, or indolent pressure sores (decubitus ulcers). ROM procedures should not be performed on nonstabilized legs after a severe orthopedic injury (e.g., fracture, ligament rupture). Bandaging to prevent or reduce edema needs to be performed carefully to prevent vascular compromise of the limb. Exercise regimens and active ROM procedures must start slowly and increase gradually in length and frequency.

POSTOPERATIVE ANALGESIA

Pain assessment is very subjective, and the technician will usually employ a number of techniques when assessing a postoperative animal. The ease and success of managing postoperative pain are directly related to preoperative analgesia. That is, the more successful the attempts to preempt surgical pain, the easier it is to control postoperative pain with minimal additional analgesics. Assuming adequate preemptive analgesia, the overall goal of postoperative pain management should be to maintain the analgesic plane achieved throughout the procedure.

Increases in heart rate, respiratory rate, blood pressure, and capillary refill time (CRT) can indicate that an animal is in pain. Remember, an animal should never be required to prove that it is in pain before the pain is addressed. There are a number of veterinary-specific pain scoring systems that can be employed to provide a more objective assessment of an individual animal's pain level.

The patient should recover quietly and calmly without displays of overt signs of pain (e.g., vocalization, excessive movement, abnormal body posturing). Some patients experience

pain that persists or develops despite adequate doses of analgesics and must be treated with additional analgesia or analgesic techniques. This type of pain is termed *breakthrough pain* because it has "broken through" the usual analgesic barriers.

Postoperative pain management also includes medications dispensed for home use. This is a service and level of care that veterinary medicine has not sufficiently advocated until recently. Now, with veterinarians' increased awareness of the options available for take-home pain medication and the benefits to the patient, effective pain management can continue throughout the at-home recovery period.

Common Analgesic Classes

The two classes of analgesia most often used postoperatively are opioids and nonsteroidal antiinflammatory drugs (NSAIDs). These two classes of agents can be used individually, but the drugs may be most efficacious when used in combination with each other. For animals with severe pain, or whose pain is not fully controlled by these two classes of drugs, two other classes of analgesics are available. These are N-methyl-d-aspartate (NMDA) agonists and α_2-agonists. Postsurgical pain should be managed aggressively for anywhere from 24 hours up to a full week or more, depending on its severity. In general, experts agree that most patients with soft tissue elective surgery should receive opioids for 24 hours and NSAIDs for 3 to 4 days postoperatively. Patients that have emergency or nonroutine soft tissue procedures (e.g., thoracotomy, gastric dilation–volvulus repair) may be managed initially with opioids alone until cardiovascular health is restored. A major concern is the effect of opioids on GI motility. Although morphine may slow GI motility, the benefit of opioids outweighs the risk of altered GI function because stress and pain are likely to play a larger role in decreasing GI motility than short-term postoperative opioid administration. Patients with severe GI disease may benefit from the addition of a CRI of lidocaine for systemic analgesia, provided that the patient does not have cardiovascular disease.

Patients may also benefit from postoperative local anesthetics, such as bupivacaine, which can be instilled through indwelling chest tubes or by soaker catheter.

Patients undergoing orthopedic procedures should receive postoperative opioids for the first 24 to 72 hours after surgery and NSAIDs for at least 1 week. The exact type of opioid is matched to the expected level of pain and the species of the animal.

Wind-Up

Patients who do not respond satisfactorily to the maximum dose and frequency of opioids and require additional analgesia may have experienced the phenomenon known as **wind-up**. In this condition the spinal cord has become hypersensitized to incoming pain signals as a result of constant bombardment. Once hypersensitization occurs, traditional analgesia may no longer be adequate. There are several effective techniques for managing wind-up, including CRI of morphine, ketamine, or lidocaine. Ketamine blocks the sensitization of neurons in the spinal cord, essentially "unwinding" it, and may allow the patient to become responsive to usual dosing regimens, as described earlier.

Epidural and Block Analgesia

Local anesthetics such as lidocaine and bupivacaine act by preventing conduction of nerve impulses. They are helpful for topical anesthesia, infiltrative anesthesia, peripheral nerve blocks, and epidural injections. Although all of these techniques require some level of skill, they are all easily learned by a dedicated technician and provide further pain relief for our patients.

Dispensed Analgesia

Nonsteroidal Antiinflammatory Drugs

The availability of veterinary NSAIDs has greatly improved outpatient pain management. These relatively inexpensive analgesics provide long-lasting perioperative and chronic pain relief in convenient oral formulations. Once-daily administration tends to improve owner compliance. NSAIDs provide adequate pain relief for many patients during the at-home recovery period, especially if therapy was instituted preoperatively. Some patients require additional take-home medications, most often opioids.

Opioids

Several oral opioids are available for take-home use; however, because of the potential for human abuse of these controlled drugs, care must be taken in prescribing them. Sustained-release morphine is available and can be used in dogs, but morphine is difficult to obtain in sufficiently small doses to administer safely to cats. On the basis of research at the University of Florida, buprenorphine can be safely and efficaciously administered to cats by the transbuccal (sublingual) route. Small, single-dose aliquots can be prepared for administration by owners at home. The opioid fentanyl is available in a transdermal patch (Duragesic, Janssen Pharmaceuticals, Titusville, NJ), which can be applied in the hospital to provide up to 3 days of postoperative analgesia for hospitalized as well as discharged patients. A fentanyl patch does require up to 24 hours to become fully effective, so additional forms of pain relief may be necessary to cover this period adequately.

Butorphanol tablets are not recommended for take-home analgesia because of butorphanol's extremely short duration of action. Just because an animal is sedated does not mean that its pain has been addressed.

The synthetic opioid tramadol is available in tablet form. Tramadol has gained popularity for long-term use in dogs and cats as an effective take-home analgesic. The latest research in dogs shows that while tramadol does provide analgesia, it is likely through a nonopioid mechanism as dogs do not produce high levels of the metabolite responsible for the opioid effect of the drug. Research has consistently failed to show analgesic effects with oral administration in both acute and chronic pain settings. Cats appear to make more of the effective metabolite than do dogs, but drug palatability has limited its use in cats. Tramadol can be used as an adjunct to NSAIDs for the treatment of moderate to severe pain. Because of recent changes in the law, tramadol is now a Schedule IV drug and must be recorded and reported the same way as the other scheduled analgesics.

■ KEY POINTS

1. When monitoring recovery of a patient intubated with an endotracheal (ET) tube, the technician must be prepared for the animal to awaken quickly. The ET tube is untied from the head or muzzle. All limbs should be untied and the patient placed in lateral recumbency. A syringe is at hand if needed to deflate the ET tube cuff. The technician should never leave the patient unattended on the table, and it is best to have a hand on the patient at all times.

2. The ET tube should not be removed until the patient has regained the ability to swallow.

3. Extubation of a brachycephalic breed should be delayed until the patient can raise its head without assistance.

4. All patients should be closely monitored until fully recovered.

5. When the body temperature is less than 97° F, immediate and active measures should be taken to warm the patient. Additional postoperative opioid analgesics should not be given until the patient's temperature is greater than 98° F.

6. When treating an animal for hypothermia, do not assume that the measures are successful. Monitor the patient's body temperature and confirm that the body temperature is rising.

7. A patient thrashing in a cage during recovery must be protected from injury. Measures must be taken so that the animal does not cause injury to itself or others and to ensure that pain is adequately managed that may contribute to thrashing activity.

8. The technician who thinks a patient is not recovering as expected should notify the attending veterinarian. The cause of the delayed recovery needs to be identified and corrected.

9. Attention to the surgical wound is an important part of the recovery process. Any change in the wound's condition should be reported immediately to the surgeon.

10. Débridement and lavage are important steps in the wound cleansing process.

11. Bandages, casts, splints, and slings must be monitored closely for displacement, patient mutilation, wetness, and odor.

12. A drain must be kept clean so that drainage can continue as long as needed and the skin around the exit wound for the drain does not become irritated by the draining fluid.

13. Indwelling IV and urinary catheters need regular inspections to ensure that they are functional and have not been disturbed by the patient.

14. A patient that will not eat will not heal quickly and is predisposed to development of complications.

15. Enteral tube feeding may be necessary to meet nutritional needs.

16. Any food that can be blenderized can be fed through a feeding tube of a large enough diameter.

17. Feeding of a raw or uncooked diet through a feeding tube is not recommended because of the possibility of bacterial contamination of the food.

18. Use of a gastrostomy tube should be delayed for 12 hours after it is placed to allow a temporary stoma to form internally between the visceral peritoneum and parietal peritoneum.
19. Physical therapy techniques used during the recuperative period can greatly improve patient outcome and enhance client satisfaction.
20. Providing adequate preoperative analgesia ("preemptive analgesia") makes it easier to achieve successful postoperative pain management.
21. Postoperative pain management should continue at home. Oral analgesics and transdermal analgesic patches can provide continued pain relief after the patient leaves the veterinary hospital.
22. The best pain relief is achieved by combining different classes of analgesics that block or prevent pain by different mechanisms of action. Postoperatively, these typically include oral opioids and NSAIDs.

REVIEW QUESTIONS

1. What constitutes the recovery period of anesthesia?
   a. Cessation of anesthesia to extubation
   b. Cessation of anesthesia to patient discharge from hospital
   c. Extubation to the time the patient's vital signs and level of consciousness return to normal
   d. Cessation of anesthesia to the time the patient's vital signs and level of consciousness return to normal
2. As a general rule, extubation of which of these dog breeds should be delayed until they are able to lift their head?
   a. Pug
   b. Collie
   c. Greyhound
   d. Yorkshire terrier
3. Shivering in a patient recovering from anesthesia indicates
   a. severe pain.
   b. severe hypothermia.
   c. the patient's body is attempting to produce heat.
   d. the patient is still in a surgical plane of anesthesia.
4. Rewarming should be considered when the body temperature is
   a. <96.7 °F.
   b. <97.6 °F.
   c. <98.6 °F.
   d. <100 °F.
5. Rewarming efforts should be decreased as the patient's body temperature returns to normal to avoid
   a. rebound hypothermia.
   b. rebound hyperthermia.
   c. damage to the patient's skin.
   d. slowing the recovery process.
6. Which of these is a patient-related cause of prolonged recovery from anesthesia?
   a. Hypotension
   b. Hyperthermia
   c. Hypertension
   d. Hyperglycemia
7. Which breed of dog is more likely to have postoperative bleeding related to Von Willebrand disease?
   a. Greyhound
   b. English bulldog
   c. Yorkshire terrier
   d. Doberman pinscher

8. The process of autotransfusion is administering
   a. packed red blood cells from a blood bank.
   b. blood donated from another animal of the same species to the patient.
   c. blood from a patient that is taken prior to surgery and stored for use if needed.
   d. blood aseptically collected from a patient's body cavity back to the patient.
9. Premature loss of sutures that allows the surgical site to open is called
   a. seroma.
   b. dehiscence.
   c. pétrissage.
   d. débridement.
10. The forceful rinsing of a wound is called
    a. lavage.
    b. pétrissage.
    c. dehiscence.
    d. débridement.
11. Which material is an example of an occlusive dressing?
    a. Natural cellulose
    b. Cotton gauze pads
    c. Petroleum jelly-coated gauze pads
    d. Antibiotic ointment-coated polyethylene sponges
12. If a patient's wound is left open for 2 days and protected with a dressing, then surgically closed, what type of wound closure was performed?
    a. Primary closure
    b. Secondary closure
    c. Delayed primary closure
    d. Second intention healing
13. The primary layer of a bandage is also known as
    a. outer layer.
    b. contact layer.
    c. padded layer.
    d. adherent layer.
14. A catheter placed in which vein allows monitoring of central venous pressure?
    a. Jugular
    b. Cephalic
    c. Medial saphenous
    d. Lateral saphenous

15. What is the FDA-approved appetite stimulant for dogs?
    a. Diazepam
    b. Mirtazapine
    c. Capromelin
    d. Cyproheptadine
16. Which type of physical therapy limits swelling by causing vasoconstriction?
    a. Pétrissage
    b. Cryotherapy
    c. Thermotherapy
    d. Passive range of motion exercises
17. Intervention for nutritional support should be provided when a patient has been completely anorexic for
    a. 2 days.
    b. 3 days.
    c. 4 days.
    d. 5 days.
18. List three methods to prevent an animal from causing self-trauma to an incision postoperatively.
19. List 3 things that contribute to hypothermia in a perisurgical patient.
20. List 3 clinical signs that may indicate postoperative internal bleeding.
21. When bandaging a distal extremity, how can limb be monitored for swelling?
22. What is the benefit of feeding a commercially prepared diet instead of a homemade diet when feeding a patient via a tube?

BIBLIOGRAPHY

Bassert JM, Beal AD, Samples OM, editors: *McCurnin's clinical textbook for veterinary technicians*, ed 9, St Louis, 2018, Elsevier.

Millis D, Levine D, editors: *Canine Rehabilitation and Physical Therapy*, ed 2, St. Louis, 2014, Elsevier Saunders

Duffy T: Thermoregulation of the perioperative patient. *Proc Am College Vet Surgeons* :707–712, 2007.

Fossum TW, et al: *Small animal surgery*, ed 4, St. Louis, 2013, Elsevier Mosby.

Thomas JA, Lerche P. *Anesthesia and Analgesia for Veterinary Technicians*, ed 5, St. Louis, 2017, Elsevier

Norkus C: *Veterinary technician's manual for small animal emergency and critical care*, ed 2, Ames, Iowa, 2018, Wiley-Blackwell.

Simpson AM, Radlinsky M, Beale BS: Bandaging in dogs and cats: basic principles. *Compend Contin Educ Pract Vet* 23:1, 2001.

Slatter D: *Textbook of small animal surgery*, ed 3, Philadelphia, 2003, Saunders. Not updated since 2003

Tabor B: Heatstroke in dogs. *Vet Tech* 28:228, 2007.

Taylor R, McGehee R: *Manual of small animal postoperative care*, Baltimore, 1995, Williams & Wilkins.

Wortinger A, Burns K: *Nutrition and disease management for veterinary technicians and nurses*, ed 2, Ames, Iowa, 2015, Wiley-Blackwell.

The Technician's Role in Pain Management

Marianne Tear

LEARNING OBJECTIVES

After completion of this chapter, the reader will be able to:
- Define *pain*.
- Discuss the importance of pain management.
- Discuss the physiologic effects of pain.
- Understand key terms associated with pain and pain management.
- Discuss the importance of preoperative, intraoperative, and postoperative pain management.
- Identify painful procedures.
- Distinguish the difference between dysphoria and pain.
- Describe behavioral changes associated with pain.

KEY TERMS

Acute pain
Adaptive pain
Allodynia
Analgesia
Anesthesia
Breakthrough pain
Central sensitization
Chronic pain
Hyperalgesia

Hyperesthesia
Hypoalgesia
Hypoesthesia
Maladaptive pain
Multimodal analgesia
Neuroplasticity
Nociception
Pain threshold
Pain tolerance level

Pathologic pain
Physiologic pain
Preemptive analgesia
Regional anesthesia
Somatic pain
Visceral pain
Wind-up

This chapter is not meant to be a stand-alone text on pain management. There are many excellent books whose entire content is devoted to the subject of analgesia. One such text is the *Handbook of Veterinary Pain Management* by Gaynor and Muir. Several dedicated veterinarians and technicians have spent almost their entire careers advocating for the recognition, prevention, and treatment of animal pain. One has only to Google the names Nancy Shaffran or Mary Ellen Goldberg to receive multiple references on pain management. The purpose of this chapter is to discuss the technician's role in recognizing and helping to prevent pain in our animal patients. It is meant to complement Chapter 4's discussion on the general mechanism of pain transmission and general classes of drugs used to prevent pain.

As advances in veterinary medicine continue, the role and responsibility of the veterinary technician will increase. Technicians will be expected to know more, do more, and be more in almost every hospital setting. Although this addition of duties will be gratifying, it is imperative that the primary role of the technician not be lost or pushed to the side. Regardless of the clinical setting, the technician is first and foremost the patient advocate. No single person in the hospital spends more time with the patients than the technician. Nowhere is this strong, compassionate, knowledgeable advocacy more essential than in the realm of pain management.

As the primary caregiver, it is the technician who needs to communicate the animal's needs to the veterinarian. The doctor is ultimately responsible, but it is the technician's job to ensure that the doctor has the most current information to facilitate the best medical care.

In addition to physical condition, an animal's mental state can contribute to the level of pain being experienced. With the growing inclusion of Fear Free and Low Stress Handling in the veterinary clinic, fear, anxiety, and stress (FAS) should also be assessed and treated. The signs associated with FAS can mimic pain. Many of the drugs that are used to treat pain are also used to help an animal that is experiencing a stress response. Dr. Sally Foote, DVM, CABC-IAABC, and Fear Free® have fantastic resources that discuss reducing stress to reduce discomfort in our patients. While it is recommended that those resources be utilized in conjunction with pain management, this chapter does not cover those aspects.

UNDERSTANDING PAIN

What is pain, and how can it be quantified? The International Association for the Study of Pain classifies it as "an unpleasant sensory and emotional experience associated with actual or potential tissue damage or described in terms of such damage." The inability to communicate this discomfort in no way negates the experience, nor should it exclude the patient from receiving pain-relieving treatment. It has been argued by some that animals do not feel pain the same way as humans. On a physiologic level, pain is processed in a similar fashion in all mammals.

"It is possible that animal pain is worse than human pain because lacking the language and sophisticated reasoning skills and temporal concepts, animals cannot understand the reasons for and causes of pain, and thus lack the ability to hope for and anticipate its cessation," says Bernard Rollin, in *Handbook of Veterinary Pain Management.*

Pain creates adverse physiologic changes that can delay healing and even lead to a patient's decline or demise. With this realization, more and more concerned professionals are advocating the concept of preemptive analgesia—to prevent as much of the pain as possible rather than trying to alleviate it once it has already occurred. The American Animal Hospital Association (AAHA) encourages veterinary professionals to consider pain a vital sign, requiring that all hospitals seeking its accreditation have a comprehensive pain management protocol in place (Box 12.1).

Communication, whether it be among the health care team or with clients, is the best way to ensure that pain management is initiated. Having a standardized vocabulary will help ensure that the team is on the same page and working together toward the common goal (Box 12.2).

BOX 12.1 American Animal Hospital Association (AAHA) Pain Standards

- Pain assessment for every patient regardless of presenting complaint.
- Assessment recorded in the patient's record.
- Utilization of preemptive pain management.
- Appropriate pain management for the anticipated level and duration of pain.
- Pain management with all surgical procedures.
- Reassessment throughout the procedure.
- Written protocols.
- Teaching clients to recognize pain in their pets.

BOX 12.2 Definitions of Pain-Related Terms

Acute pain: pain that follows some bodily injury, disappears with healing, and tends to be self-limiting.

Adaptive pain: normal response to tissue damage; includes inflammatory pain.

Allodynia: pain caused by a stimulus that does not normally cause pain.

Analgesia: the loss of sensitivity to pain.

Anesthesia: total or partial loss of sensation.

Breakthrough pain: a transient flare-up of pain in the chronic pain setting, which can occur even when chronic pain is under control.

Central sensitization: an increase in the excitability and responsiveness of nerves in the spinal cord.

Chronic pain: pain that lasts several weeks to months and persists beyond the expected healing time, when nonmalignant in origin.

Hyperalgesia: an increased response to a stimulation that is normally painful either at the site of injury or in surrounding undamaged tissue.

Hyperesthesia: increased sensitivity to sensation.

Hypoalgesia: decreased sensitivity to pain.

Hypoesthesia: decreased sensitivity to stimulation.

Maladaptive pain: hypersensitivity to pain resulting from abnormal processing of normal input; can also occur if adaptive pain is left untreated.

Multimodal analgesia: the use of multiple drugs with different actions to produce optimal analgesia.

Neuroplasticity: the idea that the nervous system can be changed by the effect of the environment, external stimuli, and the effects of physiologic stimuli, such as pain.

Nociception: the transaction, conduction, and central nervous system processing of nerve signals generated by the stimulation of certain receptors.

Pain threshold: the minimal amount of pain that a patient can recognize.

Pain tolerance level: the greatest level of pain that a patient can tolerate.

Pathologic pain: pain that has an exaggerated response beyond its protective usefulness. It is often associated with tissue injury incurred at the time of surgery or trauma.

Physiologic pain: pain that acts as a protective mechanism that incites individuals to move away from the cause of potential tissue damage or to avoid movement or contact with external stimuli during a reparative phase.

Preemptive analgesia: the administration of an analgesic drug before painful stimulation to prevent sensitization of neurons, or wind-up, thus improving postoperative analgesia.

Regional anesthesia: the loss of sensation in part of the body caused by interruption of the sensory nerves that conduct impulses from that region of the body.

Somatic pain: pain that originates from damage to bone, joints, muscle, or skin and is described by humans as localized, constant, sharp, aching, and throbbing.

Visceral pain: pain that arises from stretching, distension, or inflammation of the viscera and described by humans as deep, cramping, aching, or gnawing without good localization.

Wind-up: temporal summation of painful stimuli in the spinal cord. Mediated by C fibers and responsible for "second" pain.

Adapted from Gaynor J, Muir W: Handbook of veterinary pain management, St Louis, 2002, Mosby.

THE TECHNICIAN'S ROLE IN PAIN MANAGEMENT

The role of the technician in pain management encompasses everything from assessing the patient to providing the veterinarian with information, administering and logging the drugs prescribed, and educating the owner on proper home analgesia. Box 12.3 gives a brief overview of some of the pain management tasks technicians perform daily. It is by no means an exhaustive list.

Communicating With Clients

Pain management should begin before the animal enters the clinic. Elective procedures are planned, painful events and should be prepared for as such. Communicating the need for analgesia and stress/anxiety management with the client *before* the animal comes in or at the time of admission helps lay the foundation for quality care. Analgesia should not be considered optional treatment. This gives the client a mixed message that "pain management is important only if you can afford it." Educating the client on the process of pain and the importance of preventing it should be standard operating procedure. Most owners want to do what is best for their pets; they just lack an understanding of why something is being recommended.

Many animals mask signs of pain in the hospital, so owners need to be advised as to what to watch for once the patient is discharged. Client education should include verbal and written orders along with hospital contact information in case additional questions arise. At-home pain management should be tailored to the animal and the home situation; this includes the type of medication and the route and frequency of administration.

Anticipating Painful Procedures

All tissue damage, including that caused by surgery, has the potential to cause pain. It is in the best interest of the pet to start analgesics before, rather than after, the painful event. Preemptive therapy can reduce the likelihood of wind-up: Progressive stimulation of pain receptors leads to hyperexcitability, hyperalgesia, and allodynia. Once wind-up has occurred, treatment becomes exponentially more difficult and, in some cases, impossible.

BOX 12.3 Technician's Role in Pain Management*

Administer medications and perform analgesic techniques.
Anticipate painful procedures.
Assess the patient postoperatively.
Communicate with clients.
Log controlled substances.
Monitor and treat drug effects.
Recognize signs of pain.
Request appropriate analgesia.

*Not listed in order or according to frequency that tasks are performed.

When assessing the amount of postoperative pain a patient may experience, several factors should be considered: the expectation of pain associated with the procedure to be performed, the individual animal's response to the procedure, and its response to the analgesic protocol. Although two of the three factors cannot be assessed until the animal awakens, the expectation of pain can be anticipated. It should be stressed that this is just estimation and should not be used as a reason to deny pain medications.

Pain is often increased in anxious or stressed animals, so tranquilizers or sedatives should be included in the premedication process. See Chapter 4 for premedication discussion. Many pain management protocols take into consideration home administration of antianxiety medications prior to arriving at the hospital.

Administering Intraoperative Pain Management

Good preemptive pain management protocols are designed to transition the patient through the surgical period and into the recovery phase. However, patients undergoing surgical procedures of more than several hours' duration often require additional analgesia intraoperatively. In addition, patients undergoing procedures necessitating major tissue or nerve damage (e.g., back, knee, or hip procedures; amputation; multiple anastomoses; and ear or rectal procedures) will benefit from intraoperative analgesia and analgesic techniques. Finally, patients with poor tolerance for gaseous anesthesia can be effectively managed with constant-rate infusions (CRIs) of opioids, which can greatly decrease the inhalant requirements.

In any of these cases, increased duration or intensity of surgical pain, often evidenced by sudden elevation in heart or respiratory rate, should not be addressed by merely increasing the concentration of inhaled anesthesia. Although turning up the gas will keep the patient immobile on the table, it will not manage acute pain, which will become evident as soon as the patient returns to consciousness.

Administration of additional bolus doses of opioids is determined by the patient's response to surgical stimulation. Such responses include movement; audible sounds such as growling or crying (if the patient is not intubated); and increases in heart rate, blood pressure, or respiratory rate. Intraoperative boluses should be delivered intravenously for fastest onset of action. The full opioid agonists, morphine, hydromorphone, and oxymorphone, are optimum choices. Fentanyl is not recommended for one-time bolus use because of its short half-life, and it is best administered as a CRI.

Intraoperative analgesia is best administered by CRI. Many agents can be delivered by this method, but the drug groups most often given by CRI are local anesthetics (lidocaine), opioids (morphine or fentanyl), and N-methyl-d-aspartate (NMDA) antagonists (ketamine). Regardless of the drug, a loading dose is typically given immediately before CRI is begun. These drugs can be used as single agents or in combination with one another. For other procedures, regional local anesthesia, or nerve blocks, can aid in pain management. Ring blocks can be used to add additional analgesia during declaw procedures by blocking nerve impulses before they enter the central nervous system. Subcutaneous injections of bupivacaine or bupivacaine/lidocaine can be used to block the three major nerves in the forelimb. Blocking the infraorbital and mandibular foramen enables the animal's entire muzzle to be anesthetized; this approach greatly reduces the pain association with dental extractions. Each of these blocks can be successfully administered by the technician.

Assessing the Postoperative Patient

The ease and success of managing postoperative pain are directly related to preoperative analgesia. That is, the more successful the attempts to preempt surgical pain, the easier it is to control postoperative pain with minimal additional analgesics. Assuming adequate preemptive analgesia, the overall goal of postoperative pain management should be to maintain the analgesic plane achieved throughout surgery.

The patient should recover quietly and calmly without displays of overt signs of pain (e.g., vocalization, excessive movement, abnormal body posturing). At no time should the patient be required to return to a painful state and request additional analgesics during the immediate postoperative period. Some patients experience pain that persists or that develops despite adequate doses of analgesics and must be treated with additional analgesia or analgesic techniques. This type of pain is termed *breakthrough pain* because it has broken through the usual analgesic barriers.

Postoperatively, pain and dysphoria, a state of restlessness with or without vocalization, can occur at the same time. It is important to differentiate between the two. An animal that is experiencing pain can be temporarily quieted with a calm voice and reassuring petting. Painful behavior resumes when the human interaction stops. On the other hand, an animal experiencing dysphoria or emergence delirium cannot be quieted by interaction.

Once the animal is completely recovered from the effects of anesthesia, change in behavior is often the most common sign of pain. Every animal that is admitted to the hospital for a surgical procedure should undergo a complete physical examination. That examination should include an assessment of the animal's behavior: Is it outgoing and inquisitive or hesitant and shy? Having the "normals" on behavior can help in monitoring the animal's pain response postoperatively.

Physiologic signs, such as increased heart rate and respiratory rate, can be good indicators of pain or stress in the recovering animal. They should not be the sole indicator of whether pain medication should be administered. Rather, these changes and the behavioral changes should be looked at in combination in an attempt to objectively determine pain.

BOX 12.4 Components of a Comprehensive Pain Scoring System

- Physiologic parameters
- Anticipated pain associated with the procedure
- Behavior
- Patient's response to current therapy

There are many different types of pain scoring systems, each with advantages and disadvantages (Box 12.4). It is important that the clinic have a standard method to assess all patients that is comprehensive but easy to use (Fig. 12.1).

Each animal should be treated as an individual, regardless of the scoring scale used. Animals undergoing the same procedure with the same preemptive analgesia protocol may exhibit different levels of pain. This variation can reflect differences in genetics or other underlying conditions. For example, a geriatric dog may experience more pain during a routine spay than a younger dog, because of the onset of arthritis and positioning during the procedure. Some animals are also naturally more stoic than others; reluctance to show pain should not penalize the animal.

Pain should be assessed at least every 2 hours postoperatively, and treatment should be adjusted according to the patient's response.

Requesting Appropriate Analgesia

Although technicians are the primary caregivers, they lack the authority to initiate therapy without the veterinarian's approval. This can prove to be daunting and frustrating. Technicians can leverage their knowledge and skill set to advocate for their patients. Giving the veterinarian objective details about the patient's conditions, including heart rate, respiratory rate, and food intake, balanced with a detailed summary of what has already been implemented allows the technician to more effectively argue the case for (increased) analgesia.

Understanding the pharmacology of different pain medications is also an advantage for a skilled technician. Explaining to the veterinarian how monitoring and assessment of the patient will change with the addition of or a change in pain management protocol will increase the likelihood of cooperation. In the end, pain management is the responsibility of the team. The veterinarian relies on the technician's keen observation and nursing skills to ensure that adequate analgesia is on board. By working together, the animal is the ultimate winner.

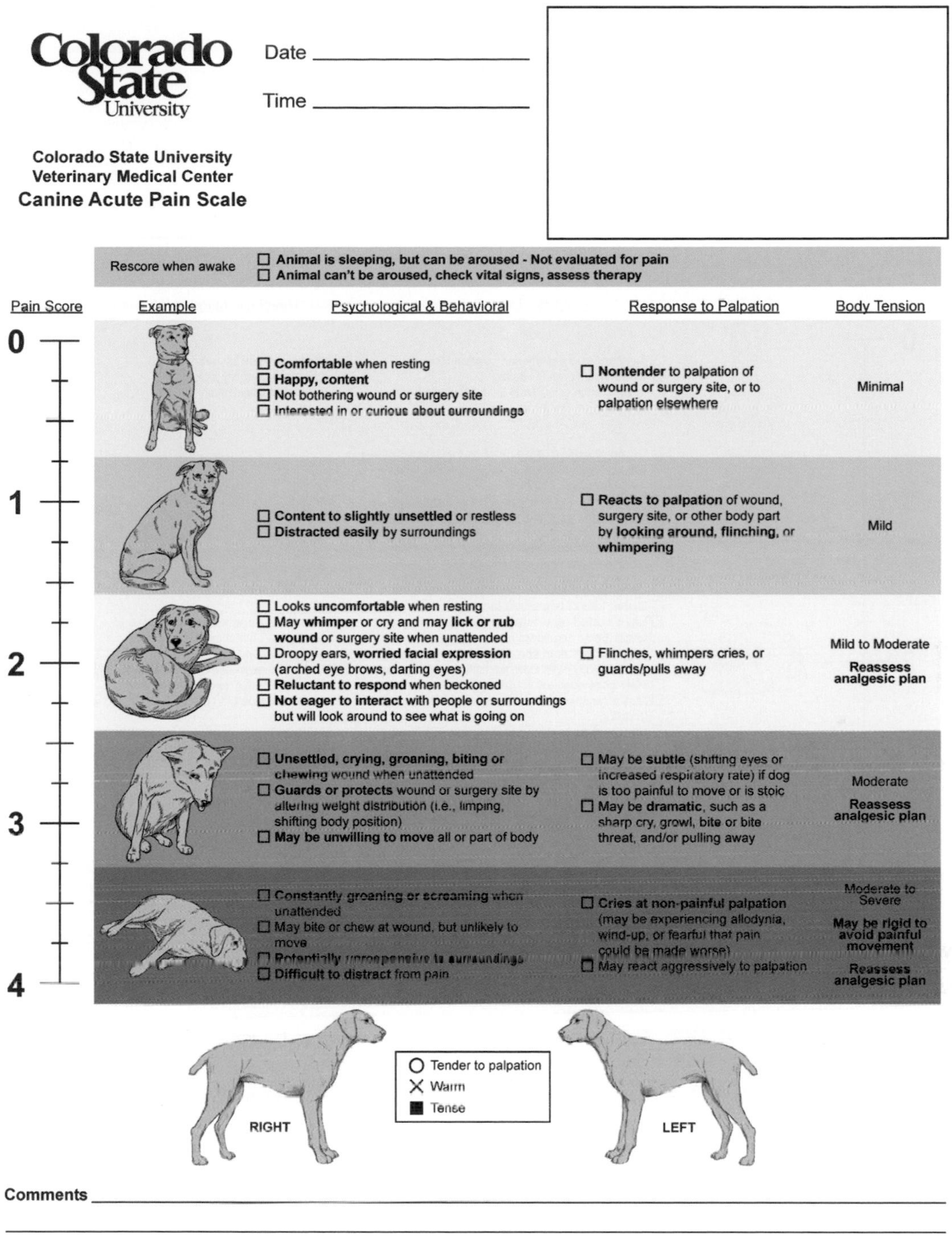

Colorado State University

Date _____

Time _____

**Colorado State University
Veterinary Medical Center
Canine Acute Pain Scale**

Rescore when awake	☐ **Animal is sleeping, but can be aroused - Not evaluated for pain** ☐ **Animal can't be aroused, check vital signs, assess therapy**

Pain Score	Example	Psychological & Behavioral	Response to Palpation	Body Tension
0		☐ **Comfortable** when resting ☐ **Happy, content** ☐ Not bothering wound or surgery site ☐ Interested in or curious about surroundings	☐ **Nontender** to palpation of wound or surgery site, or to palpation elsewhere	Minimal
1		☐ **Content to slightly unsettled** or restless ☐ **Distracted easily** by surroundings	☐ **Reacts to palpation** of wound, surgery site, or other body part by **looking around, flinching,** or **whimpering**	Mild
2		☐ Looks **uncomfortable** when resting ☐ May **whimper** or cry and may **lick or rub wound** or surgery site when unattended ☐ **Droopy ears, worried facial expression** (arched eye brows, darting eyes) ☐ **Reluctant to respond** when beckoned ☐ **Not eager to interact** with people or surroundings but will look around to see what is going on	☐ Flinches, whimpers cries, or guards/pulls away	Mild to Moderate **Reassess analgesic plan**
3		☐ **Unsettled, crying, groaning, biting or chewing** wound when unattended ☐ **Guards or protects** wound or surgery site by altering weight distribution (i.e., limping, shifting body position) ☐ **May be unwilling to move** all or part of body	☐ May be subtle (shifting eyes or increased respiratory rate) if dog is too painful to move or is stoic ☐ May be dramatic, such as a sharp cry, growl, bite or bite threat, and/or pulling away	Moderate **Reassess analgesic plan**
4		☐ Constantly groaning or screaming when unattended ☐ May bite or chew at wound, but unlikely to move ☐ Potentially unresponsive to surroundings ☐ Difficult to distract from pain	☐ Cries at non-painful palpation (may be experiencing allodynia, wind-up, or fearful that pain could be made worse) ☐ May react aggressively to palpation	Moderate to Severe **May be rigid to avoid painful movement** **Reassess analgesic plan**

RIGHT   **LEFT**

○	Tender to palpation
✕	Warm
■	Tense

Comments _____

Fig. 12.1 Colorado State University (CSU) pain scales for (A) dogs and (B) cats. Acute animal pain scales were developed by P. Hellyer and colleagues at CSU for assessing pain in dogs and cats. They are available at www. IVAPM.org. (From Bassert JM, McCurnin DM, editors: *McCurnin's clinical textbook for veterinary technicians*, ed 9, St Louis, 2018, Elsevier.)

Colorado State University

Date _____

Time _____

**Colorado State University
Veterinary Medical Center
Feline Acute Pain Scale**

Rescore when awake	☐ **Animal is sleeping, but can be aroused - Not evaluated for pain** ☐ **Animal can't be aroused, check vital signs, assess therapy**

Pain Score	Example	Psychological & Behavioral	Response to Palpation	Body Tension
0		☐ **Content and quiet** when unattended ☐ **Comfortable** when resting ☐ Interested in or **curious** about surroundings	☐ **Not bothered** by palpation of wound or surgery site, or to palpation elsewhere	Minimal
1		☐ **Signs are often subtle and not easily detected in the hospital setting**; more likely to be detected by the owner(s) at home ☐ Earliest signs at home may be <u>withdrawal from surroundings or change in normal routine</u> ☐ In the hospital, may be content or slightly unsettled ☐ **Less interested** in surroundings but will look around to see what is going on	☐ May or may not react to palpation of wound or surgery site	Mild
2		☐ Decreased responsiveness, **seeks solitude** ☐ **Quiet**, loss of brightness in eyes ☐ **Lays curled up or sits tucked up** (all four feet under body, shoulders hunched, head held slightly lower than shoulders, tail curled tightly around body) with eyes partially or mostly closed ☐ **Hair coat appears rough** or fluffed up ☐ May intensively groom an area that is painful or irritating ☐ Decreased appetite, **not interested in food**	☐ **Responds aggressively or tries to escape** if painful area is palpated or approached ☐ Tolerates attention, may even perk up when petted as long as painful area is avoided	Mild to Moderate **Reassess analgesic plan**
3		☐ Constantly **yowling, growling, or hissing** when unattended ☐ May bite or chew at wound, but **unlikely to move** if left alone	☐ **Growls or hisses at non-painful palpation** (may be experiencing allodynia, wind-up, or fearful that pain could be made worse) ☐ **Reacts aggressively** to palpation, adamantly pulls away to avoid any contact	Moderate **Reassess analgesic plan**
4		☐ Prostrate ☐ Potentially **unresponsive** to or unaware of surroundings, difficult to distract from pain ☐ Receptive to care (even mean or wild cats will be more tolerant of contact)	☐ **May not respond** to palpation ☐ **May be rigid** to avoid painful movement	Moderate to Severe **May be rigid to avoid painful movement** **Reassess analgesic plan**

○ Tender to palpation	
✕ Warm	
■ Tense	

RIGHT   LEFT

Comments _____

Fig. 12.1, cont'd

KEY POINTS

1. The technician is first and foremost the patient advocate.
2. It is the technician's job to ensure that the doctor has the most current information to facilitate the best medical care.
3. Pain is considered one of the five parameters that should be monitored.
4. Animals should not have to prove that they are in pain to receive analgesia.
5. On a physiologic level, pain is processed in a similar fashion in all mammals.
6. Pain can delay healing and even lead to a patient's decline.
7. Communication is the best way to ensure that pain management is initiated.
8. The role of the technician encompasses everything including assessing the patient, providing the veterinarian with

information to administer and log the drugs prescribed, and educating the owner on proper home analgesia.
9. Pain management should begin before the animal enters the clinic.
10. Analgesia should not be considered optional.
11. Many animals mask the signs of pain in the hospital.
12. All tissue damage has the potential to cause pain.
13. Pain is often increased in anxious or stressed animals.
14. Increased duration or intensity of surgical pain should not be addressed by increasing the concentration in inhaled anesthesia.
15. Postoperatively pain and dysphoria can occur at the same time; care must be taken to differentiate between the two.

REVIEW QUESTIONS

1. When advising client's on pain management the technician should
   a. allow the client to decline all pain medication to save money.
   b. assume the client understands how to monitor their pet for pain.
   c. provide only verbal instructions regarding pain management.
   d. educate the client about clinical signs of pain to monitor for in their pet.
2. Breakthrough pain can be defined as pain that develops
   a. due to emergence delirium.
   b. as a normal response to tissue damage.
   c. despite administration of adequate preemptive pain control.
   d. due to administration of insufficient preemptive pain control.
3. A ring block is used as preemptive analgesia for which type of procedure?
   a. Onychectomy
   b. Dental extraction
   c. Pelvic fracture repair
   d. Surgery in or around the anus
4. Postoperative dysphoria is also known as
   a. allodynia.
   b. breakthrough pain.
   c. emergence delirium.
   d. central sensitization.
5. Pain that arises from stretching, distention, or inflammation of an abdominal organ is called
   a. somatic pain.
   b. visceral pain.
   c. pathologic pain.
   d. physiologic pain.
6. A physiological change that can indicate pain in a postoperative patient is
   a. tachypnea.
   b. bradycardia.
   c. hypotension.
   d. hypothermia.
7. In the veterinary practice setting, who has the authority to order pain medications for patients?
   a. Veterinarian
   b. Client/owner
   c. Veterinary technician
   d. All of the above
8. Which of these surgical procedures is likely to be most painful for a patient?
   a. Castration
   b. Mastectomy
   c. Nephrectomy
   d. Tooth extraction
9. According to the American Animal Hospital Association Pain Standards, pain assessment should be done on
   a. all patients.
   b. all surgical patients.
   c. patients outlined in hospital protocols.
   d. a patient when the client requests a pain assessment.
10. An increased response to a stimulation that is normally painful at the site of injury is called
    a. hyperalgesia.
    b. hypoesthesia.
    c. physiologic pain.
    d. central sensitization.
11. List four behavioral responses you might note in a painful patient.
12. List three variations in patients that may cause varying levels of pain for the same procedure.
13. How can a technician distinguish between pain and dysphoria?
14. Tranquilizers or sedatives are included in the premedication process for procedures because:
15. At a minimum, how often should pain be assessed postoperatively?

BIBLIOGRAPHY

Allen DG, Dowling PM, Smith DA et al.: *Handbook of veterinary drugs*, ed 3, Baltimore, 2005, Lippincott Williams & Wilkins.
Anderson C: *Introduction to pain management*, Lansing, 2010, Michigan Veterinary Conference proceedings.
Bassert JM, McCurnin DM, editors: *McCurnin's clinical textbook for veterinary technicians*, ed 9, St Louis, 2018, Elsevier.
Carter, Heather: Is it pain or dysphoria? How to tell the difference and what to do about it., March 6, 2020. http://www.dvm360.com/views/is-it-pain-or-dysphoria-hot-to-tell-the-difference-an what-to-do-about-it

Dyson DH: Perioperative pain management in veterinary patients. *Vet Clin North Am Small Anim Pract* 38:1309, 2008.

https://fearfreepets.com/https://www.drsallyjfoote.com/veterinary-professional/publications-free-resources/

Fossum TW, Hedlund CS, Hulse DA, et al.: *Small animal surgery*, ed 5, St Louis, 2018, Mosby.

Gaynor JS, Muir WW: *Handbook of veterinary pain management*, ed 3 St Louis, 2014, Mosby

Hellyer P, Rodan I, Brunt J, et al: American Animal Hospital Association, American Association of Feline Practitioners, AAHA/AAFP Pain Management Guidelines Task Force Members. AAHA/AAFP pain management guidelines for dogs & cats. *J Am Anim Hosp Assoc* 43:235, 2007.

Merskey H, Bogduk N: Part III: Pain terms, a current list with definitions and notes on usage. In *Classification of chronic pain*, ed 2, Seattle, 1994, ISAP Task Force of Taxonomy, IASP Press.

Plumb DC: *Plumbs' veterinary drug handbook*, ed 5, Ames, IA, 2005, Blackwell.

Shaffran N: Pain management: the veterinary technician's perspective. *Vet Clin North Am Small Anim Pract* 38:1415, 2008.

Shaffran N: The psychology of animal pain management. In Proceedings of the International Veterinary Emergency and Critical Care Symposium, September 11-15, 2010, San Antonio, TX.

Thomas JA, Lerche P: *Anesthesia and analgesia for veterinary technicians*, ed 5, St Louis, 2017, Elsevier.

Client Education for Postoperative Care

Marianne Tear

LEARNING OBJECTIVES

After completion of this chapter, the reader will be able to:

- Provide instructions to the owner describing the proper care of a patient after anesthesia.
- Provide instructions to the client describing proper care of a patient with postoperative drains.
- Describe client education for postoperative care of a patient with a bandage, splint, or cast.
- Provide instructions to the owner describing proper care of a patient after the following common surgical procedures:
  Tooth extraction

Gastrointestinal surgery
Feeding tube placement
Cystotomy
Declaw
Aural hematoma
Ear canal resection or ablation
Orthopedic surgery
Cesarean section

KEY TERMS

Enteral feeding
Dehiscence
Hematoma

Ileus
Inappetence
Peritonitis

Seroma

DISCHARGE INSTRUCTIONS

The role of the veterinary technician does not end when the patient is ready to go home; the owner must be taught how to properly provide care in the home environment. The responsibility for explaining the patient's aftercare to the owner is usually assigned to the veterinary technician. This is a logical policy because the technician has been the postoperative caregiver and understands the patient's needs and reactions. The technician knows the patient, can advocate for the patient, and can best educate the owner on how to care for the patient. Each patient should be treated as an individual, and home care should be tailored accordingly. The approach to providing the prescribed treatments is dictated by the patient's needs, reactions, and willingness to cooperate. The veterinary technician assigned to care for the patient should have determined what method to use to administer medication and how effective the analgesic drugs have been for the patient. Areas to discuss with the client include timing of drug administration, wound care, nutrition, and exercise. For example, antibiotics and analgesics may or may not be administered with a meal. The wound care should be delayed for about an hour after the analgesic is given.

Postoperative education can begin before the actual procedure is started. Providing the clients with a generalized handout on the procedure (Fig. 13.1) can give them the opportunity to become familiar with the condition. By having information on

Dystocia in Dogs and Cats

Ronald M. Bright, DVM, MS, DACVS

BASIC INFORMATION

Description

Dystocia is the inability to initiate the act of labor or the delivery of pups or kittens at the end of a pregnancy. Dog breeds at increased risk for dystocia include the Yorkshire terrier, miniature poodle, Pomeranian, English bulldog, dachshund, Chihuahua, and Scottish terrier.

Causes

The causes of dystocia can generally be classified into those caused by the mother and those caused by the fetus.

Uterine inertia is a condition in which the uterine muscles either do not contract (primary uterine inertia) or become fatigued during labor (secondary uterine inertia) from persistent straining against an obstruction within the birth canal. Secondary uterine inertia is almost never the sole cause of dystocia.

A narrow birth canal caused by a previous fracture of the pelvis can prevent passage of the fetus. The head of the fetus may be too large to pass through the birth canal, or the fetus may be oversized or malformed. Sometimes an improper position of the fetus as it approaches the birth canal makes passage difficult.

Psychological stress can delay the onset of labor. A rare cause of dystocia is twisting of the uterus on itself (uterine torsion).

Clinical Signs

The following are signs of dystocia:

- Active straining has occurred for more than 30-60 minutes without the birth of a fetus.
- Straining for 2 or more hours has not resulted in delivery of a fetus.
- The resting stage between expulsion of fetuses is greater than 4 hours and there is no sign of straining even though it is known that more fetuses remain in the uterus.
- Signs of systemic illness, such as vomiting, weakness, or fever, are present.
- Abnormal vaginal discharge, such as frank blood or pus, is present.
- The pregnancy is known to be a high risk (predisposed breed); only one, large fetus is present; or narrowing of the birth canal has occurred from a prior pelvic fracture.
- Attempts to expel a fetus are painful.
- Obvious signs of distress are present.

Diagnostic Tests

The diagnosis of dystocia is often derived from the clinical signs and a thorough physical examination. Other tests that may be recommended include x-rays, an abdominal ultrasound, and laboratory tests, such as measurement of blood calcium levels. Low blood calcium may be associated with uterine inertia. Commercially available external whelping monitors can be used to detect diminished fetal viability (fetal stress) and abnormal patterns in the uterine contractions.

TREATMENT AND FOLLOW-UP

Treatment Options

The treatment of dystocia varies, depending on the underlying cause. If a fetus has passed part of the way through the birth canal but is now caught, it may be possible to dislodge the fetus through cautious use of fingers or instruments. Administering a tranquilizer to relieve stress in an apprehensive bitch or queen may be helpful.

If uterine inertia is diagnosed, medical therapy may be attempted, provided that the birth canal is a normal size, the cervix is open, the fetus is not too large to pass through the canal, and no other obstruction is identified. Medical therapy involves administration of the hormone, oxytocin, to stimulate uterine contractions. If calcium levels are low, supplementation of calcium is indicated, because it enhances uterine contractions and increases the effects of oxytocin.

If medical therapy fails, surgery to perform a cesarean section (C-section) is indicated. Your veterinarian may discuss the option of spaying the mother at the time of the cesarean section. If there are no further plans for breeding the mother or if a uterine rupture is present, ovariohysterectomy (spaying) may be recommended.

Follow-up Care and Prognosis

Following resolution of the current dystocia, emphasis must be placed on preventing dystocia during future pregnancies. Such measures include providing consistent and adequate amounts of exercise during the pregnancy and making sure the mother is fed a well-balanced diet.

To increase the chances of an optimal litter size, it is often recommended that bitches be bred 2 days after ovulation. All queens and bitches should be provided a quiet, dark, stress-free, and sanitary birthing environment.

Fig. 13.1 Example of a client handout explaining dystocia in dogs and cats.(From Morgan R: Small animal practice: client handouts, St Louis, 2010, Saunders Elsevier.)

the causes, signs, and follow-up care, the clients will feel more actively involved. Many clients then come to the discharge with questions of their own.

In addition to the verbal discussion, written instructions explaining how to care for the postoperative patient should be sent home with the client. The hospital often has generic instructions that are prepared for all routine postoperative patients. Special instructions are added for certain nonroutine surgical procedures or medical conditions. However, each patient is an individual, and each client appreciates and deserves an explanation of the specific observations of the patient's reactions and the specific care techniques used. The veterinary technician personally discharging the patient to its owner can provide this communication. It is best to explain the discharge instructions in a quiet area of the clinic, like an exam room. The client's full attention needs to be directed to the technician's instructions, so the patient should not be brought to the client until all the information has been provided. Alternatively, the veterinary technician can write out special instructions and add these to the generic instructions (Fig. 13.2).

DISCHARGE INSTRUCTIONS
Elsewhere Veterinary Clinic
123 Street Road
Somewhere, USA
123-555-1234

Client name:_____ Patient's name: _____

Date admitted: _____ Date discharged: ____ _____

Procedure or diagnosis: _____

Medications:
- ☐ None dispensed
- ☐ Dispensed—directions on medication bottle
- ☐ Start medication _____

Food and water:
- ☐ Only offer ___ cup water and _____ food today
- ☐ Offer normal meal tonight
- ☐ Normal feeding may resume _____

    Special diet _____

Exercise:
- ☐ Restrict running, jumping, playing until _____
- ☐ If cat, confine indoors for _____ days
- ☐ If dog, leash walk only for _____ days

Sutures:
- ☐ Discourage your pet from licking or chewing at incision site

    If excessive licking or chewing occurs, please call the clinic for a collar to prevent this.

- ☐ Check the incision daily for swelling, redness, or discharge.

    If it appears irritated, swollen, or bleeding please notify us.

- ☐ **Please make an appointment for suture removal in ____ days.**
- ☐ Sutures are absorbable and do not need to be removed.
- ☐ No sutures.

Please notify the clinic if any of the following occur:

- ☐ Loss of appetite for more than ____ days
- ☐ Pain
- ☐ Straining to urinate/defecate

- ☐ Excess drainage from incision
- ☐ Excessive vomiting/diarrhea
- ☐ Depression

*Special instructions: _____
_____
_____
_____
_____
_____

Emergency clinic numbers:_____

Veterinarian's signature: _____

Fig. 13.2 Example of general postoperative instructions for clients (owners) after a veterinary patient's discharge.

Regardless of the type of procedure that was performed, the technician must be certain that all the client's questions have been answered. In a busy hospital, a technician may discharge 10 animals who have undergone spay procedures in a single day. It is easy to talk at the client rather than with them. The technician should include the owner in the discussion by asking nonleading questions to make sure the information has been understood. "What time will you be feeding Fluffy tonight?" allows for more interaction than "You understand what time to feed Fluffy, right?" The client's response to the first question allows the technician to gauge the client's understanding of postoperative feeding.

GENERAL POSTANESTHESIA INSTRUCTIONS

All patients that have been under sedation or general anesthesia should go home with instructions regarding their care for at least the first 24 hours. The instruction sheet should address (1) confinement, (2) feeding, (3) medications, (4) signs of possible adverse reactions, and (5) how to reach the hospital or 24-hour emergency clinic. If possible, a contact person, such as the technician, should also be listed. This helps personalize the treatment and makes the client feel more comfortable contacting the clinic with questions or concerns.

The client may need to confine the patient to a recovery crate or room. The patient may still be sedated and unable to walk normally. The patient may need to be accompanied or carried up and down stairs. Other pets in the household may disturb the patient, and it may be preferable to have the patient isolated from other animal housemates for a specified time. Over the long term, it may be necessary to keep cats inside and to walk dogs only with a leash.

The owner needs specific instructions regarding when and how much to feed the animal after returning home. The time to resume the normal feeding schedule should also be addressed. The technician should take the time to discuss the possibility of nausea after anesthesia. The owner should be instructed to start with smaller meals offered more frequently to the patient. Special diets may be prescribed and may be introduced gradually. The technician should give detailed examples of how to mix the new food in with the old to prevent gastrointestinal (GI) upset. Typically for a therapeutic diet, a 7- to 10-day transition once the animal is at home and eating well is recommended. Days 1 to 3, ¼ new diet, ¾ old diet; days 4 to 6, ½ new diet, ½ old diet; days 7 to 10, ¾ new diet, ¼ old diet; day 11, 100% new diet. Also, the owner should be given some helpful suggestions on how to make the new food more palatable— warming slightly, adding water, and so on. Specific instructions regarding a special diet should be written in the space provided on the postoperative discharge form.

Medications may be sent home with the patient. Specific instructions regarding their administration are written on the label of the medication bottle. The instructions are repeated on the discharge instructions with more details, including whether the medication should be administered with food or on an empty stomach. It is also a good idea to indicate what class of drugs each medication is (e.g., antibiotic, antiinflammatory,

pain medication). In addition, the necessity of giving one medication at a separate time from other medications can be explained to the owner at discharge. Colored labels can be pre-printed and placed on the medication bottles to help the owner remember specific requirements. Possible side effects of the medication should be addressed.

Patients that have undergone anesthesia or sedation may experience undesirable side effects. GI motility may be slowed (ileus), which may cause inappetence, vomiting, constipation, or bloating. Lethargy, ataxia, or depression may be symptoms of prolonged recovery from anesthesia. These symptoms should be discussed with the client or listed on the instruction sheet. The informed owner will be an observant advocate for the patient.

Finally, instructions should be clearly provided regarding how to reach the hospital or a referral emergency center 24 hours a day and which situations would require emergency contact.

GENERAL POSTOPERATIVE INSTRUCTIONS

In addition to the postoperative instructions already mentioned, the client should be instructed on the need to observe the patient's surgical site. The integrity of the surgical site should be monitored at least twice daily. If skin sutures are present, the number of sutures should be counted. The client should observe the area for swelling, redness, and discharge. If sutures are missing or if excessive swelling, discharge, or redness is noted, the owner should be instructed to call the veterinary hospital. Calling for advice regarding the management of the patient or with any concerns should be encouraged. If possible, the owner should be shown pictures of a normally healing incision and then pictures of seromas (a collection of fluid [serum] that builds up under the skin), hematomas (a collection of blood under the skin), and inflamed incisions. This knowledge will allow the owner to better understand the terms and conditions being described.

Specific instructions on confining the patient should be discussed with the owner. Each situation is unique, and residences vary, for example, in the presence and number of stairs to the outside. Other pets in the household may necessitate new routines regarding feeding, litter boxes, and walks outside. Children may need to be restricted from handling the pet until the patient is fully recovered. During the pet's recuperative phase at home, the family's routines and lifestyle will be disrupted, which can be stressful. The technicians should remind the client that the patient cannot articulate its pain or discomfort. It is vital for the client to track changes, improvements, or declines in behavior. These small clues can help the veterinary staff determine whether the animal is progressing as anticipated or there might be underlying complications.

If the patient is sent home with an Elizabethan collar (E-collar) or a BiteNot Collar (BiteNot Products, Inc., San Francisco), the technician needs to stress the importance of leaving the collar in place. Removing the collar for even a short period can lead to disaster; it only takes a matter of seconds for the patient to remove the skin sutures or completely open the incision, dehiscence. The owner should also be advised that the collar will not prevent the other animals in the household from licking the site and causing damage. An E-collar can also impede the patient's ability to eat or drink. Even properly fitted collars can touch the floor around the food bowl before the animal can reach the food with its mouth or can hit the bowl itself and prevent eating. If this occurs, the animal should be provided with elevated bowls or bowls with a smaller diameter.

If possible, before leaving the hospital, appointments should be scheduled for rechecks, suture removal, and drain removal. The hospital should also have a policy on calling the client to check on the patient's progress. Many clients assume that abnormal behavior is common after surgery. Having the technician call 24 hours after discharge and then at a preset time (or times) after that can put clients at ease. They will also be more likely to voice what they may feel are minor concerns.

Postoperative Care of Patients With Drains

Many surgical procedures involve the implanting of drains. These devices are temporarily placed to channel unwanted fluid or gas from a wound or body cavity. Often the patient is sent home with a passive drain. The owner is required to clean the discharge from the drain site and ensure that the drain is not disturbed by the patient. Clear, detailed instructions regarding drain care are important. Owners should also be informed that the discharge from an unbandaged drain can get on furniture, carpet, and clothing. In multipet households the owner should also be reminded that the E-collar will not prevent the other animals from licking at the site or removing the drain.

Written instructions as well as a demonstration regarding the care of the drain site can facilitate owner compliance. Warm soaks to loosen and remove dried serous discharge will be necessary (Fig. 13.3). The skin may need to be protected from the development of a moist dermatitis caused by contact with the discharge. A thin film of petroleum jelly can be spread over the area where the discharge tends to dry to the skin. The petroleum jelly serves as a protective barrier helping to prevent skin irritation or serum scald and facilitates skin cleaning.

The veterinary technician must emphasize to the client the importance of proper and thorough cleaning of the drain site. Inadequate cleaning of discharge can prevent the drain from functioning and block further discharge. Fluid becomes trapped under the wound or in the body cavity. This will slow the healing process or compromise a successful outcome in other ways.

The client also needs instructions about effective restraint of the pet while the drain is being cleaned. The technician who has been caring for the patient knows the most effective means to restrain the patient safely and effectively. These customized instructions can be written on the discharge information form in the area for special instructions.

If the pet pulls out the drain, the owner should report this to the clinic. The owner should search for any parts or pieces of the drain. These pieces can help the veterinary technician determine whether a portion of the drain is still in the patient. If a piece of the drain remains deep in the wound or body cavity, it will need to be surgically retrieved because it will prevent adequate healing of the wound.

Postoperative Care of Patients With a Bandage, Splint, or Cast

When a bandage, splint, or cast has been applied to a limb, the patient should be kept quiet. Cats are confined indoors and restricted from jumping. Dogs may need to be confined in a recovery crate. Play with other pets and humans in the household must be suspended. Dogs are walked only by leash. Depending on the number of stairs in the house, the dog may require assistance or need to be carried up and down the stairs.

Weekly in-hospital rechecks should be scheduled. The owner is instructed to examine the patient carefully each day and note the condition of the bandage and the extremity (Box 13.1). Toes should be checked for smell, warmth, and color. Foul odor can indicate tissue damage under the bandage; if swelling is present, the toes will move apart, or if the bandage is too tight, the toes may become cyanotic or extremely pale. In the event that any abnormalities are noted, the owner should be instructed to

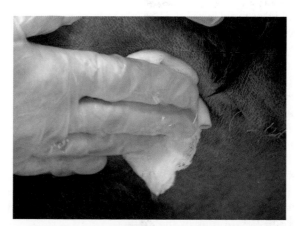

Fig. 13.3 Care of postoperative drains. Clean the area where the drain exits the wound with a warm compress of gauze. Apply warm soaks to the area to soften the discharge. Once the discharge is soft and loose, wipe the area clean.

BOX 13.1 Client Postoperative Instructions for Animals With a Bandage, Cast, or Splint

1. Position of bandage. Check to be sure that the bandage, cast, or splint has not slipped or shifted.
2. Irritation of adjacent skin. Check the skin adjacent to the edge of the bandage, cast, or splint by parting the fur and looking for redness or feeling for moisture.
3. Discoloration of bandage. The bandage, cast, or splint can become discolored because of staining from wetness on the outside or discharge soaking through from the inside.
4. Moisture. A wet bandage, cast, or splint should be replaced immediately.
5. Odor. A foul odor associated with the bandage, cast, or splint may be caused by infectious discharge.
6. Signs of chewing on bandage. Torn areas of tape or spots of discoloration or moisture are telltale signs of chewing. The patient chewing at the bandage, splint, or cast may have discomfort or pain. Replacement of the bandage (splint, cast) may be necessary, and an Elizabethan collar may be needed for the animal.

contact the hospital for bandage removal and or replacement. The client should be made aware of the serious complications that can arise from a damaged bandage.

The owner should be given instructions regarding how to protect the cast, bandage, or splint from wet grass, snow, puddles, and other sources of moisture. A plastic bag taped to the limb can effectively cover and protect the bandage (cast, splint) while the pet is outside. Empty fluid bags are made of heavy plastic that holds up well to repeated use. The bag should be removed as soon as the pet is back inside because the animal's body heat can create condensation within the bag, leading to a moist bandage.

POSTOPERATIVE INSTRUCTIONS FOR COMMON PROCEDURES

Gastrointestinal Enterotomy or Anastomosis

Surgery of the GI tract is indicated to remove foreign body obstructions, collect tissue biopsy samples, remove growths, and resect diseased areas of intestine (e.g., cancer, necrosis, intussusception). Fluid therapy is continued until the animal is drinking and not vomiting. Feeding is resumed after the animal is able to consume water without vomiting. Prophylactic antibiotic therapy is typically discontinued within hours postoperatively.

Animals recovering from GI surgery need to be observed with great care. If the intestinal surgical site does not hold and intestinal contents leak into the abdominal cavity, a serious infection will ensue. This complication, peritonitis, can occur within hours or days after surgery. Peritonitis is an extremely painful condition that responds only slightly to analgesics. The patient will also have a fever, so postoperative monitoring of body temperature is important. If the patient spikes a fever, laboratory procedures (e.g., complete blood cell count) may be ordered. As peritonitis progresses, fluid accumulates in the abdominal cavity and the patient appears bloated. An abdominocentesis procedure may be performed to obtain a sample for cytologic testing to evaluate cells present in the fluid and for culture if bacteria or white blood cells are found; abdominal ultrasound may be helpful in diagnosing the presence of fluid in the abdomen, which could indicate peritonitis. The owner should be instructed to monitor the patient closely at home immediately after and for several weeks postoperatively for signs of peritonitis (Box 13.2).

Two other postoperative concerns may not appear for weeks or months. First, the intestinal lumen may narrow because of scar formation causing a stricture. Second, a small, slow leak from the enterotomy site can lead to an abdominal abscess. Both complications may cause clinical signs associated with an obstruction. If an abdominal abscess has formed, vomiting, anorexia, lack of bowel movements, and abdominal pain may occur.

Spay (Ovariohysterectomy)

In female dogs and cats, the typical practice is to surgically remove the ovaries, uterine horns, and uterine body to the level of the cervix to prevent pregnancy and pyometra. Although this is an elective procedure, it is still a major abdominal surgery and must be treated with the same care as any other abdominal procedure. Each surgeon will determine at what age the procedure will be performed. Care must be exercised during the surgical prep and scrub to not cause undo skin irritation that could exacerbate healing and encourage licking afterward. Exercise restrictions and pain medications are typically done after this procedure to ensure the animal is comfortable and as pain free as possible. Although complications are not common, infections, wound dehiscence, and trauma to the surgical site can all occur.

Cesarean Section

After a cesarean section, the mother and newborns are kept apart until all have completely recovered from anesthesia. The neonates are at risk of being crushed if introduced to a mother that is still heavily sedated or ataxic. Even when fully recovered, the mother may reject the newborns. The staff must watch the mother carefully for any sign of aggression toward the neonates.

The newborns should be weighed at least once daily. Each one should be steadily gaining weight every day. If any newborn is not gaining weight, it should have extra time by itself on the mammary glands. If the newborn is not nursing, the owner should be shown how to supplement the neonate's feeding with milk replacer (e.g., KMR, Esbilac).

The mother's surgical incision is at risk of irritation and injury from her licking or the newborns' suckling. The owner should inspect the incision daily. A bloody, mucous discharge is expected from the vulva for several days postoperatively. The color of the discharge may change from red to brown as the days pass. A foul odor to the discharge is not normal, and the hospital should be notified.

It is common for the new mother to have loose stools after giving birth. The mother's appetite should be good. It is important that the new mother have plenty of high-calorie food because she must eat enough for herself and all her offspring. Typically puppy or kitten food is recommended for the mother while she is nursing. The new mother that is not eating will not heal promptly and cannot produce enough milk to feed the newborns. Access to plenty of clean, fresh water is imperative for production of milk by the mother.

The owner should be shown how to express milk from each mammary gland to check it for milk production and color and consistency. Colostrum (the first milk, generally rich in

---

BOX 13.2   Client Postoperative Instructions After Gastrointestinal or Anastomosis Surgery

1. Check the abdominal incision daily for redness, swelling, discharge, and tenderness.
2. Monitor the pet's temperature twice daily, if possible. If a fever is detected, the hospital should be notified.
3. Alert the hospital if vomiting, diarrhea, constipation, or inappetence occurs.
4. Alert the hospital if the patient appears unusually lethargic or in excessive pain.
5. Alert the hospital if the patient appears bloated.

antibodies) is usually slightly yellow and sticky. After the newborns have nursed for approximately 24 hours, the milk becomes thinner and whiter. If the mammary glands stop releasing milk or become painful or red, or if the milk is thick or discolored (any color other than white), the owner must contact the veterinarian. The mother will need to be treated, and the newborns will need to be fed milk replacer. The veterinary technician often must instruct clients on how to bottle-feed or tube-feed the newborns.

Pet supply stores carry milk replacers for puppies and kittens. Bottles with nipples of appropriate size for the newborn should be purchased at the same time. Milk replacers come in canned as well as powdered forms. The process of tube or bottle feeding neonates can be very labor intensive. The technician should discuss the pros and cons of both options with the owner. Detailed description and hands-on demonstrations will be necessary to ensure that the young animals get the proper nutrition with minimal complications.

There are several veterinary textbooks dedicated to the pediatric patient; *Small Animal Pediatrics: The First 12 Months of Life* is one example.

Castration (Orchiectomy)

Surgical removal of the testicles is a common elective procedure in dogs and cats. In dogs this is seen as a sterile procedure, whereas in cats is it usually seen as a nonsterile procedure. Techniques will vary based on the surgeon's preference. Care must be taken when doing the surgical prep in this delicate area so as to not cause clipper burn or skin irritation from the surgical scrub. Especially in dogs, the owners must be informed to watch for any signs of licking or chewing and to restrict activity for a predetermined period. Excessive activity can lead to seroma formation or breakdown in the suture line. Cats do not usually require sutures at the scrotal incision, so activity does not need to be restricted.

Cystotomy

One major concern after bladder surgery is bladder distension. To prevent the bladder from becoming overly distended, the patient needs to be able to and allowed to empty its bladder frequently. While in the hospital, a urinary catheter is often placed to help prevent bladder distension. Because this is not possible at home, frequent access to the outdoors or a litter box is necessary. See Box 13.3 for postoperative instructions for the owner of a patient that has undergone a procedure involving surgical incision of the bladder

Perianal Surgery

The removal of tumors, debridement and drainage of fistulas and anal sacs, removal of anal sacs, and creating new urethra openings all require surgery around the anus. In addition to the general postoperative instructions, special instructions should be given to the client (Box 13.4). It is imperative that the surgical site be kept as clean as possible. The use of warm water–soaked cloths can help to remove any discharge, and applying petroleum jelly to the site can help to prevent serum scald and make future cleanings easier.

> **BOX 13.3 Client Postoperative Instructions After a Cystotomy**
>
> 1. Expect bloody urine (hematuria) for 12 to 36 hours. The amount of blood in the urine should diminish as time passes. The owner can monitor the color of the urine by lining the litter box with a white paper towel or placing a white paper towel under the pet when it urinates. Blood in the urine is more easily observed when soaked into a white paper towel.
> 2. A special diet may be prescribed. Instructions may recommend a gradual change to the new diet by mixing the previous and new diets together for several days.
> 3. Antibiotic therapy may be prescribed. The choice of antibiotic may change when the results of the urine culture and sensitivity test are known.
> 4. The dog should be walked outside frequently, and the amount and color of the urine should be monitored. Having the dog urinate on a white paper towel is helpful.
> 5. If the pet is straining to urinate or exhibiting pain when urinating, the hospital should be notified.
> 6. If the pet is not passing urine, it should be immediately examined. This is an emergency. Stones remaining in the bladder or blood clots in the bladder can cause obstructions.

> **BOX 13.4 Client Postoperative Instructions After Perianal Surgery**
>
> 1. A special diet high in fiber may be prescribed to keep the stools soft. The diet may or may not be a permanent change.
> 2. Stool softeners such as lactulose may be prescribed for short-term therapy.
> 3. If diarrhea occurs, the veterinary hospital should be notified. Discontinue the stool softener, and clean the surgical site by flushing thoroughly with warm tap water. Do not scrub the site.
> 4. Observe the pet while it passes a bowel movement. If the pet is straining or crying in pain, the veterinary hospital should be notified. Fecal incontinence (inability to stop or leakage of feces) also warrants hospital contact.

Aural Hematoma

Aural hematomas are typically messy (Fig 13.4), and the bandaging can be quite distressing to the owner. The technician needs to stress the importance of treating the underlying cause of the hematoma, such as yeast, bacterial, or parasitic infections, as well as keeping the pinna clean (Box 13.5).

Lateral Ear Canal Resection or Ablation

The ear canal is ablated, or surgically removed, when it is so chronically diseased that medical treatment is unable to establish a healthy canal. This surgery is a last resort. The theory is that if the diseased part is removed, the pain and discomfort will disappear. Part or all of the ear canal can be removed. If the entire ear canal is removed, the pet may be rendered deaf in that ear.

The pet is usually not released to the owner's care until the need for daily bandage changes has passed and all drains have been removed. Postoperative infection may be caused by preexisting disease or contamination during surgery. Facial nerve paralysis is a well-recognized complication that usually resolves within 2 weeks. In some patients the vestibular system can be adversely affected when the entire ear canal is ablated. In these cases the pet exhibits a head tilt, nystagmus, and difficulty walking. Overall,

BOX 13.5   Client Postoperative Instructions After an Aural Hematoma

1. The area where the drain exits the pinna needs to be cleaned of discharge. Warm water and a clean face towel or gauze work well. The drains usually stay in for 2 to 3 weeks (Fig. 13.4).
2. Some animals may also need to have an infected ear canal treated with topical drops and ear cleansers. The pinna may be sore to the touch, so take extra care when instilling medication into the ear canal.
3. Some patients may have their head wrapped in a bandage. The same observations outlined earlier for extremity bandages apply to head bandages. Watch for soiling, slipping, moisture, foul odor, and skin irritation along the edges of the bandage.

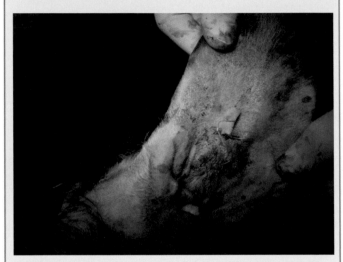

Fig. 13.4 Aural hematoma repair using soft Penrose drain.

BOX 13.6   Client Postoperative Instructions After an Orthopedic Procedure

1. The pet will need to be confined. Dogs are walked only by leash. Cats must stay indoors during the recuperative period. Excessive activity and exercise can slow the healing process by allowing weight bearing too early or causing excessive movement of the affected joint or fracture site.
2. Dogs especially may need help standing and walking. A bath towel can be placed under the abdomen or chest to act as a sling (Fig. 13.5).
3. If a bandage or cast has been applied, the owner receives specific instructions regarding its care (see Box 13.1).
4. If the patient has an external fixation device, the stainless steel pins and connecting pieces need particular attention, as follows:
- The site where the pin exits the skin will not heal while the pin is in place. Dried discharge is cleaned from the area once or twice daily as needed. An antimicrobial ointment can be applied to the skin around the exit site.
- The connecting pieces are covered with tape to prevent sharp edges from catching on furniture or the opposite limb.

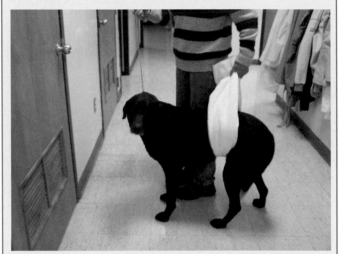

Fig. 13.5 Towel sling. Place a towel under the dog's abdomen. Pull up with one or both arms. The towel sling takes some of the weight off the dog's hind end, allowing the animal to walk more easily.

many complications may occur, and intensive nursing care in the hospital setting is needed for a variable time after ear canal resection or ablation surgery.

The patient typically tries to scratch at the surgical site. An Elizabethan collar is an important piece of equipment used to help protect the integrity of the surgical site. Postoperative pain often drives the pet to self-trauma. Lateral ear canal resection or ear canal ablation tends to be very painful. Administration of analgesic medication and close observation of the surgical site are the owner's primary directives.

Orthopedic Procedures

The client with a pet that underwent orthopedic surgery should receive postoperative instructions specific to that procedure. The animal may need additional support such as a bandage, cast, or non–weight-bearing sling (Fig 13.5). Exercise and even moderate activity may be severely restricted for weeks or months. Extensive pain management may also be indicated. See Box 13.6 for general home care instructions after orthopedic procedures.

Feline Declaw (Onychectomy)

An onychectomy is a painful procedure regardless of the method used. Pain management preoperatively, perioperatively, and

postoperatively will ensure that the patient recovers quickly and with few complications. Owners need to understand that jumping must be forbidden, because the force of even the smallest jump could damage the paws. This may mean confining the cat to a small bathroom or even a kennel during the healing processes. Even though the site of the phalange removal is covered or closed, it still needs to be treated like any other surgical incision. The paws should be checked daily for swelling, redness, discharge, and odor. Clay or clumping litter should be replaced with newspaper pellets or shredded paper. Clay litter can leave material in the surgical site that could predispose the patient to an infection (Box 13.7). Once healing has occurred (10–14 days), the cat can be transitioned back to its normal litter.

Dental Extraction

While the mouth is healing after a tooth extraction, the pet will have a soft-food diet, such as canned, semimoist pet food or dry food soaked in water until mushy. The socket will heal in

1 to 2 weeks. During the healing phase the pet may be gradually returned to its usual dry-food diet.

The client should watch the patient for a number of specific signs. For the first day the owner may see the water in the bowl tinged red after the pet drinks. If this does not subside, the veterinarian should be notified. Long-term bleeding from the mouth indicates delayed healing, infection, or a coagulation problem. The pet rubbing or pawing at its face is an indication of pain, and the veterinarian should be notified. Crying out while eating or refusing to eat any hard food after several days to weeks have passed indicates an ongoing problem. The patient that refuses to eat will not heal promptly or properly.

Feeding Tube Placement

An **enteral feeding** tube may be placed for many reasons to aid in the patient's nutritional support (see Chapter 11). This tube may stay in place for many weeks to months. Because of the critical support the feeding tube provides and the possible long-term need for it, the client caring for the patient at home requires detailed instructions on the tube's use and care (Box 13.8; Fig. 13.6).

Commercially prepared liquid diets (e.g., CliniCare, Carnivore Care) are mandated when the tube has a very small diameter (less than 10 French). Gastric and esophageal tubes are often large enough in diameter that therapeutic recovery diets or canned pet foods can be used. It is important that large chunks of food be eliminated during preparation and not be forced down the tube; this can result is tube obstruction and loss of function. Using a therapeutic recovery diet will ensure that no large chunks of food are present. If a blenderized food is chosen, ensure that it is blended exceptionally well before feeding. Water can be added to all diets to ease passage through the tube. If adding water, ensure that the volume of food being delivered is adjusted accordingly. Although medications can be administered through the feeding tube, they should either be in a liquid form or ground into a very fine powder and suspended in water before administration. Medications should always be given separately from the food to prevent undesirable interactions.

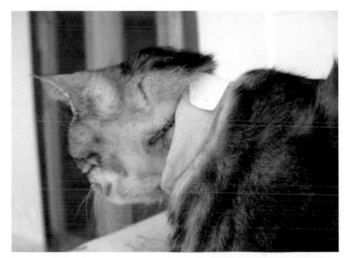

Fig. 13.6 Patient relaxing at home with an unbandaged feeding tube.

KEY POINTS

1. As the primary caregiver in the hospital setting, the veterinary technician is the best team member to discharge the patient to the owner's care.
2. Instructions for all postanesthesia patients address confinement, feeding, medication, possible adverse reactions, and hospital contact information.
3. The client should receive written instructions as well as a demonstration of cleaning steps for passive drains.
4. To prevent distraction, all discharge instructions should be given in a quiet area where there will be minimal distractions. The pet and owner should not be reunited until after all home care has been thoroughly discussed.
5. It is important to ask nonleading questions to assess the client's understanding of home care.
6. The client should be given a point-of-contact person, typically the technician, so that he or she feels more comfortable calling with questions.
7. The technician or other staff member should call the owner 24 hours after discharge to see how the patient is doing and then again at set intervals during the recovery.
8. Patients with a bandage, cast, or splint need to be strictly confined. The owner must understand the importance of this measure.
9. The owner needs to report any change in the appearance or position of the bandage, splint, or cast to the veterinary hospital.
10. If a patient is sent home with an E-collar, the owner must make sure that the animal is able to eat and drink normally.
11. Owners in multipet households should be reminded that the E-collar will not prevent the other animals from licking the patient's incision and causing damage.
12. Within a week, the patient that has undergone one to several tooth extractions should be pain free, and the tooth sockets should be almost healed.
13. The patient exhibiting signs of unrelenting pain hours to days after gastrointestinal surgery most likely has peritonitis.
14. The patient recovering from a cesarean section must heal and also raise a litter. The newborns' feeding may have to be supplemented with milk replacer.
15. Though they are routine procedures, castrations and spays are still surgical procedures, and complications can occur.
16. The bladder of the patient recovering from a cystotomy should be kept small by allowing the patient to void every few hours.
17. After aural hematoma surgery, passive drains usually remain in place for several weeks. The pinna may heal with scar tissue and significant wrinkling.
18. Insufficient confinement of the patient after an orthopedic procedure is the most common reason for delayed healing.
19. The heavier and older the cat, the longer it will take for the cat to recover from declaw surgery. Confining the cat to an indoor lifestyle is ideal after onychectomy because the animal no longer has the ability to defend itself.
20. A feeding tube may be needed for several weeks, so the owner must care for the tube properly.
21. To assess the necessity of maintaining the feeding tube, the patient must have food available when it is ready to eat.

REVIEW QUESTIONS

1. How often should the client monitor the surgery incision after the patient is discharged?
   a. Once daily
   b. Twice daily
   c. Every other day
   d. The surgical site does not need to be checked after discharge.
2. Clinical signs of prolonged recovery from anesthesia include
   a. hyperactivity, pacing, and ataxia.
   b. lethargy, anorexia, and depression.
   c. vomiting, constipation, and bloating.
   d. inappetence, diarrhea, and vomiting.
3. Infection within the abdominal cavity after surgery is called
   a. seroma.
   b. stricture.
   c. peritonitis.
   d. dehiscence.
4. At what age should an ovariohysterectomy be performed on a dog?
   a. 12 weeks
   b. 6 months
   c. 1 year
   d. When recommended by the veterinarian

5. A client called to ask about vaginal discharge from her bull dog that had a caesarean section 3 days ago. What would be considered a normal discharge for this patient?
   a. Bloody and mucousy
   b. Black and malodorous
   c. White and foul smelling
   d. No discharge should be noted
6. What is the typical appearance of colostrum when expressed from the mammary gland?
   a. Red and thick
   b. White and thin
   c. White and thick
   d. Yellow and sticky
7. When can a cat be transitioned back to clay or clumping litter post-onychectomy?
   a. 2–3 days
   b. 5–7 days
   c. 7–10 days
   d. 10–14 days
8. Commercially fed liquid diets should be fed via feeding tubes that are less than what diameter?
   a. 3 French
   b. 5 French

    c. 8 French

    d. 10 French

9. How long should hematuria be expected post-cystotomy?

    a. No longer than 12 hours

    b. No longer than 24 hours

    c. Up to 36 hours

    d. Up to 48 hours

10. Approximately how long should a patient be self-feeding before a feeding tube is removed?

    a. 2–3 days

    b. 1 week

    c. 2 weeks

    d. 1 month

11. List three reasons a patient should be rechecked post-perianal surgery.

12. What is a simple way to help clients monitor for migration of a feeding tube?

13. What feeding recommendations should be made post-dental extraction?

14. List three postoperative complications of a lateral ear resection.

15. List two methods of preventing or removing discharge around a perianal incision clean.

16. List the five items that should be addressed in a general postanesthesia instruction.

BIBLIOGRAPHY

Bassert JM, Beal AD, Samples OM, editors: *McCurnin's clinical textbook for veterinary technicians*, ed 9, St Louis, 2018, Elsevier.

Peterson ME, Kutzler M: *Small animal pediatrics: the first 12 months of life*, St Louis, 2011, Saunders.

Piermattei DL, Flo GL, DeCamp CE: *Handbook of small animal orthopedics and fracture repair*, ed 4, St Louis, 2006, Elsevier.

Wortinger A, Burns K: *Nutrition and disease management for veterinary technicians and nurses*, ed 2, Ames, IA, 2015, Wiley Blackwell.

Postoperative Cleaning

Ann Wortinger

OUTLINE

LEARNING OBJECTIVES

After completion of this chapter, the reader will be able to:

- Describe the ideal cleaning procedure for a surgery room.
- Identify the different types of disinfectants and the microorganisms they target.
- Describe the cleaning methods used for preparing instruments for sterilization.
- Identify which method is best for sterilizing particular instruments.

- Demonstrate how to wrap a pack for sterilization.
- Describe the types of expiration dating.
- Explain the different types of sterilization indicators.
- Identify the supplies that should be stocked in a surgery room.
- Explain supply rotation in the surgery room.

KEY TERMS

Biological indicator
Cavitation
Chemical indicator
Chlorine-based
Cold sterilization
Decontamination
Disinfectant
Disposable supplies
Enzymes
Ethylene oxide (gas) sterilization

Event-related expiration
Flash sterilization
Gravity air-displacement
High-level disinfection
High-vacuum sterilizer
Indicator tape
Mechanical friction
Movable equipment
Phenol-based
Plasma sterilization

Precleaning
Preparation area
Presoaking
Quaternary amine–based
Recipe
Reusable supplies
Shelf-life expiration
Sterilization
Surfactant
Terminal cleaning

CLEANING OF THE SURGERY ROOM

Equipment used to clean the surgery room should be designated for use only in the surgery room to prevent cross-contamination from other areas of the veterinary facility. Various agencies and organizations that evaluate human medical facilities provide recommendations that the veterinary facility can use when setting up a protocol for the cleaning and maintenance of the surgery room.

Infection Control Today has stringent guidelines addressing a surgical conscience in the operating room that encompasses a heightened awareness of intraoperative transmission pathogenic organisms and a comprehensive environmental hygiene program. Although these recommendations may be difficult to meet in all veterinary practices, it is important to the veterinary patient's health that guidelines for cleanliness and disinfection of the surgical area include as many recommended practices as possible.

The U.S. Centers for Disease Control and Prevention (CDC) provides guidelines for environmental infection control in health care facilities. The primary recommendation for infection control is to effectively prevent opportunistic, environmentally related infections in immunocompromised individuals. Proper use of disinfectants, proper maintenance of medical equipment that utilizes water, and proper ventilation standards will minimize healthcare-associated infection risks and reduce the frequency of pseudo-outbreaks. Research has demonstrated that interactions between the patient's body surfaces, operating personnel hands, and the operating room environment play a role in the transmission of bacteria. Significant areas of contamination in the surgical suite included the anesthetic machines, the floors, intravenous (IV) poles, and the operating room (OR) entry door handle. Wet vacuuming the surgery room floor is recommended at the end of the day. The CDC also states that the actual physical removal of microorganisms and soil by scrubbing is more important than the antimicrobial effect of the cleaning agent used.

Current recommendations are that high-traffic areas in the surgical suite be cleaned between patients and the entire floor cleaned at the end of each day. The following Association of periOperative Registered Nurses (AORN) recommendations, including a rationale (purpose) to clarify some practices, may be useful as a protocol for the cleaning of a surgery area in a veterinary facility.

1. Cleaning is performed on a regular basis to reduce the amount of dust, organic material, and microbial presence in the surgery room.
2. The surgery room should be cleaned before and after each surgical procedure.
3. All horizontal surfaces in the surgery room should be damp-dusted before the first surgery of the day. In "damp dusting," a lint-free cloth dampened with disinfectant is used to wipe down the horizontal surfaces.
Rationale: Proper cleaning of horizontal surfaces helps reduce airborne contaminants that may travel on dust and lint.

4. Surgical room equipment and furniture that are visibly soiled should be cleaned at the end of each procedure.
Rationale: Items used for surgery are considered contaminated through contact with the patient's blood, tissue, and body fluids and should be cleaned before admittance of the next patient to the surgery room.
5. Surgery rooms should be "terminally cleaned" daily. **Terminal cleaning** is cleaning that is performed at the completion of the daily surgery schedule. It includes all the equipment in the surgery and prep areas and all the permanent and **movable equipment.**
6. Surgery rooms should be cleaned daily whether they are used or not.
Rationale: A clean surgical environment reduces the number of microbial flora present.
7. **Mechanical friction** (a scrubbing motion) should be used to clean all surfaces, including (but not limited to) the following:
   - Surgical lights
   - Any fixed equipment
   - All furniture and equipment, including wheels, casters, step stools, foot pedals, telephones, and light switches
   - Handles of cabinets
   - Ventilation faceplates
   - Horizontal surfaces (doorway ledges)
   - Areas adjacent to surgery room
   - Scrub sinks
8. Refillable soap dispensers are not recommended because they can harbor bacterial growth. Single-use containers are recommended to prevent growth of resistant bacteria in the bottom of the containers.
9. Surgery rooms should be wet-vacuumed at the end of the day.
Rationale: Terminal cleaning in the surgery room reduces the number of microorganisms, dust, and organic debris in the environment.
10. Cleaning equipment (mops, wet vacuums) should be disassembled, cleaned, and dried before storage.
Rationale: This practice prevents growth of microorganisms during storage and subsequent contamination of the surgery room.

DISINFECTANTS

Definitions

The basic definitions in Box 14.1 can aid in understanding how the different disinfectants work and interact with bacteria, viruses, spores, and even one another. The ideal disinfectant should have the following characteristics:
- Broad spectrum
- Nonirritating
- Nontoxic
- Noncorrosive
- Inexpensive

Effectiveness

The effectiveness of any disinfectant depends on the following factors:

Type of microorganism: Some microorganisms are more resistant to certain types of disinfectants.

Degree of contamination: This may affect the length of time and the amount of chemical disinfectant necessary to disinfect effectively.

Amount of protein in area: Proteins may absorb or inactivate the disinfectant.

Organic matter: Hair, feces, litter, and other organic matter decrease the effectiveness or render the disinfectant ineffective. All organic matter should be removed from the area, and the area should be sanitized before the disinfectant is applied.

Additional sanitizing compounds: Other compounds used to sanitize the area may inactivate or react with the disinfectant. Thorough rinsing and drying after sanitizing should be attempted before a disinfectant is applied.

Concentration and quantity of chemical: Improper dilution or inadequate amount of the correct dilution may result in ineffective disinfection.

BOX 14.1   Disinfectant Terms

Anionic detergent: Soap that has free, negatively charged ions that precipitate when combined with calcium and magnesium in hard water.

Antiseptic: Chemical that inhibits or prevents the growth of microbes on living tissue; compare with **disinfectant**.

Bactericide: Agent that destroys (kills) bacteria.

Bacteriostat: Agent that inhibits the growth of bacteria.

Biocide: Agent that kills living organisms.

Cationic detergent: Contains positively charged ions that remain suspended in solution (e.g., quaternary ammonium).

Detergent: Chemical that contains free ions and leaves a film on surfaces.

Disinfectant: Chemical used to inhibit or prevent the growth of microbes on inanimate objects; compare with *antiseptic*.

Fungicide: Agent that kills fungi.

Sanitize: To reduce the number of microbes to a safe level.

Sporicide: Agent that kills spores.

Sterilize: To eliminate all microbes by killing or inactivation.

Viricide: Agent that kills viruses.

Contact time and temperature: Incorrect contact time or the temperature of the surface may result in ineffective disinfection.

Types of Disinfectants

Many types of disinfectants are commercially available for use in a veterinary facility. Each facility should research the product information and determine the best policy for the facility based on the disinfection needs of the facility. Most disinfectants require some form of dilution. The manufacturer's recommendations for dilution should be followed so that each disinfectant is used at its maximum effectiveness against bacteria, viruses, and other infective agents. Table 14.1 compares types of various disinfectants.

An example of a chlorine-based disinfectant is bleach (Fig. 14.1). It can be used for cleaning as well as disinfecting. Bleach does corrode metals and causes fabrics to deteriorate. It can be irritating to eyes, mucous membranes, and skin. Bleach can be deactivated by fecal matter. Decreased temperature and the pH of the water in which the bleach is diluted may alter its efficacy.

Phenol-based disinfectants include common household disinfectants (e.g., Lysol™, Pine-Sol™). Phenols are able to work in the presence of organic material. These disinfectants are relatively safe but can cause skin irritation. They are infrequently used in veterinary medicine. Phenols can cause toxicities in cats; therefore, caution should be used when cleaning with phenols in the veterinary clinic.

An example of a quaternary amine–based disinfectant is Dual-Quat (Vetoquinal, Delaware,) (Fig. 14.2). Quaternary amine–based disinfectants, or quats, provide broad-spectrum disinfection and are often germicidal, viricidal, and fungicidal. These disinfectants bind to and are inactivated by organic material, so the area must be cleaned of organic debris before disinfection. They also react with soaps, so the area must be well rinsed after sanitizing. Hard water may also deactivate quaternary amine–based disinfectants.

Iodine disinfectants such as povidone-iodine are not generally used as disinfectants, but in veterinary medicine they are often used as antiseptics (Fig. 14.3). The iodines can stain skin, fabric, and floors and can irritate tissue. They are also corrosive. Iodines are inactivated by organic material.

TABLE 14.1   Common Disinfectants Used in Veterinary Practice

Agent	Practical Use	Disinfectant Properties	Antiseptic Properties	Mechanisms of Action	Precautions
Alcohol: isopropyl alcohol (50%-70%); ethyl alcohol (70%)	Spot cleaning; injection site preparation	Good	Very good	Protein denaturation, metabolic interruption, and cell lysis	Corrosive to stainless steel; volatile
Chlorine compounds: hypochlorite	Cleaning floors and countertops	Good	Fair	Release of free chlorine and oxygen	Inactivated by organic debris; corrosive to metal
Iodine compounds: iodophors (7.5%) scrub solution	Cleaning dark-colored floors and countertops	Good	Good	Iodination and oxidation of essential molecules	Stains fabric and tissue
Glutaraldehyde: 2% alkaline solution	Disinfection of lenses and delicate instruments	Good; sterilizes	None	Protein and nucleic acid alkylation	Tissue reaction odor (rinse instruments well before using)

From Fossum TW: Small animal surgery, ed 4, St Louis, 2012, Mosby.

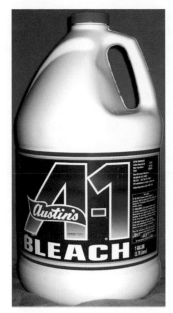

Fig. 14.1 Chlorine-based disinfectant.

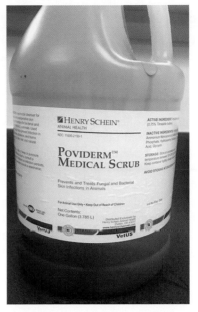

Fig. 14.3 Povidone-iodine disinfectant.

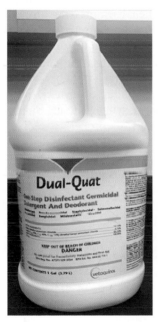

Fig. 14.2 Quaternary amine–based disinfectant.

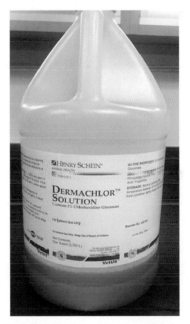

Fig. 14.4 Chlorhexidine diacetate disinfectant.

Chlorhexidine disinfectants are widely used in veterinary medicine as disinfectants for examination tables and for the disinfection of instruments for minor procedures (Fig. 14.4). They are also used as an antiseptic. Chlorhexidine maintains its effectiveness in the presence of organic material but is not as effective against some bacteria and viruses as other disinfectants. It also has residual activity, which can be important. One drawback is that chlorhexidine must have sufficient contact time to be effective.

Technician Notes

- Disinfectants should be used according to the manufacturer's instructions.
- There is no ideal disinfectant, but many good disinfectants meet most of the criteria of an ideal disinfectant.
- The effectiveness of a disinfectant depends on many factors (e.g., microorganisms, contamination, and organic matter).
- No disinfectant will kill all contagious organisms. Know which disinfectants are effective on which organisms.

INSTRUMENT CLEANING

Cleaning, decontaminating (or sanitizing), and sterilizing are the three cornerstones to providing sterile instruments in the surgery room. Each of these processes contributes to the overall destruction of microorganisms that could cause serious postoperative complications, including the death of the patient.

Basic cleaning procedures for instruments include presoaking, decontaminating, and ultrasonic cleaning. It is imperative to begin the process of presoaking immediately after a surgery.

Presoaking of Instruments

Presoaking or precleaning can make the cleaning process more efficient. Presoaking involves placing the soiled instruments in distilled water mixed with a detergent solution that is specifically approved for use with surgical instruments (e.g., HAEMO-SOL; HAEMO-SOL, Baltimore) (Fig. 14.5), without using mechanical agitation. Tap water can contribute to staining and rust formation because of its high iron content and therefore should not be used for prolonged presoaking. The purpose of presoaking is to soften dried blood and debris on the instruments and to further prevent blood and debris from drying on the instruments.

Precleaning involves rinsing the instruments in distilled water to rid them of tissue and blood. If this is not done, processing the instruments may take longer. Allowing tissue and blood to dry on the instruments makes cleaning much more difficult, especially in hinged areas and box locks. Debris can build up and harden in crevices, making decontamination more difficult as well. The distilled water should be cold because heating contributes to the proteins in blood and tissue adhering to the surgical instruments, thus making precleaning more difficult.

Decontamination of Instruments

The decontamination process is the manual cleaning of an instrument in a commercial instrument detergent solution to assist in the breakdown of biological debris. The commercial instrument detergent solution should be diluted with cold distilled water. Because this may be the only cleaning before sterilization, the instruments must be cleaned thoroughly. When cleaning instruments by hand, the technician must take care not to damage the more delicate items and must pay special attention to cleaning areas such as teeth, ridge, and box locks or joints to ensure they have been thoroughly cleaned. Instruments should be decontaminated using the following procedural steps:

1. Prepare a basin with warm water and a detergent approved for use on surgical instruments.
2. Open all box locks and unlock ratchets as each instrument is gently placed in the basin.
3. Wash all surfaces of each instrument with a soft bristle brush. Pay special attention to box locks, joints, and serrations because biological debris builds up in these areas. Use a brushing motion, directed away from you, to scrub the instruments; this method prevents biological debris from splashing back toward you.
   - Never use a wire brush on instruments because it will damage the instruments' surfaces and cause microscratches that can harbor pathogens (microorganisms).
   - Instruments have a protective coating of chromium oxide to extend their usefulness as properly functioning devices. If the coating is removed, the instrument will be compromised, and then its surface can harbor pathogens that can adversely affect the patient's health.
4. Rinse each instrument thoroughly with distilled water. This will prevent the buildup of scale on the instruments. If tap water is used, scale will eventually build up on instruments and they will not work properly.
5. With locks and ratchets opened, place the instruments flat on a lint-free, absorbent surface.
6. When the instruments are clean, check each for its general condition and its ability to function properly. Box locks should open and close smoothly, ratchets should engage and disengage easily, scissors should cut easily and smoothly, and the jaws and teeth should mesh as designed. One way to check the integrity of ratchets is to close them and firmly tap the ringed end of the instrument against a firm, smooth surface. If the ratchets pop open when tested, they cannot be trusted to hold the target tissue in surgery and should not be included in the surgery pack.

Instruments with broken or missing parts, malfunctioning parts, pitted or discolored parts, or rusted surfaces should be set aside for repair or replacement. It is best to buy high-quality instruments that will withstand repeated and excessive use.

Ultrasonic Cleaning of Instruments

After the decontamination process has been completed, the next step is ultrasonic cleaning with a solution of distilled water and chemicals (enzymes) (Fig. 14.6). Several brands of enzymatic solutions are available, and the solution chosen should contain a surfactant, a product that reduces surface tension. An example of a surfactant solution is MetriClean 2 (Metrex, Orange, CA) (Fig. 14.7). Enzymes are organic substances that

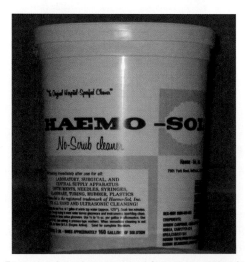

Fig. 14.5 Example of product approved for use as a cleaning solution for surgical instruments.

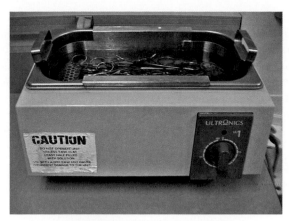

Fig.14.6 Ultrasonic cleaning unit.

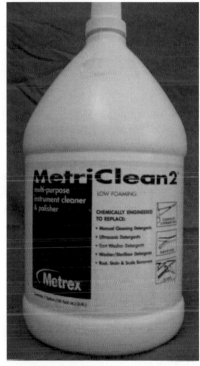

Fig. 14.7 Example of enzymatic cleaning solution used in ultrasonic cleaning unit.

The benefit of ultrasonic cleaning is best demonstrated with hinged instruments or those with inaccessible areas (e.g., box lock), including hinged retractors and bone-cutting instruments. These devices should be in the open position for cleaning. An ultrasonic cleaner uses sound waves higher than those heard by the human ear, which create tiny bubbles. These bubbles form and collapse thousands of times each second, producing a scrubbing effect, known as **cavitation,** on the surface of items immersed in the liquid. Particles that have been agitated from the instruments are suspended in solution and are subjected to negative pressure or suction. As a result, proteins are coagulated, the cell walls are disrupted, and microorganisms are destroyed.

The typical processing time of instruments in the ultrasonic machine is 3 to 6 minutes. Based on the manufacturer's recommendation, the temperature of the solution should be maintained in the range of 110°F to 130°F (43°C to 54°C). The temperature at which the chemical has greatest effect varies with the enzyme used. The instrument may be damaged if the enzyme is kept at too high of a temperature. Additionally, if the solution is not maintained at the correct temperature, contaminants may be heat set on the instrument, making it more difficult to clean.

After the ultrasonic cleaning is complete, the instruments are rinsed with distilled water to remove mineral deposits left behind. If tap water must be used, make sure to blot the instruments to prevent mineral deposits, or scale, from being deposited. At this point, application of an instrument lubricant to prolong the life of the instruments and help prevent rust and corrosion is appropriate. Many different types of instrument lubricants are available. Some are used as a bath for soaking the instruments; other lubricants are sprayed on opened instruments spread out on a lint-free towel, then left to air-dry. Regardless of the type used, it is important to use only fresh, clean lubricant and to follow the manufacturer's directions. Lubricants can penetrate into difficult-to-reach areas such as box locks and leave a lubricating, microscopic film on the instrument. Most lubricants are steam permeable and do not interfere with the sterilization process. The instruments are now ready for wrapping.

PACK WRAPPING

Recipes

Typically, each instrument pack has a **recipe,** which details pertinent pack information that is kept in a procedure manual. The recipe should include the names of all the instruments contained in each pack and the quantity of each type of instrument required to complete the pack. Additionally, the recipe should include the types and quantity of supplies that are necessary for pack completion, such as the number of gauze squares, or size of drape, if any are included. It should contain a photo or illustration of each instrument and should specify whether linen or paper material should be used to wrap the pack. The procedure manual should also include the manufacturer's guidelines for any instrument in the pack that requires special handling and maintenance, any warranty that may be

cause a particular chemical reaction. Enzymes assist in the breakdown of biologic contaminants and are generally formulated with a surfactant to improve their penetration into dried contaminants. Enzymes work most effectively when kept in water at a temperature recommended by the manufacturer. If the temperature is too high or too low, the enzymes may be inactivated. Some ultrasonic cleaners have a variable temperature control; adjust the temperature setting on the ultrasonic cleaner as recommended by the enzymatic cleaner manufacturer's instructions as needed to ensure effective cleaning of instruments. Enzymes can clean without mechanical action and are therefore used to clean instruments with lumens, such as endoscopes, as well.

appropriate for items in the pack, and the manufacturer's telephone number.

Wrapping Material

Wraps used for sterilizing instruments are usually made of cotton or linen textiles or paper. These materials are able to sustain the heat and moisture of steam sterilization. For technicians working in a small animal facility that relies on steam sterilization for in-house procedures, the choice is usually linen or paper. The ideal wrap should have the following qualities:

Selective permeability: Steam or gas must be able to penetrate the wrapping for sterilization to occur and must be easily exhausted from the pack once the sterilization process is completed. Microbes and dust particles must not be able to penetrate from the outer surface of the wrap to the inner surface.

Resistance: The material should be resistant to damage when handled. Rips, punctures, or worn areas should be readily visible to help ensure that contaminated packs will not be used.

Flexibility: The material should be able to conform to the shape of the pack.

Memory: After the pack has been opened, the wrapping material should return to the original flat position. This feature helps prevent accidental contamination of the pack contents.

Textile wraps traditionally are cotton with a thread count of 140 to 288 threads per square inch. Textile wraps must be laundered separately from nonsurgical laundry, dried, and inspected for any damage before reuse as instrument pack wraps. The advantage of using textile wraps is that they are more resistant to rips and punctures than paper and generally have a higher degree of flexibility and memory. Cotton is the best option for textile wrappers. Synthetic wrap may contribute to static electricity in the operating room. Gray, light tones of green, and medium tones of blue are often preferred because they result in less eyestrain over time than white. Fabric should be selected by thread count, not by its weight or texture.

Disadvantages of textile wraps are that they must be laundered after each use, and personnel may be reluctant to discard textile wraps that have become torn or ripped and may attempt to mend them because of the costs associated with replacement. Continued use of damaged textile wrap is not recommended because each stitch in the wrap creates a passage for microbes. If heat-sealed patches are used, steam cannot penetrate the patches during sterilization as easily as it penetrates the body of the wrap.

There are many types of paper wraps, but crepe paper is preferred over the non-crepe papers. Crepe paper should not be reused because continuous autoclaving can destroy the integrity of the paper fiber. Packs are usually wrapped with two layers of fabric or paper wraps.

A sterilization indicator strip should be placed in the middle of the pack, typically on top of the instruments, and under the gauze or drape packets. This strip will change colors once the correct temperature and pressure are reached inside the middle of the pack. Packs can be wrapped with one wrap (single-wrapped) or with two wraps (double-wrapped). If a pack is double-wrapped, only the outer layer is sealed with steam indicator tape. Generally, when a pack is double-wrapped, the circulating technician unwraps the outer layer and the scrubbed-in assistant unwraps the inner layer. If inadvertent contamination occurs when the outer layer (circulating technician accidentally touches the outer surface of inner wrap) is unwrapped, a double-wrapped pack has the advantage of an additional layer of material protecting the instruments. The circulating technician may then open the interior layer, and as long as contamination does not occur, the surgeon can still use the pack. The disadvantage of double-wrapping is the additional cost of the material used to wrap the pack.

Sealing of the Pack

Steam indicator tape is recommended when securing the wrapping material in place. Pretreated strips on the steam indicator tape change color from a pale yellow to black when the pack has been autoclaved. This indicates that conditions were met for sterilization.

When securing a wrapped pack, personnel may attempt to use ordinary masking tape instead of indicator tape. This is not advisable because the adhesive on masking tape will not adhere adequately during steam sterilization nor will it indicate that appropriate sterilization has occurred.

Once the instrument recipe has been followed, the indicator strip included, and the two wraps applied, the pack needs to be identified. Usually this is done by labeling the indicator tape on the outside of the pack with the name/initials of the person who prepared it, the date it was sterilized, and the type of pack that is contained within (Fig. 14.8). An indelible marker is preferred, as it won't be damaged by the heat and steam of the autoclave.

The following guidelines should be followed in the preparation of packs:

1. All items to be sterilized must be clean and in good condition.
2. The wrap material used must be durable enough for the sterilization process.

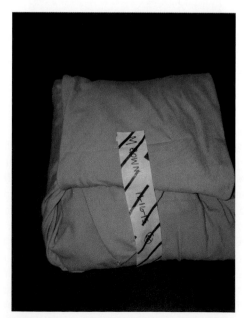

Fig. 14.8 Sterilized pack with labeling information. Black strips along the indicator tape show that this pack has been autoclaved.

3. Contents of frequently used packs should be standardized so that the same pack can be used for the same surgical procedure from session to session (e.g., spay pack).

4. Pack size must be compatible for the size of the autoclave chamber.

5. Soft items such as towels and drapes should be folded using the accordion pleat technique (Fig. 14.9). Items that have been folded in this manner can be lifted by one corner and allowed to fall open. No elaborate unfolding or shaking is necessary, reducing the potential for air currents that may circulate microbes.

6. All packs should be wrapped using the same method so that they can be unwrapped in the same way. One common method uses angled wrapping (Fig. 14.10).

7. A sterilization indicator strip should be placed in the middle of the pack to verify that appropriate conditions were met for sterilization.

8. The outer wrap should be sealed with indicator tape to indicate the pack has been autoclaved and unopened (Fig. 14.11).

Each step of this process is critical in providing sterile instruments; that is, each method used in these steps fulfills a particular function that cannot be omitted. Box 14.2 provides directions on how to wrap a surgical gown and towel pack.

Expiration Dating

Debate surrounds the issue of how long an item can be stored and can still be considered sterile. Shelf-life expiration and event-related expiration are the two types of dating for sterilized items. **Shelf-life expiration** includes a predetermined date that identifies how long an item should be considered sterile (Table 14.2).

In contrast, **event-related expiration** is determined from an environmental perspective. A pack is deemed sterile until an "event" occurs. If damaged in any way, the pack would be considered nonsterile. Excessive handling of the pack, causing it to fall onto the floor, or accumulation of dust on the pack would lead personnel to question whether the pack is still sterile. Even under these conditions, packs have been found to be sterile after 50 weeks. However, whenever a pack's sterility is in question, it must be assumed that the pack is contaminated. Products that break down or alter over time, such as latex tubing, require expiration dating.

A study on small metal instruments found that autoclaved packages in double-wrapped linen or plastic/paper combinations can be safely stored for at least 96 weeks (2 years). The study stored the instruments in open shelves, about 30 cm above the floor. Some hospitals continue to date every sterilized

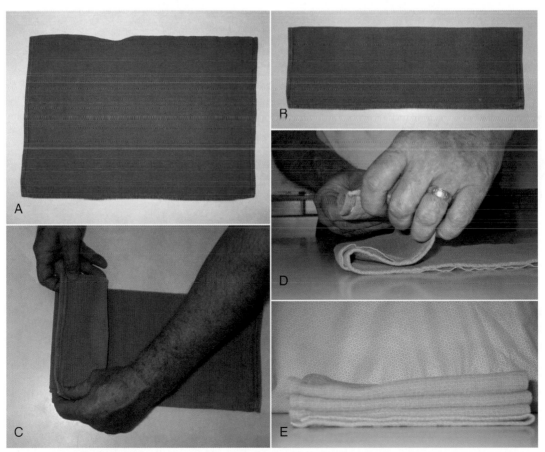

Fig. 14.9 Steps in accordion pleat folding of a hand or field towel. A, Spread towel flat on table. B, Fold towel in half lengthwise. C, Make first fold of accordion. D, Lateral view of first accordion fold. E, Completed accordion folding.

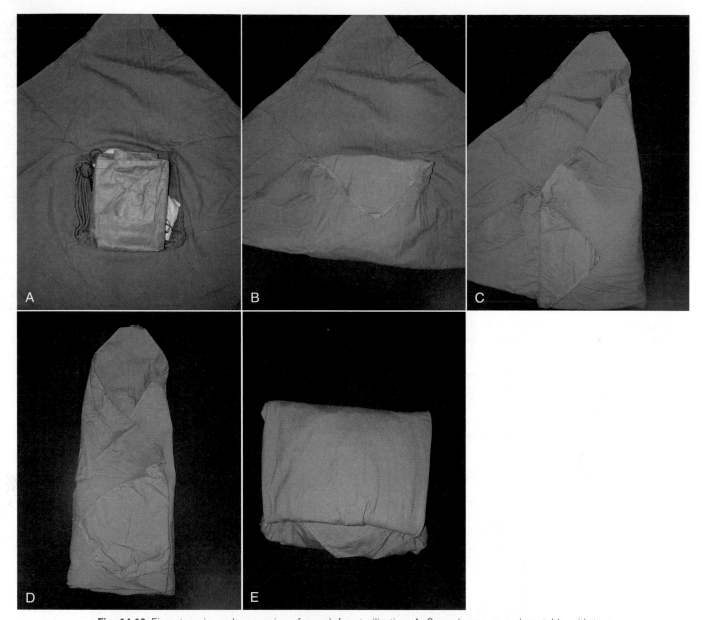

Fig. 14.10 Five steps in angle wrapping of a pack for sterilization. A, Spread wrap on a clean table with tray centered in the middle of the wrap. B, Bring bottom flap on top of tray, and fold back the corner to create a tab. C, Bring first side flap to center, and fold back the corner to create another tab. D, Bring second side flap to center, and fold back the corner to create another tab. E, Make final fold of pack wrap, and tuck under other flaps, leaving a short tab untucked to allow for easier unwrapping of the pack when opened for surgery.

product and use the time-related shelf-life practice. Many hospitals have switched to an event-related shelf-life practice. The event-related practice recognizes that the product should remain sterile until some event causes the item to become contaminated (e.g., tear in packaging, packaging becomes wet, seal is broken). Event-related factors that contribute to the contamination of a product include the amount of contamination in the environment, air movement, traffic through and around the room, location, humidity, insects, vermin, flooding, storage area space, open versus closed shelving, environmental temperature, and the properties of the wrap material. Contamination of a sterile package is event-related,

and the probability of contamination increases with increased handling.

STERILIZATION

The last step in the cleaning process after presoaking/precleaning, decontamination, and wrapping is sterilization. Sterilization is defined as the use of a process to rid an object of all living microbes. Two types of sterilizers (autoclaves) are typically used in small animal practices: gravity air-displacement autoclaves and high-vacuum sterilizers (also known as prevacuum sterilizers). Both types use steam under pressure to kill

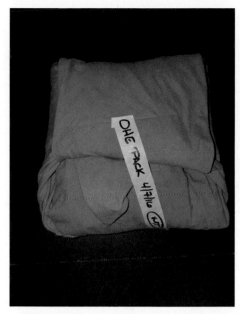

Fig. 14.11 Wrapped and taped pack, ready for sterilization. Yellow strips on the indicator tape used to seal this pack have not yet changed to black, indicating that this pack has not yet been autoclaved.

BOX 14.2 Wrapping Gowns and Hand Towels

Gowns
1. Place a clean gown flat on a surface with the outer surface facing up.
2. Straighten out the sleeves and cuffs.
3. Fold the near edge of the gown to the center.
4. Fold the far edge of the gown toward the center to meet the near edge.
5. Fold the gown in half lengthwise.
6. Fold the gown lengthwise in accordion fashion into thirds.
7. Ensure that neck ties are easily accessible on the uppermost surface of the gown.

Hand Towels
1. Place a clean hand towel flat on a clean surface.
2. Use the accordion pleat technique to fold the towel on its long axis.
3. Fold the towel in accordion fashion into thirds or quarters.
4. Fold back a corner tab

Gowns and Towels Together
1. Flatten out a clean outer wrap on a clean surface (single-layer wrap).
2. Place the folded gown in the center.
3. Place the folded hand towel on top of the gown.
4. Place an indicator strip inside the towel.
5. Wrap in same fashion as an instrument pack.*
6. Seal with tape, label "gown pack," note gown's size and the date, and initial.

*Most instrument packs are wrapped in two layers (double-wrapped). Gown packs typically are wrapped with one layer (single-wrapped).

microorganisms. Some autoclaves are capable of performing both methods of sterilization. With both types of sterilizers, proper sterilization depends on the following three factors:
- Proper operation of the sterilizer
- Proper preparation of the packs
- Proper loading of the sterilizer

TABLE 14.2 Safe Storage Times for Sterile Packs

Wrapper	Closed Cabinet	Open Cabinet
Single-wrapped muslin	1 week	2 days
Double-wrapped muslin	7 weeks	3 weeks
Single-wrapped crepe paper	At least 8 weeks	3 weeks
Single-wrapped muslin sealed in 3-mL polyethylene		At least 9 months
Heat-sealed paper and transparent plastic pouches		At least 1 year

From Bassert JM, Thomas JA, editors: McCurnin's clinical textbook for veterinary technicians, ed 9, St Louis, 2018, Elsevier.

Gravity Air-Displacement Sterilizer

The **gravity air-displacement** sterilizer found in most small animal hospitals is typically a tabletop-sized autoclave (Fig. 14.12). Distilled water is placed in the bottom of the sterilizer and then heated electrically. As the water turns to steam, the steam forces air out of the sterilizer through a port. Once the air is out of the sterilizer, the steam pressure builds up until the operating temperature is reached. Once the cycle has been completed, the steam is removed and condenses back to water.

Several settings can be used in gravity air-displacement sterilization. The temperature range is 250°F to 270°F (121°C to 132°C), and pressure range is 15 to 27 pounds per square inch (psi). The cycle runs approximately 15 minutes to achieve the proper temperature and sterilizes in 3 to 15 minutes depending on the item (250°F [121°C], 15 psi for 13 minutes). At the completion of the cycle, the machine can be vented automatically, or the door should be cracked open for approximately 15 minutes to allow any moisture to evaporate and prevent condensation on the pack. Some autoclaves will have a dry cycle that can be set to prevent condensation on the pack.

High-Vacuum Sterilizer

High-vacuum sterilizers are most commonly found in busy referral/specialty hospitals and teaching hospitals. They require additional plumbing and specialized installation. Proper operation of a high-vacuum gravity air-displacement sterilizer includes setting the sterilizer between 250°F and 272°F (121.1°C and 133.3°C) for 4 minutes at 32 psi (Fig. 14.13). The sterilizer should run through (1) a conditioning phase for about 17 minutes, (2) a sterilization phase for 4 minutes, (3) a high-vacuum exhaust for about 4 minutes, and (4) a drying cycle for about 20 minutes. The total sterilization process should take about 45 minutes. To ensure proper settings for specific types of packs (e.g., instruments, soft items), the user should consult the manufacturer's operating manual.

The main difference between gravity air-displacement and high-vacuum sterilizers is that the high-vacuum sterilizer forces steam into the sterilizing chamber, which causes steam to penetrate the pack more quickly. Additionally, after the sterilization cycle has been completed, the steam is vacuumed out of the chamber. This pulls the steam out of the pack to prevent condensation in or on the pack. This avoids a wet pack, which could compromise the pack's sterility.

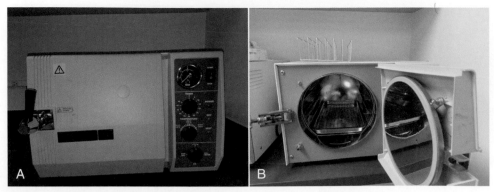

Fig. 14.12 A, Tabletop gravity air-displacement sterilizer, with door closed. B, Same autoclave, with door opened.

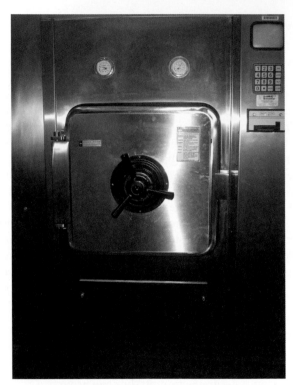

Fig. 14.13 High-vacuum sterilizer.

Preparation and Loading

Proper pack preparation should be done in an area reserved for this purpose. For many small animal practices, however, this is not always possible. An acceptable alternative is to combine both the pack preparation area and the area used for preparation of operating room personnel. Traffic to and from this area should be minimized, and routine cleaning procedures should be in place to reduce the microbial load in the area as much as possible.

Proper loading of the autoclave is a critical step in the sterilization process. The chamber of the sterilizer must not be overloaded. The outer wraps of the packs should not touch the inner surface of the chamber. Steam will not be able to penetrate the packs effectively if they are crammed too tightly into the chamber. The goal is not to see how much can be fit in the machine but to ensure adequate sterility of the items.

Flash Sterilization

Flash sterilization is an abbreviated version of a regular sterilization cycle. Instruments sterilized by this method are not wrapped and are usually sterilized one or two instruments at a time. Special flash sterilization autoclaves are available, or the autoclaves just discussed can also be used to flash sterilize individual, unwrapped instruments. The autoclave settings should be 272°F (133°C), for 2 to 3 minutes. The conditioning phase is approximately 10 minutes, with a 4-minute sterilization phase. This is followed by a gravity exhaust of approximately 1 minute, then a 1-minute dry cycle. The dry cycle is shortened because no linen or paper is present for the steam to penetrate.

Typically, this process is used for individual instruments that have been dropped during surgery. Flash sterilization should not take the place of regular steam sterilization. Care must be exercised when flash sterilizing, as patients and staff can be burned from instruments sterilized in this manner that are not allowed to cool sufficiently before use.

Ethylene Oxide (Gas) Sterilization

Another form of sterilization uses ethylene oxide (EtO), a colorless gas at room temperature. EtO is a toxin that can cause skin and mucous membrane irritation, however, and it is therefore considered a health hazard.

EtO penetrates paper and plastic film packaging without melting these materials. EtO destroys metabolic pathways in the cells and is capable of killing all microorganisms. Effective sterilization with EtO depends on the concentration of gas, exposure time, temperature, and relative humidity. Moisture is necessary for the lethal action of EtO, and optimal relative humidity for this type of sterilization is 40%. Exposure time varies from 48 minutes to several hours, but 3 to 4 hours of exposure is typically used for sterilizing at room temperature. After EtO sterilization, materials should be quarantined in a well-ventilated area for a minimum of 24 hours. The aeration time can be reduced to 4 hours with the use of aerators that vent the gas outside the work environment (Fig. 14.14). The Occupational Health and Safety Administration does require special training for all personnel exposed to or using EtO sterilization methods.

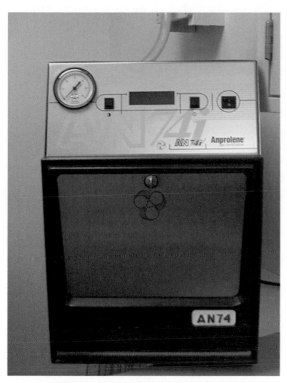

Fig. 14.14 Ethylene oxide sterilizer.

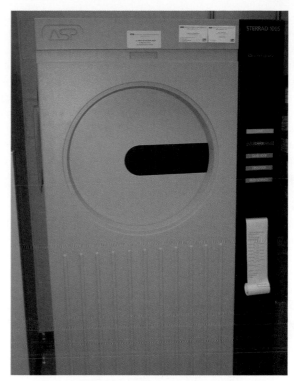

Fig. 14.15 Plasma sterilizer.

Plasma Sterilization

The three most common states of matter are solid, liquid, and gas. The fourth, plasma, often occurs in nature, as lightning and the aurora borealis (northern lights). The plasma state of matter is produced through the action of a strong electric or magnetic field.

Low-temperature plasma sterilization with hydrogen peroxide (H_2O_2) gas is produced when the gas is stimulated under a deep vacuum with radiofrequency (RF) or microwave energy. The plasma system uses H_2O_2 to form the reactive components to kill microorganisms. After a liquid solution of H_2O_2 is vaporized in a chamber, RF energy is applied to create an electric field that then creates low-temperature gas plasma (Fig.14.15). Within the plasma, H_2O_2 is broken into reactive components, including hydroperoxyl-free and hydroxyl-free radicals. These radicals interact with cell membranes, killing the microorganisms in the process. After the components lose their energy, they recombine to form harmless by-products of oxygen and water. The process operates in the range of 98.6°F to 111°F (37°C to 44°C) with a cycle time of 75 minutes. If any moisture is present on the objects being sterilized, the vacuum will not be achieved, and the cycle will abort.

One limitation to gas plasma sterilization is that it cannot penetrate the walls of an instrument with a lumen, and thus the area within the lumen is not sterilized.

Sterilization Indicators

Chemical and biological indicators help determine whether items have been properly sterilized. Chemical indicators come in the form of strips or tape. Strips are placed inside the pack next to the instruments or inside the towel of the surgical gown pack, whereas the tape is placed on the outside of the pack. The strips and tape change color if the conditions for sterilization have been met. This does not mean that the instruments or surgical gown are sterile, but only that the conditions were met for sterilization to have occurred.

Biological indicators, on the other hand, demonstrate that the sterilizer has met all the sterilization parameters. A vial of *Bacillus stearothermophilus* is typically placed in the sterilizer with the first load to be sterilized for the day. At the end of the sterilization cycle, the vial is removed and placed in an incubator for 24 hours and checked for microbial colony growth. The vial should demonstrate that all the microorganisms have been killed, providing reassurance that the sterilizer worked appropriately at that time.

SPECIALTY INSTRUMENT CLEANING

High-Level Disinfection

Cold sterilization is more of a high-level disinfection (see later discussion) process than a true sterilization process. Cold sterilization is defined as the practice of immersing items in a disinfectant solution to reduce the level of contamination. Some instruments are cold-sterilized because they will not withstand repeated exposure to high-temperature steam sterilization.

Alcohol, when used properly, exhibits strong bactericidal properties because of its ability to coagulate protein. Ethanol and isopropanol can be effective in a wide variety of applications. If used properly, alcohol solutions are effective against vegetative bacterial cells, including the bacterium that causes tuberculosis. However, alcohol cannot be relied on to kill bacterial spores or viruses and therefore should be used with caution.

Glutaraldehyde solution is considered a high-level disinfectant but not a sterilizing agent (Fig. 14.16). Glutaraldehyde is bactericidal, tuberculocidal, and viricidal with an exposure time as short as 10 minutes. If exposure time is increased to several hours, the action is considered sporicidal. Prolonged exposure may adversely affect items made of rubber and plastic. Because it is so effective in killing germs, it can also be harmful to other living organisms, including the patient and staff members.

Drill Cleaning

Power drills are commonly used in orthopedic surgery. Drills are not to be submerged in water or ultrasonically cleaned. Disposable components, such as bits, burrs and saw blades, should be removed and discarded at the point of use (e.g. surgical suite). Single-use items should not be reused! The equipment should be disassembled and inspected for any tissue or blood debris. If there is dried debris on the instrument, a foam disinfectant cleaner or dampened cloth can be used on the drill. The foam is allowed to loosen the debris so that it can be removed with a clean, lint-free towel. The drill should then be wiped with a clean, lint-free cloth moistened with isopropyl alcohol. Generally, power drills are wrapped and autoclaved according to the manufacturer's instructions in preparation for their use in orthopedic surgery. Often this involves doubling the standard sterilization time used for soft tissue instrument packs. The drill's battery must be removed before sterilization and either sterilized separately using EtO sterilization or kept unsterile pending the manufacturer's recommendations. Some pieces of equipment come with a container specifically designed for the device and its components; if this is not provided, a generic mesh tray can be used to protect the delicate components and to ensure all pieces are kept together.

Laparoscopic Instrument Cleaning

Laparoscopic equipment is expensive and should be handled gently according to the manufacturer's recommendations. The scope and fiber optic light cables can be easily damaged. These items can be cleaned with gauze and alcohol after each procedure and stored in their cases. The scope and light cable can then be gas-sterilized (**ethylene oxide**) or cold-sterilized (also known as high-level disinfection) before the procedure. Acceptable cold sterilization consists of the use of 2% glutaraldehyde (Cidex; CIVCO Medical Solutions, Kalona, IA).

A common alkylating agent approved by the U.S. Food and Drug administration (FDA) is 0.55% ortho-phthalaldehyde (Cidex OPA; CIVCO). It has a strong mycobactericidal activity level, strong stability over a wide pH range of 3 to 9, and requires no activation. Pentax and Olympus (two companies that manufacture laparoscopes) list Cidex OPA as a disinfectant compatible with flexible and rigid endoscopes for manual cleaning. Cidex states that 12-minute soaks are required to destroy all pathogenic organisms, but guidelines change and the manufacturer's instructions should be checked periodically. Gloves and eye protection should be worn to handle Cidex OPA because it is a potential respiratory and dermal irritant. Cidex OPA should be used in a well-ventilated area. The technician should always refer to the manufacturer's detailed warnings and recommendations in the packet insert for further information. Once the instruments have been sterilized in Cidex OPA, they should be rinsed thoroughly with sterile saline before entering the abdominal cavity. Laparoscopes and light cables should never be autoclaved unless the manufacturer states that they are autoclave safe.

Endoscope Instrument Cleaning

Properly maintaining endoscopes and their accessory instruments is extremely important. Failure to adequately clean and disinfect endoscopes and their accessory instruments could lead to iatrogenic transmission of infection between patients.

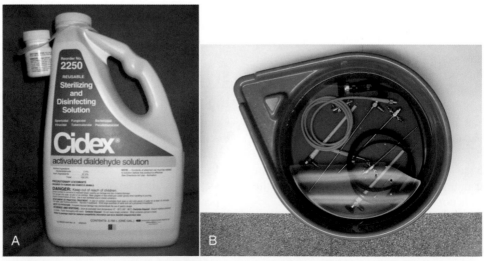

Fig. 14.16 A, Example of glutaraldehyde solution used for high-level disinfection. B, Instruments soaking in high-level disinfectant.

There are a variety of methods for cleaning and disinfecting endoscopes and instruments. Referring to the manufacturer's recommendations helps establish the cleaning protocol. This section covers the author's preferred method for cleaning and disinfecting endoscopic equipment.

Every patient should be considered a potential source of infection, and all endoscopes should be decontaminated following every endoscopic procedure. Endoscopes should be cleaned and disinfected immediately after the completion of any procedure. If this is not possible, abundant amounts of clean distilled water should be suctioned to remove as much gross debris as possible from the interior channel of the scope. This practice prevents the adherence of large pieces of organic material to the channels and allows for easier cleaning once time permits.

To maximize the effect of the water moving through the suction channel, (1) the insertion tube is placed in a bowl of water, (2) the suction button is depressed for approximately 5 seconds while aspirating up the water, and (3) the suction button is released, breaking the suction and causing the water to jump or swish back and forth in the channel (like water being agitated in a washing machine). Afterward, the outer sheath should be gently wiped down with wet gauze sponges to remove gross debris.

Endoscopes should be inspected for damage before being submerged in solutions that may damage parts not designed for exposure. A leak test should be performed to ensure that the internal and external parts of the endoscope did not incur damage during a procedure.

Because of the gastrointestinal endoscope's delicate design, holes and tears of the inner lumen of the scope make it possible for water and other debris to contact otherwise impermeable areas of the scope. If the endoscope fails the leak test, it should not be submerged or used, and the manufacturer should be contacted immediately for inspection and repair. To perform a leak test, the technician places the appropriate soaking caps and then attaches the leak tester and uses it according to the manufacturer's instructions (Fig. 14.17). The cleaning and disinfecting protocol then can be completed.

The most important step in prevention of infection during endoscopy is manual cleaning. Organic soil (blood, feces) may contribute to the failure of disinfection by harboring embedded microbes and preventing the penetration of germicides. Also, some disinfectants are inactivated by organic material. After the endoscope has been disassembled and passed the leak test, the following channels should be cleaned with a cleaning brush: suction, air/water, and biopsy, including the detachable suction and air/water valves, the biopsy channel cover, and the whole exterior of the endoscope. This cleaning process should take place in an enzymatic cleaner designed to clean organic material by breaking down proteins and enhancing the efficacy of brushing and flushing. Endozime (Ruhof Corporation, Mineola, NY), a bacteriostatic enzymatic cleaner, is a unique formulation of protease and amylase enzymes, digesters, and buffers that can clean in 2 to 3 minutes. Allowing the endoscope to be submerged in Endozime for at least 10 minutes after precleaning is sufficient. Endozime needs to be diluted, and as with any enzymatic solution, dilution protocols specified by the manufacturer should be followed.

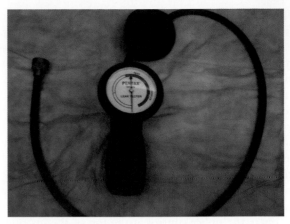

Fig. 14.17 Leak testers are manufacturer specific. This Pentax leak tester is compatible with all Pentax endoscopes. (Courtesy MJK-VHUP, Philadelphia.)

After the appropriate time has elapsed with the endoscope submerged in the enzymatic cleaner, the exterior should be rinsed off with distilled water, including the appropriate channels that do not need soaking caps, and then purged with air before being exposed to the disinfectant. The endoscope should be purged with distilled water, followed by air, before disinfection. This helps prevent contamination of the disinfectant with the enzymatic solution and dilution of the disinfectant itself.

High-level disinfection (HLD) is recommended for endoscopes because they cannot withstand available sterilization methods. HLD is a cleaning process that kills all microorganisms except large numbers of bacterial spores. Because they are not rendered sterile, endoscopes cleaned using HLD are considered semicritical items. These endoscopes may contact broken skin or mucous membranes, which are usually resistant to common spores, but they should not contact vascular or other sterile body tissue. The FDA-approved alkylating agent Cidex OPA is often used, as discussed earlier for laparoscopes. Submerging an endoscope in Cidex OPA for 40 minutes is sufficient, and it should not be submerged for longer than 60 minutes. After it is removed from Cidex OPA, the interior and exterior portions of the endoscope should be thoroughly rinsed and flushed with sterile or filtered water. If tap water is used for rinsing, 70% alcohol should be the final rinse, because tap water may contain microbes (e.g., *Pseudomonas, Mycobacterium*). The endoscope can then be purged with air and allowed to hang to dry either on a wall mount or in a well-ventilated storage cabinet.

As with the endoscope, failure to adequately clean the biopsy and retrieval instruments can spread disease. With inadequate cleaning, instruments also may not open or may break when opened. Not only should instruments be precleaned with distilled water followed by an enzymatic cleaner with a brush, but detachable parts (e.g., valves, biopsy channel covers) should be cleaned as well. The same cleaning protocol used on the endoscope can be used on the biopsy instruments. Cleaning brushes are usually disposable, but if they are thoroughly cleaned by HLD, they can be reused. Water bottles and tubes used for endoscopic irrigation are difficult to clean and disinfect, so sterile water should be used rather than tap water.

NOTE: Reported iatrogenic infections from endoscopes not thoroughly disinfected include *Escherichia coli, Pseudomonas, Klebsiella, Serratia,* and *Salmonella.* Other organisms of concern in gastroenterology settings include *Campylobacter, Clostridium difficile,* and *Helicobacter pylori,* as well as many viral pathogens.

Biopsy forceps cups tend to lock in the position in which they dry after cleaning, which will require releasing any tension before use. If locked in a closed position, cups can be soaked in warm water or mineral oil for several seconds and then gently separated with a small-gauge needle. Once the biopsy forceps cup is open, the finger control at the top of the instrument is used to open and close the cup several times to ensure free movement. If locked in an open position, cups can be soaked for several seconds in warm water, and then gentle digital pressure can be applied to the cups to work them closed. The finger control is used to ensure that the cups are moving freely.

ROTATING AND RESTOCKING SUPPLIES

Supplies in the surgery room should be limited to an amount that would be used over a short time. Necessary supplies in the surgery room vary greatly among veterinary facilities, depending on the number and types of procedures performed and what is needed for each one. Supplies should not be stocked in excess because increased inventory can tie up the facility's money unnecessarily. The veterinary technician plays a vital role in communicating with the veterinarians on staff about their needs for the surgery area. The veterinary technician is often the person who restocks and organizes the room and frequently practices inventory controls such as ordering. It is important to keep lines of communication open and to closely monitor the supplies used in the room. Supplies can be broken down into two categories: disposable and reusable.

Disposable Supplies

Disposable supplies consist of the supplies purchased for single-time use, such as scalpel blades, suture material, and surgical gloves. These items are purchased as sterile items and usually are labeled with a date specifying when they should be "used by" or when they are considered "outdated." These items need to be checked and rotated each time the surgery area is stocked. Items with expiration dates that are shortest (or closest) should be rotated so that they are used before items with longer (further) dates. If too much stock of one item is kept in the area, the potential for outdating increases. For this reason, keep only a minimum of what is needed in a day. This practice keeps the stock rotated, and the potential for outdated items decreases.

Reusable Supplies

Reusable supplies are the items that the veterinary facility uses and resterilizes between patients. These items consist of surgery packs, clean and laundered reusable cloth drapes, hand towels, and individual instruments. These items are often cleaned after surgery, repackaged, sterilized, and placed back in the storage cabinets of the surgery room. For reusable supplies, as with disposable items, the oldest packs should be placed so that they are used first and the stock is continually rotated. If the veterinary facility has more than one spay pack, it is important to rotate the packs so that they do not fall out of the rotation.

Current practice in human medicine is that packs do not automatically become outdated after a certain number of days. An event must occur to cause the item to become nonsterile. An "event" is something that occurs to cause a breach of the item's sterility. Examples of events are opening of the pack, the pack's coming in contact with moisture, and the pack's being dropped on the floor.

Many veterinary facilities still operate on the assumption that an item is outdated after a certain arbitrary period, such as 30 days. For items sterilized in a veterinary facility, is it necessary to keep everything wrapped and sterilized, just in case it might be needed? It would be a better practice for the facility to sterilize only the items that will be needed in the next few days or weeks. Although the veterinary profession is not always predictable and emergencies do occur, not all the spay packs need to be sterile unless multiple spays are scheduled for the next day. This practice would save on storage of sterile items in the surgery room and facilitate a more organized rotation of supplies.

The veterinary profession has few legal guidelines in surgery room cleanliness and supply rotation in comparison with the human medical profession, but this does not mean these areas can be ignored. For the well-being of the patients and the financial well-being of the veterinary facility, it is important that veterinary technicians take a proactive role in establishing protocols for cleanliness, stock rotation, and sterilization of surgical items. A breakdown in any of these areas can be costly for the veterinary facility. By being organized, efficient, and detail-oriented, the veterinary technician can serve the best interests of the patient, the client, and the veterinary facility.

▮ KEY POINTS

1. Surgery rooms should be spot-cleaned after each procedure.
2. Surgery rooms should be terminally cleaned at the end of each day.
3. Mechanical friction should be applied during cleaning.
4. Disinfectants should be used according to the manufacturer's instructions.
5. There is no "ideal disinfectant," but there are many good disinfectants that meet most of the criteria of an ideal disinfectant.
6. The effectiveness of a disinfectant depends on many factors (e.g., microorganisms, contamination, and organic matter).
7. The stock of disposable surgical supplies should be limited so that expiration does not occur.

8. Reusable supplies are items that are cleaned and resterilized.

9. All surgical supplies should be rotated so that the items are used in a rotating order (oldest first).

10. In event-related contamination, an event must occur to cause an item to become nonsterile (contaminated).

11. Appropriate cleaning procedures begin with a thorough presoaking of instruments to rid the items of any blood or tissue.

12. Decontamination of instruments is vital in removing debris from the instrument's box locks and hinges.

13. Lubricants make instruments easier to open and close and aid in the prevention of the buildup of protein on the instruments.

14. Ultrasonic cleaning is a critical step in removing microbes from instruments.

15. Enzymes are used to assist in the breakdown of debris to allow more thorough ultrasonic cleaning of instruments.

16. Each instrument pack should contain a "recipe" that specifies the types of instruments, quantity of each, type of wrapping material, manufacturers' guidelines, and any warranty.

17. Pack wraps are made of linen or paper and should have selective permeability, flexibility, memory, and resistance to damage.

18. Textile wraps are selected based on thread count (140-288 threads/square inch), not weight or texture.

19. Torn wraps repaired by stitching can allow an avenue for microbes to penetrate the pack, and patches can hamper steam penetration during sterilization; torn wraps should be discarded and replaced.

20. Steam indicator tape is used in securing wraps; a black stripping effect indicates that conditions were met for sterilization.

21. Guidelines for preparing a pack for sterilization address the items' condition, wrap material, standardization of contents, compatibility with autoclave, folding of soft items, use of similar wrapping methods, placement of indicator strips, and sealing of the outer pack.

22. Expiration dating may be used for packs with items that degrade over time (e.g., latex tubing).

23. Sterilization takes place after presoaking, decontaminating, and ultrasonic cleaning. The sterilization process rids the instruments of any living microbes.

24. Sterilization depends on three factors: proper sterilizer operation, proper pack preparation, and proper loading.

25. Gravity air-displacement sterilization is typically done on a tabletop. Steam enters the chamber by gravity and is set at a lower pressure.

26. High-vacuum sterilizers force steam into the sterilizer chamber for quicker penetration.

27. If a separate area is unavailable for proper pack preparation, it can be done in the preparation area for surgical personnel.

28. Flash sterilization is used for items dropped in the surgery suite.

29. Use of ethylene oxide is an excellent means to sterilize instruments and supplies wrapped in paper and plastic, but health and environmental risk factors have decreased its use over the years.

30. Plasma sterilization offers a safe technique for sterilization, but it is not an effective means of sterilizing items with lumens.

31. Chemical and biological indicators determine whether items have been properly sterilized. Biological indicators show that the sterilizer has met all the sterilization parameters.

32. Alcohol exhibits strong bactericidal properties but may not kill spores or viruses. Glutaraldehyde is considered a high-level disinfectant and is bactericidal, tuberculocidal, and viricidal.

33. Orthopedic drills should not be immersed in liquid and should be cleaned with a foaming disinfectant and alcohol before sterilization.

34. Maintaining endoscopes involves proper cleaning and disinfection, leak testing and inspection, microbial monitoring, and storage.

REVIEW QUESTIONS

1. Cleaning equipment and agents for the surgery room should be
   a. used only in the surgery room.
   b. disinfected prior to using in the surgery room.
   c. cleaned and stored in the surgery room.
   d. used throughout the hospital to save money.

2. The Centers for Disease Control and Prevention (CDC) states elimination of microorganisms from the surgery room is best accomplished by
   a. a dilute bleach solution.
   b. physical removal by scrubbing.
   c. using the strongest disinfectant possible.
   d. preoperative antibiotics for all surgical patients.

3. How should the cleaning equipment for the surgery room be handled prior to storage at the end of the day?
   a. Disassembled, cleaned, and dried
   b. Disassembled, sterilized, and dried

   c. Disinfected and dried without disassembling
   d. Cleaned, sterilized, and dried without disassembling

4. Which disinfectants are toxic to cats?
   a. Phenol-based
   b. Chlorine-based
   c. Quaternary amine–based
   d. Chlorhexidine disinfectants

5. Which disinfectant may be inactivated by hard water?
   a. Phenol-based
   b. Chlorine-based
   c. Quaternary amine–based
   d. Chlorhexidine disinfectants

6. Presoaking of surgical instruments involves placing the soiled instrument in
   a. tap water.
   b. distilled water.

c. a commercial detergent solution.

d. distilled water mixed with a detergent.

7. What product is used in ultrasonic cleaning of instruments to reduce surface tension?

   a. Enzyme

   b. Phenols

   c. Surfactant

   d. Iodine disinfectant

8. What product is used in ultrasonic cleaning of instruments to assist in the breakdown of biologic contaminant?

   a. Enzyme

   b. Surfactant

   c. Quaternary amines

   d. Iodine disinfectant

9. Which of these items should not be used in the cleaning of surgical instruments?

   a. Enzymes

   b. Wire brush

   c. Soft bristle brush

   d. Chlorhexidine disinfectant

10. The scrubbing effect caused by ultrasonic cleaners is called

    a. cavitation.

    b. surfactant.

    c. flash sterilization.

    d. gravity airdisplacement.

11. The last step in instrument cleaning, prior to wrapping in a pack, is

    a. drying.

    b. soaking.

    c. lubrication.

    d. ultrasonic cleaning.

12. Selective permeability is the quality of a pack wrapping material that

    a. makes it resistant to damage when handled.

    b. allows the wrap to conform to the shape of the pack.

    c. allows the wrap to return to its original flat position.

    d. allows steam or gas to penetrate the wrap for sterilization to occur.

13. What information should the label of a pack include?

    a. Name/initials of preparer, sterilization date, and type of pack

    b. Clinic name, sterilization date, and type of pack

    c. Name/initials of preparer, expiration date, and type of pack

    d. Clinic name, sterilization date, and expiration date

14. The process to rid an object of all living microbes is

    a. cleaning

    b. disinfection

    c. sterilization

    d. decontamination

15. When performing ethylene oxide sterilization, how long should the sterilized instruments be aired out if an aerator is not used?

    a. 48 minutes

    b. 3 hours

    c. 4 hours

    d. 24 hours

16. What compound is used to clean a laparoscope and its fiber optic light cables?

    a. Alcohol

    b. Chlorhexidine

    c. Ethylene oxide

    d. Iodine compounds

17. Which compound is used for cold sterilization and is viricidal?

    a. Ethanol

    b. Isopropanol

    c. Ethylene oxide

    d. Glutaraldehyde

18. What type of disinfectant inhibits the growth of bacteria?

    a. Biocide

    b. Fungicide

    c. Bactericide

    d. Bacteriostat

19. Which of these is an example of a disposable surgical supply?

    a. Cloth drape

    b. Paper drape

    c. Hand towels

    d. Needle holders

20. Which disinfectant kills all microorganisms?

21. Why are most textile wraps gray, light tones of green, and medium tones of blue?

22. Where should the sterilization indicator strip be placed?

23. How are textile wraps superior to paper wraps?

24. What is an advantage of a high-vacuum sterilizers versus a gravity air-displacement sterilizer?

25. What is the recommended technique for folding towels and drapes?

BIBLIOGRAPHY

Association of Surgical Technologists (AST). *Standard of Practice for the Decontamination of Surgical Instruments.* 2009. accessed 11/6/19 http://www.ast.org/uploadedFiles/Main_Site/Content/About_Us/Standard_Decontamination_%20Surgical_Instruments_.pdf

Bassert JM, Beal AD, Samples OM, editors: *McCurnin's clinical textbook for veterinary technicians,* ed 9th, St Louis, 2018, Saunders.

Bhumisirikul W, Bhumisirikul P, Pongchairerks P. *Long-term Storage for Small Surgical Instruments in Autoclaved Packages.* In Asian Journal of Surgery Vol 26, No 4, October 2003. Accessed 11/6/19 https://core.ac.uk/download/pdf/82309919.pdf

Castro MC, Lind N. *Powered Surgical Instruments* in Instrument Continuing Education (ICE) CIS Self-Study Lesson Plan Purdue University. Accessed 11/6/19 https://www.iahcsmm.org/images/Lesson_Plans/CIS_Plans/CIS254.pdf

Centers for Disease Control and Prevention (CDC). *Environmental Infection Control Guidelines.* accessed 11/6/19 https://www.cdc.gov/infectioncontrol/guidelines/environmental/index.html

Centers for Disease Control and Prevention (CDC). *Flash Sterilization.* accessed 11/6/19 https://www.cdc.gov/hicpac/Disinfection_Sterilization/dS_includes/13_02ds_FlashSterilization.html

Centers for Disease Control and Prevention (CDC). *Guideline for Disinfection and Sterilization in Healthcare Facilities,* 2008, updated 2019. access 11/6/19 https://www.cdc.gov/infectioncontrol/pdf/guidelines/disinfection-guidelines-H.pdf

Centers for Disease Control and Prevention (CDC). *Hydrogen Peroxide Gas Plasma. Guideline for Disinfection and Sterilization in Healthcare Facilities* 2008. Accessed 11/6/19 https://www.cdc.gov/infectioncontrol/guidelines/disinfection/sterilization/hydrogen-peroxide-gas.html

Centers for Disease Control and Prevention (CDC). *Low-Temperature Sterilization Technologies.* accessed 11/6/19 https://www.cdc.gov/infectioncontrol/guidelines/disinfection/sterilization/low-temp.html

McReynolds, T. *A Practical Guide to Veterinary Hospital Design* in AAHA Publications. 10/31/18 accessed 11/6/19 https://www.aaha.org/publications/newstat/articles/2018-10/a-practical-guide-to-veterinary-hospital-design/

Muscarella LF. *The Benefits of Ultrasonic Cleaning* in Infection Control Today. May 1, 2001. Accessed 11/6/19 https://www.infectioncontroltoday.com/environmental-hygiene/benefits-ultrasonic-cleaning

Pyrek KM *Updated Environmental Cleaning RP Addresses OR Imperatives* in Infection Control Today.2014 accessed 11/7/19 https://www.infectioncontroltoday.com/environmental-hygiene/updated-environmental-cleaning-rp-addresses-or-imperatives

Schumway R, Broussard J: Maintenance of gastrointestinal endoscopes. *Clin Tech Small Anim Pract* 18:254, 2003.

Society of Gastroenterology Nurses and Associates Practice Committee. *Standards of Infection Control in Reprocessing of Flexible Gastrointestinal Endoscopes.* 2012. Accessed 11/6/19 https://www.sgna.org/Portals/0/Education/PDF/Standards-Guidelines/sgna_stand_of_infection_control_0812_FINAL.pdf

Quick Reference for Common Intravenous Infusions and Analgesic Protocols

INTRAVENOUS FLUID FLOW RATE

Occasionally it is necessary to administer intravenous (IV) fluids without an infusion pump. The following table is a quick reference that allows the veterinary technician to count the number of seconds between drops of fluid (not the number of drops per second) into the drip chamber of the administration set to estimate the hourly infusion rate, as long as the type of fluid administration set is known.

15 Drops/mL	60 Drops/mL
1 drop/sec = 240 mL/hr	1 drop/sec = 60 mL/hr
1 drop/2 sec = 120 mL/hr	1 drop/2 sec = 30 mL/hr
1 drop/3 sec = 80 mL/hr	1 drop/3 sec = 20 mL/hr
1 drop/4 sec = 60 mL/hr	1 drop/4 sec = 15 mL/hr
1 drop/5 sec = 48 mL/hr	1 drop/5 sec = 12 mL/hr
1 drop/6 sec = 40 mL/hr	1 drop/6 sec = 10 mL/hr
1 drop/7 sec = 35 mL/hr	1 drop/7 sec = 8.8 mL/hr
1 drop/8 sec = 30 mL/hr	1 drop/8 sec = 7.5 mL/hr
1 drop/9 sec = 27 mL/hr	1 drop/9 sec = 6.7 mL/hr
1 drop/10 sec = 24 mL/hr	1 drop/10 sec = 6 mL/hr

mL/hr, Milliliters per hour; *sec,* second(s).

MAINTENANCE FLUID FLOW RATE

Determining a patient's fluid flow rate is achieved with the following formula:

$$\text{Total fluids} = \text{Maintenance fluids} + \text{Replacement fluids} + \text{Ongoing losses}$$

Many formulas are available for calculating a patient's maintenance fluid requirements. However, a simple, easy-to-remember formula for estimating an animal's hourly maintenance fluid requirements is 1 mL per pound of body weight (lb BW); two times (or twice) the maintenance requirement is 2 mL/lb BW.

Body Weight (lb)	Maintenance Fluids	Twice Maintenance Fluids
1	1 mL/hr	2 mL/hr
10	10 mL/hr	20 mL/hr
20	20 mL/hr	40 mL/hr
40	40 mL/hr	80 mL/hr
80	80 mL/hr	160 mL/hr

"SPIKING THE BAG" WITH POTASSIUM CHLORIDE

- Patients undergoing fluid diuresis are at risk for hypokalemia.
- To prevent hypokalemia, the IV fluids can be "spiked," or supplemented, with potassium chloride (KCl).
- To figure out how much KCl supplementation is needed, it is necessary to know the patient's serum potassium level.
- Normal serum potassium level = 3.5 to 5.5 mEq/L.
- Failure to correct hypokalemia can result in muscle weakness, lethargy, and vomiting.
- KCl must be given in a slow drip, diluted in another fluid.

Serum Potassium Level (mEq/L)	Supplemental Potassium Chloride (per 250 mL Fluid)*
3.5–5.5 (normal)	5 mEq (20 mEq/L)
3.0–3.4	7 mEq (28 mEq/L)
2.5–2.9	10 mEq (40 mEq/L)
2.0–2.4	15 mEq (60 mEq/L)
<2.0	20 mEq (80 mEq/L)

mEq/L, Milliequivalents per liter.
*Never administer fluids supplemented with potassium chloride faster than twice the maintenance rate; with more potassium, adjust the rate even slower.

"SPIKING THE BAG" WITH DEXTROSE

- If a patient is prone to hypoglycemia, debilitated, septic, or anorectic, a dextrose supplement may be required.
- If the blood glucose (BG) is less than 40 mg/dL, dextrose should be added to fluids to make a 2.5% dextrose solution.
- If BG continues to remain at or below 40 mg/dL, the solution should be increased to a 5% dextrose solution.

Size of Fluid Bag*	To Make 2.5% Dextrose Solution	To Make 5% Dextrose Solution
250 mL	Add 12.5 mL of 50% dextrose	Add 25 mL of 50% dextrose
500 mL	Add 25 mL of 50% dextrose	Add 50 mL of 50% dextrose
1000 mL	Add 50 mL of 50% dextrose	Add 100 mL of 50% dextrose

*Before adding dextrose to fluid bag, withdraw an amount of fluid from bag equal to the amount of dextrose to be added.

HEPARINIZED SALINE ("HEP-SALINE," "FLUSH")

Size of Fluid Bag of 0.9% Sodium Chloride (NaCl)	Amount of Heparin (1000 Units/mL) to Add
250 mL	1.25 mL (1250 units)
500 mL	2.5 mL (2500 units)
1 L	5 mL (5000 units)

SAMPLE CALCULATIONS FOR CONSTANT-RATE INFUSION OF ANALGESICS

Constant pain requires a constant-rate infusion (CRI) of analgesics. The following sample calculations show how to determine the number of milliliters (mL) of the different analgesics to add to different sizes of fluid bags to deliver a CRI of analgesics through an intravenous (IV) drip.

Overview

1. Give an initial loading dose as a bolus to the desired effect.
2. Begin a CRI of one of the analgesics discussed below either in a syringe pump or as an IV drip.
3. Monitor for signs of inadequate pain control, and evaluate the following behavioral categories hourly while the patient is receiving CRI:
   a. Posture:
      - Painful signs: hunched back, tense muscles, anxious facial expression, withdrawn, cowering.
      - Managed pain: grooming, sleeping in normal posture.
   b. Vocalization:
      - Painful signs: whining, whimpering, growling, distressful yowling.
      - Managed pain: quiet, purring.
   c. Mobility:
      - Painful signs: unable to lie quietly (restless) or unwilling/reluctant to get up or move.
      - Managed pain: gets up, sits, lies down, walks willingly.
   d. Response to touch (specifically, palpation of wound if present):
      - Painful signs: trembling, guarding wound, baring teeth.
      - Managed pain: affectionate, relaxed.
4. Evaluate the following physiologic parameters hourly while the patient is receiving CRI:
   - Temperature, pulse, respiration.
   - Mucous membrane color and capillary refill time.
   - Blood pressure.
5. Titrate delivery rate accordingly (increase if painful).
   or
   If pain is unrelenting, a combination CRI of morphine, lidocaine, and ketamine may be needed.
6. Monitor for signs of excessive dosing:
   - Dysphoria.
   - Central nervous system (CNS) depression.
7. Titrate delivery rate accordingly (decrease or discontinue).
   or
   Consider an opioid antagonist if an opioid was administered.

Fentanyl CRI
Loading Dose
- Canine: 2 to 5 µg per kilogram body weight (µg/kg) IV
- Feline: 1 to 2 µg/kg IV
- Give to effect.

Constant-Rate Infusion

For this example, the patient is a 10-pound (10 lb) domestic short-hair cat.

1. Determine the hourly flow rate of IV fluids for the patient:
   - For this example, maintenance fluid flow rate is used as the hourly rate, as calculated by the following formula: 1 mL/pound (lb)/hour (hr):

   $$10\,lb \times (1\,mL/lb/hr) = 10\,mL/hr$$

   $$Hourly\ IV\ fluid\ flow\ rate = 10\,mL/hr$$

2. Determine the hourly analgesic dose rate:
   - Fentanyl CRI dose range, the units are micrograms (µg) for cats: **5 to 20 µg/kg/hr**.
   - *NOTE:* The low end of the given dose range is appropriate for postoperative, awake analgesia. The high end of the given dose range is more appropriate for intraoperative analgesia when very little inhaled anesthesia is desired.
   - Convert lb to kg: 10 lb × (1 kg/2.2 lb) = 4.5 kg.
   - Calculate the lower and upper limits of the dose range:

   $$4.5\,kg \times (5\,\mu g/kg) = 23\,\mu g$$

   $$4.5\,kg \times (20\,\mu g/kg) = 90\,\mu g$$

   $$Range = 23\ to\ 90\,\mu g\,/\,hr$$

   - Select a dose in the calculated range based on the patient's level of pain and purpose of analgesia (awake vs. intraoperative). For this example, select **23 µg/hr**.
3. Determine how many units of analgesic per mL of IV fluids:
   - In this case, using fentanyl, the units are micrograms (µg).
   - Use the hourly IV fluid flow rate determined in step 1 in the following formula:

   $$(23\,\mu g/hr) \times (1\,hr/10\,mL) = 2.3\,\mu g/mL\ of\ IV\ fluids$$

4. Determine how many units of analgesic to add to a 1-liter (1-L) bag of fluids:
   - In this case, using fentanyl, the units are µg:

   $$(2.3\,\mu g/mL) \times (1000\,mL/L) = 2300\,\mu g/L$$

   If using a 500-mL (half-liter; ½-L) bag of fluids, add 1150 µg of fentanyl to the bag.
   If using a 250-mL bag of fluids, add 575 µg of fentanyl to the bag.
5. Determine how many mL of analgesic to add to the bag of fluids.
   NOTE: Before adding analgesic to the fluid bag, remove an equal volume of fluid from the bag.
   - Determine concentration of analgesic, which is stated on the vial; in this case, fentanyl concentration is 50 µg/mL:

   $$(2300\,\mu g) \times ([mL/50\,\mu g]) = 46\,mL$$

- 46 mL of fentanyl should be added to a 1-L bag.
  Or add 23 mL of fentanyl to a half-liter bag (500 mL).
  Or add 11.5 mL of fentanyl to a 250-mL bag.
  Or connect the patient to a syringe pump of fentanyl and deliver IV fluids separately.

Morphine CRI

- Monitor for signs of histamine release (pruritus, hypotension) whenever morphine IV is administered.
- Morphine analgesia continues for approximately 30 minutes after CRI has been discontinued.
- Dysphoria associated with morphine may be alleviated with a low dose of a sedative.

Loading Dose

- Canine: 0.2 to 0.5 mg/kg IV
- Feline: 0.05 to 0.1 mg/kg IV
- Give to effect.

Constant-Rate Infusion

For this example, the patient is a 50-lb dog.
1. Determine the hourly fluid flow rate of IV fluids for the patient:
   - For this example, maintenance fluid flow rate is used as the hourly rate, as calculated by the following formula: 1 mL/lb/hr:

$$50\,lb \times (1\,mL/lb/hr) = 50\,mL/hr$$

$$\text{Hourly IV fluid flow rate} = 50\,mL/hr$$

2. Determine the hourly analgesic dose rate:
   - Morphine CRI dose range, the units are milligrams (mg) for canines: **0.1 to 0.3 mg/kg/hr.**
   - Convert lb to kg:

$$50\,lb \times (1\,kg/2.2\,lb) = 23\,kg$$

   - Calculate the lower and upper limits of the dose range:

$$23\,kg \times (0.1\,mg/kg) = 2.3\,mg$$

$$23\,kg \times (0.3\,mg/kg) = 6.3\,mg$$

$$\text{Range} = 2.3\,to\,6.9\,mg/hr$$

   - Select a dose in the calculated range based on patient's level of pain. For this example, select **5 mg/hr.**
3. Determine how many units of analgesic per mL of IV fluids:
   - In this case, using morphine, the units are mg.
   - Use the hourly IV fluid flow rate determined in step 1 in the following formula:

$$(5\,mg/hr) \times (1\,hr/50\,mL) = 0.1\,mg/mL\ of\ IV\ fluids$$

4. Determine how many units of analgesic to add to liter (L) bag of fluids:
   - In this case, using morphine, the units are mg:

$$(0.1\,mg/mL) \times (1000\,mL/L) = 100\,mg/L$$

   - If using a 500-mL bag of fluids, add 50 mg of morphine to the bag.

- If using a 250-mL bag of fluids, add 25 mg of morphine to the bag.
5. Determine how many mL of analgesic to add to the bag of fluids.
   NOTE: Before adding analgesia to fluid bag, remove an equal volume of fluid from the bag.
   - Determine the concentration of analgesic, which is stated on the vial; in this case, morphine = 15 mg/mL:

$$(100\,mg) \times ([mL/15\,mg]) = 6.7\,mL$$

- 6.7 mL of morphine should be added to a 1-L bag.
  Or add 3.4 mL of morphine to a half-liter bag (500 mL).
  Or add 1.7 mL of morphine to a 250-mL bag.
  Or connect the patient to a syringe pump of morphine and deliver IV fluids separately.

Lidocaine CRI
Loading Dose

- Canine: 2 mg/kg IV
- Give to desired effect.
- Feline: not recommended for use in cats.

Constant-Rate Infusion

For this example, the patient is a 50-lb dog.
1. Determine the hourly fluid flow rate:
   - For the following example, maintenance fluid flow rate is based on the formula 1 mL/lb/hr:

$$50\,lb \times (1\,mL/lb/hr) = 50\,mL/hr$$

$$\text{Hourly IV fluid flow rate} = 50\,mL/hr$$

2. Determine the hourly analgesic dose rate:
   - Lidocaine CRI dose range for canines: **20 to 50 µg/kg/min.**
   - Convert lb to kg: 50 lb × (1 kg/2.2 lb) = 23 kg.
   - Calculate the lower and upper limits of the dose range:

$$23\,kg \times (20\,µg/kg) = 460\,µg$$

$$3\,kg \times (50\,µg/kg) = 1150\,µg$$

$$\text{Range} = 460\,to\,1150\,µg/min$$

   - Select a dose in the calculated range based on patient's level of pain. For this example, select 600 µg/min.
   - Convert the minute rate to an hourly rate:

$$(600\,µg/min) \times (60\,min/hr) = 36,000\,µg/hr$$

$$36,000\,µg = 36\,mg$$

$$\text{Hourly rate} = 36\,mg/hr$$

3. Determine how many units of analgesic per mL of IV fluids:
   - In this example, using lidocaine, the units are now in milligrams (mg).
   - Use the hourly IV fluid flow rate determined in step 1 in the following formula:

$$(36\,mg/hr) \times (1\,hr/50\,mL) = 0.72\,mg/mL$$

4. Determine how many units to add to a 1-liter (1-L) bag of fluids:
   - In this example, using lidocaine, the units are now in mg:

$$(0.72 \, \text{mg/mL}) \times (1000 \, \text{mL/L}) = 720 \, \text{mg/L}$$

If using a 500-mL bag of fluids, add 360 mg of 2% lidocaine to the bag.
If using a 250-mL bag of fluids, add 180 mg of 2% lidocaine to the bag.
5. Determine how many mL of analgesic to add to a bag of fluids:
   NOTE: Before adding analgesia to fluid bag, remove an equal volume of fluid from the bag.
   - Determine the concentration of analgesic, which is stated on the vial; in this case, 2% lidocaine = 20 mg/mL.

$$(720 \, \text{mg}) \times ([\text{mL}/20 \, \text{mg}]) = 36 \, \text{mL}$$

   - 46 mL of lidocaine should be added to a 1-L bag.
   Or add 18 mL to a half-liter bag.
   Or add 9 mL to a 250-mL bag.
   Or connect the patient to a syringe pump of lidocaine and deliver IV fluids separately.

Ketamine CRI
Loading Dose
- Canine and feline: 0.5 mg/kg IV
- Give to desired effect.

Intraoperative Dose
- Canine and feline: 10 μg/kg/min

Constant-Rate Infusion (up to 24 Hours Postoperatively)
In this example, the patient is a 10-lb cat.
1. Determine hourly fluid flow rate.
   - For the following example, maintenance fluid flow rate will be based on the following formula: 1 mL/lb/hr:

$$10 \, \text{lb} \times (1 \, \text{mL/lb/hr}) = 10 \, \text{mL/hr}$$

$$\text{Hourly IV fluid flow rate} = 10 \, \text{mL/hr}$$

2. Determine the hourly analgesic dose rate:
   - Postoperative ketamine CRI dose for felines: **2 μg/kg/min**
   - Convert lb to kg: 10 lb × (1 kg/2.2 lb) = 4.5 kg

- Calculate the minute rate of ketamine:

$$(4.5 \, \text{kg}) \times (2 \, \mu\text{g/kg}) = 9 \, \mu\text{g/min}$$

- Convert the minute rate to an hourly rate:

$$(9 \, \mu\text{g/min}) \times (60 \, \text{min/hr}) = 540 \, \mu\text{g/hr}$$

$$\text{Hourly dose} = 540 \, \mu\text{g/hr}$$

3. Determine how many units of analgesic per mL of IV fluids:
   - In this example, using ketamine, the units are in micrograms (μg).
   - Use the hourly IV fluid flow rate determined in step 1 to the following formula:

$$(540 \, \mu\text{g/hr}) \times (1 \, \text{hr}/10 \, \text{mL}) = 54 \, \mu\text{g/mL}$$

4. Determine how many units to add to a 1-liter (1-L) bag of IV fluids:
   - Note shift from μg to mg in this example:

$$(54 \, \mu\text{g/mL}) \times (1000 \, \text{mL/L}) = 54,000 \, \mu\text{g/L}$$

$$54,000 \, \mu\text{g} = 54 \, \text{mg}$$

   - Add **54 mg** of ketamine to a 1-liter bag of fluids.
   Or add 27 mg to a half-liter bag.
   Or add 13.5 mg to a 250-mL bag.
5. Determine how many mL of ketamine to add to a bag of fluids:
   - Determine the concentration of analgesic, which is stated on the file; in this case, the ketamine concentration is 100 mg/mL.

$$(54 \, \text{mg}) \times ([\text{mL}/100 \, \text{mg}]) = 0.54 \, \text{mL}$$

   - **0.54 mL** of ketamine should be added to a 1-L bag of fluids.
   Or add 0.27 mL of ketamine to a half-liter bag.
   Or add 0.14 mL of ketamine to a 250-mL bag.
   Or connect the patient to a syringe pump of ketamine and deliver IV fluids separately.

GLOSSARY

Abdominocentesis puncture and aspiration of the abdominal cavity.

Ablation removal, especially by cutting.

Absorbable (suture) a strand of organic or synthetic material used for closing wounds that becomes dissolved in the body fluids and disappears.

ACL anterior cruciate ligament.

Active drain a surgically placed implant that creates negative-pressure gradients to facilitate the removal of unwanted fluid or gas.

Acute pain pain that follows some body injury, disappears with healing, and tends to be self-limiting.

Adaptive pain normal response to tissue damage; includes inflammatory pain.

Adrenergic activated by or capable of releasing epinephrine or an epinephrine-like substance, or having physiologic effects similar to those of epinephrine.

Aerophagia habitual swallowing of air.

Agonal breathing the spasmodic opening of the mouth with contraction of the diaphragm usually associated with death; no respiration is taking place.

Agonist a drug that can combine with a receptor on a cell to produce a physiologic reaction; a drug that binds to a receptor and causes it to express its function.

Allodynia pain caused by a stimulus that does not normally cause pain.

Analgesia the loss of sensitivity to pain.

Anastomosis surgical, traumatic, or pathologic formation of a connection between two normally distinct structures.

Anesthesia total or partial loss of sensation.

Anionic detergent soap that has free, negatively charged ions that precipitate when combined with calcium and magnesium in hard water.

Anticholinergic a drug that inhibits the action of acetylcholine by competing at the receptor sites; an agent that is antagonistic to the action of parasympathetic or other cholinergic nerve fibers.

Antiseptic a chemical that inhibits or prevents the growth of microbes on living tissue; compare with *disinfectant*.

Anuria complete suppression of urine formation.

A-O *Arbeitsgemeinschaft für Osteosynthesefragen,* Swiss for the Association for the Study of Internal Fixation (ASIF). These abbreviations are often seen together but separated by a slash: AO/ASIF. The AO is involved in research and development of medical devices used in orthopedic surgery. Their devices are available through a company called Synthes.

Articular pertaining to a joint.

Asepsis the absence of pathogenic microorganisms that cause infection.

Aseptic free from contamination.

Aseptic loosening breakdown of bone and loosening of prosthesis in the absence of microorganisms.

Assisted ventilation the depth of spontaneous ventilation is augmented by the anesthetist.

Atelectasis complete or partial collapse of a lobe or the entire lung.

Atraumatic not producing injury or damage.

Auscultation listening with a stethoscope.

Autotransfusion reinfusion of the patient's own blood.

Bactericide agent that destroys (kills) bacteria.

Bacteriostat agent that inhibits the growth of bacteria.

Balanced anesthesia anesthesia protocol that offsets the depressing effects of anesthetic agents on the motor, sensory, reflex, and mental aspects of nervous system function by combining different agents.

Biocide agent that kills living organisms.

Biological indicator a vial containing the spore state of a specific bacteria that is placed in a sterilizer to show that a sterilizer is functioning properly.

Blepharospasm squinting, blinking.

Bone wax a composition of beeswax and isopropyl palmitate used to seal the cut end of bone; also called *bone sealant.*

Box lock hinged part of a needle holder, tissue forceps, or hemostatic forceps.

Brachycephalic head shape that is shortened in the rostrocaudal dimension, as seen with breeds such as pugs, Boston terriers, and boxers.

Breakthrough pain a transient flare-up of pain in the chronic pain setting that can occur even when chronic pain is under control.

Butterfly catheter a small-gauge needle with a plastic set of "wings" just below the needle hub that make holding the needle easier and more stable.

Callus unorganized network of woven bone formed about the ends of a broken bone that is reabsorbed as healing is completed.

Capillarity the action by which the surface of a liquid where it is in contact with a solid is elevated or depressed.

Capnography the measurement of carbon dioxide (CO_2) concentration in the exhaled air, especially of anesthetized animals.

Cationic detergent cleaning agent that contains positively charged ions that remain suspended in solution (e.g., quaternary ammonium).

Cavitation the formation of bubbles in a liquid.

CCL cranial cruciate ligament.

Celiotomy surgical incision into the abdominal cavity.

Central sensitization an increase in the excitability and responsiveness of nerves in the spinal cord.

Central venous pressure the pressure of blood in the right atrium.

Chemical indicator an item in the form of a strip or tape that shows, by changing color, that conditions for sterilization were met.

Chief complaint the most apparent clinical sign in a patient's illness.

Chlorine-based a chemical that contains chlorine.

Chronic pain pain that lasts several weeks to months and persists beyond the expected healing time, when nonmalignant in origin.

Circulating technician a nonsterile person who opens items for the surgical team and helps maintain surgical conscience.

Closed reduction nonsurgical realignment of fracture or joint.

Closed system involves the total rebreathing of expired gases

Coaptation application of external appliance, such as a splint or cast.

Cold sterilization a misnomer for the use of a liquid disinfectant to "sterilize" instruments. The objects are clean but not truly sterile.

Conjunctivitis inflammation of the conjunctiva.

Cryotherapy therapeutic techniques to decrease tissue temperature.

Cryptorchid animal with undescended testes.

Crystalluria presence of crystals in the urine.

Cyanosis a bluish discoloration of the skin and mucous membranes caused by excessive concentration or reduced hemoglobin in the blood.

Cystectomy excision or resection of the urinary bladder.

Cystostomy surgical formation of an opening into the bladder.

Cystotomy a surgical incision into the bladder to expose the lumen or interior of the urinary bladder.

Cystourethrogram radiograph of the urinary bladder and urethra.

Débridement the removal of all foreign material and all contaminated and devitalized tissues from or adjacent to a traumatic or infected lesion until surrounding healthy tissue is exposed.

Decontamination the manual cleaning of an instrument in a detergent solution to assist in the breakdown of biologic debris.

Dehiscence a splitting open; the breakdown of a surgical incision such that the tissue layers separate from each other.

Delayed union prolonged renewal of continuity in a broken bone or between the edges of a wound.

Detergent chemical that contains free ions and leaves a film on surfaces.

Disarticulation amputation or separation at a joint.

Disinfectant chemical used to inhibit or prevent the growth of microbes on inanimate objects; compare with *antiseptic.*

Dislocation complete separation of the articular surfaces of a joint.

Dissociative anesthesia loss of perception of certain stimuli while that of others remains intact.

Dissociative anesthetic a class of anesthetic agent that cause a disruption of the nerve transmission in some parts of the brain and elective stimulation in others; this combination of actions causes the animal to appear awake but immobile and unaware of its surroundings.

Disposable supplies items that are meant for a single use and that are thrown away at the end of a procedure.

Dysuria difficulty urinating.

E

Elective referring to surgical procedure that can wait for later scheduling.

Emergence delirium delirious behavior resulting from incomplete recovery from gas anesthesia.

Endogenous contamination contamination from the patient.

Endotoxemia the presence of endotoxins in the blood.

Enophthalmos pulling back of the eye and a secondary, raised third eyelid.

Enteral feeding delivery of nutrients directly into the stomach, duodenum, or jejunum; also called *enteral nutrition*.

Enterotomy incision of the intestine.

Entropion inversion or turning inward of the margin of an eyelid.

Enzymes organic substances that assist in the breakdown of soils and are generally formulated with a surfactant to improve their penetration into dried soil.

Ethylene oxide (gas) sterilization a sterilization process used for items that cannot be steam sterilized because the heat would destroy the item.

Event-related expiration a method that uses environmental causes to determine item sterility. If a sterile item is damaged in any way, it would be considered nonsterile.

Evisceration extrusion of the viscera or internal organs.

Exogenous contamination contamination that comes from the surgical team or the environment.

F

Fenestrated to have one or more window-like openings.

Fenestration an opening in a surface.

Flash sterilization an abbreviated version of a regular sterilization cycle used for individual instruments that have been dropped during surgery.

Flexibility the state of being unusually pliant.

Fungicidal an agent that destroys fungus.

Fungicide agent that kills fungi.

Fungistatic a substance that inhibits the growth of fungus.

G

Gastrectomy excision of the stomach or a portion of the stomach.

Gastritis inflammation of the lining of the stomach.

Gastropexy surgical fixation of the stomach.

Gastrotomy the creation of an opening into the stomach.

Gravity air-displacement a method of steam sterilization that relies on gravity to assist steam in penetrating items within the chamber. It is the most common sterilization method in veterinary practices.

H

Hematoma collection of blood under the skin.

Hematuria blood in urine.

Hemostasis the arrest of bleeding by either natural (clot formation) or artificial (compression or ligation) means.

Herniation abnormal protrusion of an organ or other body structure through a defect or natural opening.

High-level disinfection immersing items in a disinfectant solution to reduce the level of contamination. Items are not sterile.

High-vacuum sterilizer a steam sterilizer that forces steam into the sterilizing chamber, causing steam to penetrate the pack more quickly; after the sterilization cycle has been completed, the steam is vacuumed out of the chamber.

Hip dysplasia abnormal development of coxofemoral joint characterized by subluxation or complete luxation of femoral head in younger patients and mild to severe degenerative joint disease in older patients.

Hyperalgesia an increased response to a stimulation that is normally painful either at the site of injury or in surrounding undamaged tissue.

Hypercarbia elevated CO_2 levels, values higher than 45 mm Hg

Hyperesthesia increased sensitivity to sensation.

Hypoalgesia decreased sensitivity to pain.

Hypocarbia lowered CO_2 levels, values less than 35 mm Hg

Hypoesthesia decreased sensitivity to stimulation.

Hypoglycemia lower than normal levels of blood glucose resulting in lack of fuel to the brain and other organ systems.

Hypotension lowered blood pressure.

Hypothermia abnormally low body temperature.

I

Iatrogenic any adverse condition in a patient caused by the action of the doctor or medical staff.

Ileus functional obstruction of the intestines or failure of peristalsis; partial or complete nonmechanical blockage of the small and/or large intestine.

Inappetence partial lack of appetite; inferred in animals with depressed food intake.

Indicator tape pretreated strips on the sterilization tape that change color when the pack has been through the sterilization process.

Injection cap a plug that fits into the end of an intravenous catheter and allows for the injection of substances into that catheter.

Insufflation blowing of a powder, vapor, or gas into a body cavity.

Interfragmentary bone fragments of a fracture that may or may not be able to be reconstructed and stabilized.

Intussusception prolapse of one part of the intestine into the lumen of an immediately adjacent part, causing intestinal obstruction.

Ischemia deficiency of blood in a part.

IVDD intervertebral disc disease associated with disc degeneration and extrusion, causing spinal cord compression and nerve root entrapment.

K

Keratitis inflammation of the cornea.

L

Lacrimation tearing.

Laparotomy flank incision into the abdominal cavity; sometimes used interchangeably with *celiotomy*.

Lavage to wash out or irrigate.

Ligate to tie off or constrict blood vessels or tissue.

Luxation complete separation of a bone from its articulation.

M

Macrodrip set an intravenous set with a drop factor of 15 drops per milliliter.

Maladaptive pain hypersensitivity to pain resulting from abnormal processing of normal input; can also occur if adaptive pain is left untreated.

Malunion incorrect anatomical alignment of the fragments of a fractured bone; faulty union and alignment of the fractured bone.

Mechanical friction a scrubbing motion used to clean all surfaces.

Memory (suture) a property of some synthetic fibers that encourages the spontaneous untying of knots.

Microbial shedding occurs when microorganisms are released into the environment from the body of surgical personnel.

Microdrip set an intravenous set with a drop factor of 60 drops per milliliter.

Movable equipment pieces of equipment that can be transported from the surgery room to other areas of the hospital.

MPL medial patellar luxation.

Multimodal analgesia the use of multiple drugs with different actions to produce optimal analgesia.

N

Neoplasia the formation of abnormal growth.

Neuroplasticity the idea that the nervous system can be changed by the effect of the environment, external stimuli, and the effects of physiologic stimuli, such as pain.

Nociception the transaction, conduction, and central nervous system processing of nerve signals generated by the stimulation of certain receptors; term used to describe three neuralgic phases of the pain pathway transduction, transmission, and modulation.

Nonelective surgical procedures that cannot wait for later scheduling.

Nonmovable (permanent) equipment pieces of equipment that are attached to the floor, wall, or ceiling in the surgery room.

Nonreducible unable to be restored to the normal place or position.

Nonunion failure of the ends of a fractured bone to unite.

Normothermia normal body temperature.

Nosocomial infection infection acquired during hospitalization or during attendance at any veterinary medical facility.

O

Occlusive wound dressing a dressing used on the skin that retains moisture and heat while increasing the concentration and absorption of medication being applied; impermeable to air and fluid.

OCD osteochondritis dissecans; inflammation of bone and cartilage that results in the splitting of cartilage pieces into the affected joint.

Onychectomy declawing; the removal of the claw and its associated third phalanx.

Open reduction surgical opening and exposure to realign a fracture or joint.

Orchiectomy castration.

Osteomyelitis bone infection.

Over-the-needle catheter an intravenous catheter system in which the needle, stylette is inside the catheter. The catheter itself sits over the needle and is advanced once the needle has entered the vessel.

P

Pain threshold the least experience of pain that a patient can recognize.

Pain tolerance level the greatest level of pain that a patient can tolerate.

Passive drain a surgically placed implant that uses gravity and overflow to facilitate the removal of unwanted fluid or gas.

Pathologic pain pain that has an exaggerated response beyond its protective usefulness. It is often associated with tissue injury incurred at the time of surgery or trauma.

Percutaneous performed through the skin.

Peripheral catheter catheter that is placed in the limbs.

Peritonitis an inflammatory process that involves the serous membrane of the abdominal cavity.

Pétrissage a type of massage that consists of kneading, rhythmic lifting, squeezing, and releasing the tissue.

Phenol-based a chemical agent that contains phenol.

Photophobia sensitivity to light.

Physiologic pain pain that acts as a protective mechanism that incites individuals to move away from the cause of potential tissue damage or to avoid movement or contact with external stimuli during a reparative phase.

Plasma sterilization low-temperature plasma sterilization with hydrogen peroxide (H_2O_2) gas used for items that cannot be steam sterilized.

Pollakiuria abnormally frequent passage of urine.

Positive-pressure ventilation increased air pressure that pushes air out of the surgical suite, reducing the influx of bacteria from the rest of the facility.

Precleaning cleaning before a subsequent process.

Preemptive analgesia the administration of an analgesic drug before painful stimulation to prevent sensitization of neurons, or *wind-up*, thus improving postoperative analgesia.

Premedication preliminary medication, particularly internal medication, to produce sedation or narcosis before general anesthesia.

Preparation area a room used for patient preparation and the storage of surgical supplies.

Presoaking placing soiled instruments in distilled water or water mixed with a detergent solution without using mechanical agitation.

Pronate to turn the palm downward or from the body to face the ground.

Pronation the rotation of the hand and forearm so that the palm faces backward or downward.

Prophylaxis use of an agent to prevent disease.

Pulse deficit the difference between the apical pulse (that heard over the heart with a stethoscope) and the arterial pulse.

Pulse oximetry an instrument that measures pulse rate and the percentage of oxygenated and reduced hemoglobin.

Pulse strength the ease or difficulty of palpating the blood flowing through the artery.

Q

Quaternary amine–based a chemical agent that contains quaternary ammonia.

R

Recipe a document that details pertinent information about surgery pack preparation and contents; often maintained in a procedures manual.

Reducible able to be restored to the normal place or relation of parts, as in a reducible fracture.

Regional anesthesia the loss of sensation in part of the body caused by interruption of the sensory nerves that conduct impulses from that region of the body.

Reusable supplies items that are cleaned, sterilized, and reused from procedure to procedure.

S

Sanitize to reduce the number of microbes to a safe level.

Scrub area an area near the surgery room with the scrub sink, autoclave, and room to gown and glove.

Semi-closed system the most common rebreathing circuit used in veterinary medicine, wherein there is partial rebreathing of expired gases

Semi-open system

Semiocclusive wound dressing bandage that allows air to penetrate and exudates to escape from the wound surface.

Sepsis the presence of pathogenic microorganisms or their toxins in blood or other tissue.

Septicemia systemic disease associated with the presence of pathogenic microorganisms and their toxins.

Seroma a serosanguineous accumulation of fluid between tissue planes.

Serrated having a sawlike edge or border.

Shank portion of a surgical instrument that connects the handle with the working end.

Shelf-life expiration a method that uses a predetermined date that identifies how long an item should be considered sterile.

Shock a condition of acute peripheral circulatory failure.

Signalment the part of the veterinary medical history dealing with the animal's age, sex, breed, and reproductive status.

Somatic pain pain that originates from damage to bone, joints, muscle, or skin and is described by humans as localized, constant, sharp, aching, and throbbing.

Sphygmomanometer an instrument for measuring blood pressure.

Splenectomy excision of the spleen.

Sporicide agent that kills spores.

Stenosis narrowing or contraction of a body passage or opening.

Sterile free from all living organisms.

Sterile field a microorganism-free area.

Sterility the absence of all living microorganisms, including spores.

Sterilization the use of a process to rid an object of all living microbes.

Sterilize To eliminate all microbes by death or inactivation.

Stranguria slow and painful discharge of urine.

Strike-through contamination contamination that occurs when liquids soak through a drape from a sterile area to an unsterile area, or vice versa.

Subluxation partial or incomplete separation of a joint.

Suction the ability to remove fluid or air from an area by using either a manual or a mechanical device.

Supination to rotate the forearm to bring the palm face upward.

Surfactant a substance, such as a detergent, that can reduce the surface tension of a liquid and thus allow it to foam or penetrate solids.

Surgery room a separate room that should be used only for surgery.

Surgical conscience the commitment of surgical personnel to adhere strictly to aseptic technique, because anything less could increase the potential risk of infection, resulting in harm to the patient.

Surgical hand rub a scrubless, brushless, waterless antiseptic hand preparation product used during the process of scrubbing in for surgery.

Surgical hand scrub process of removing as many microorganisms as possible from nails, hands, and arms by mechanical washing and chemical antisepsis before participating in a surgical procedure.

Surgical technician sterile person who assists with surgical duties such as passing instruments, retracting tissue, and maintaining hemostasis.

Swage to fuse, as suture material to the end of a suture needle.

T

Terminal cleaning cleaning performed at the completion of the daily surgery schedule.

Thermoregulatory the physiologic process controlling the balance between heat production and heat loss in the body so as to maintain body temperature.

Traumatic pertaining to, resulting from, or causing trauma.

Trichobezoar hair ball.

Trocar a sharp, pointed, needlelike instrument equipped with a cannula; used to puncture the wall of a body cavity and withdraw fluid or gas.

U

Urethrotomy incision into the urethra.

Urine scald moist irritating effect of urine in contact with the skin.

Uroabdomen presence of urine in the abdominal cavity; generally associated with a ruptured bladder.

Urolith calculus or stone found in the urine or urinary system.

Urolithiasis formation of calculi in the urinary tract.

Uveitis intraocular inflammation.

V

Vaporizer its primary function is to hold liquid anesthetic and to turn that liquid into a gas form that can be delivered to the patient in a controlled manner.

Viricidal an agent that kills viruses.

Visceral pain pain that arises from stretching, distension, or inflammation of the viscera and described by humans as deep, cramping, aching, or gnawing without good localization.

Volvulus rotation of an organ.

W

WAGs waste gases.

Wind-up alterations in the nervous system that occur as a result of untreated or inadequately treated pain and lead to untreatable pain states; temporal summation of painful stimuli in the spinal cord. Mediated by C fibers and responsible for "secondary" pain.

INDEX

Note: Page numbers followed by *f* indicate figures, *t* indicate tables and *b* indicate boxes.

A

AA. *see* Arachidonic acid (AA)
AAHA. *see* American Animal Hospital Association (AAHA)
Abdomen
 blood pooling in, 219
 clipping of, 76f
 insufflation of, achievement, 191
 systematic exploration of, 135
Abdominal cavity
 puncture of (abdominocentesis), 141
Abdominal exploratory surgery, 135, 135b
 definition of, 135
 indications of, 135
 procedure of, 135
Abdominal incision
 dehiscence of, 134f
 swelling of, 134f
 through subcutaneous tissue and linea
  alba, 147
Abdominal procedures, 132–134
 instruments in, 132–133, 132f, 133f
 patient draping in, 133, 133f
 patient positioning and preparation in, 133
 postoperative considerations and instructions
  for, 134, 134f
 surgery report in, 134, 135b
 wall closure in, 133
Abdominal skin incision, 147f
Abdominal surgery, 82, 82f, 83f
Abdominal tap (abdominocentesis), 218–219
Abdominal wall closure, 133
 for GDV, 145
 intestine and, 139
 in ovariohysterectomy, 148
Abdominocentesis (abdominal tap,
 "belly tap"), 141
 performing, 218–219
Absorbability, 28
Absorbable (suture), 28
Absorbable sutures, length cut of, 127
AccuVet Novapulse LX-$_2$0SP CO$_2$ laser, 187f
AccuVet V25 fiber-coupled diode laser system,
 187f
Activated-charcoal scavenger canister, 41f
Activated partial thromboplastin time (aPTT),
 219
Active drains, 226
Active scavenging systems, 41
Acute abdomen, curative surgery for, 135
Acute pain, 238b
Adaptive pain, 238b
Adhesions, problem of, 124
Adjustable pressure relief valve ("pop-off"
 valve), 39
Administration sets, 63
Adson-Brown thumb tissue forceps, 16
Adson dressing, 16
Adson thumb tissue forceps, 16
Adson 1 x 2 instrument, 16
Agonal ("death agony") breathing, 91
Agonist-antagonist opioids, 55

Agonists, 55–56
Alanine aminotransferase (ALT), 49, 53
Alcohol
 antimicrobial properties of, 110–111
 with bactericidal properties, 267–268
 evaporation of, 77
Alcohol-based rubs, 110
Alcohol rub (brushless technique), 110
Alkylating agent, FDA approved, 268
Allis tissue forceps, 16–17
 for gastrotomy, 136–137
 tips of, 17f
Allodynia, 238b
Alopecic eyelid neoplasms, 162
AORN. *see* Association of periOperative
 Registered Nurses (AORN)
α$_2$-adrenergic agonist, 56–57
 causing peripheral vasoconstriction, 92
α$_2$-agonists
 candidates for administration of, 57
 function of, 56
 side effects of, 56–57
ALT. *see* Alanine aminotransferase (ALT)
AMDUCA. *see* Animal Medical Drug Use
 Clarification Act of 1994 (AMDUCA)
American Animal Hospital Association (AAHA)
 pain standards, 238b
 surgical facility areas, 1
American National Standards Institute (ANSI),
 188
American Society of Anesthesiologists (ASA), for
 anesthetic risk rating system, 72, 72t
Amputation, 175–176, 175f, 176f
 pain management for, 175–176
Analgesia, 238b
 dispensed, 234
 requesting, 240
Analgesics, 54–57
 calculations for constant-rate infusion of,
  275–277
 classes of, 233
 drugs, impact of, 54f
 side effects of, 55t
Anastomosis, 140–142, 250
 completion of, 142f
 definition of, 140
 indications of, 141
 intestine and abdominal wall closure of,
  141–142, 142f
 jejunal resection and, 141f
 postoperative considerations and instructions
  for, 142
 postoperative instructions after, 250b
 procedure of, 141, 141f
 special instruments for, 141
 surgery report of, 143b
 tissue handling during, 124
Anesthesia, 238b
 breed predisposition of, 217
 complications of, 214–218
 deeper stages of, 94
 depth of, excessive, 217

Anesthesia *(Continued)*
 dextrose and, 218
 effects, recovery, 240
 fluid therapy and, 218
 form of, 72–73
  graph component of, 74f
 machine, 3, 3f
 monitoring, devices, 95–99, 95t
 patient-related causes, 217–218
 physical stimulation and, 218
 recovery from, 213–214
  food, offering, 217–218
  prolongation, 217–218
 reversal agents and, 218
 side effects of, 248
 stages of, 89t
 therapeutic measures for, 218
 ventilation and, 218
 warming measures for, 218
Anesthesia-related causes, 217
Anesthetic depth, 91, 92
Anesthetic gases, 41
Anesthetic induction, 73
 drug, IV administration, 73
Anesthetic machine, 34–45, 35f
 ability of, 34
 breathing circuits, 42–43
 components, 34–41, 39f
  function, 34–35
 configuration of, 34
 leaking, potential, 41–42
 leak testing, 41–42, 42b
 oxygen flow rates, 44
 purpose of, 34
 review questions, 44–45
 vaporizers/device storage, 35f
Anesthetic monitoring, 95t
Anesthetic risk, ASA status of, 72t
Anesthetist, in constant monitoring, 89
Angle wrapping, 263, 264f
Animal Medical Drug Use Clarification Act of
 1994 (AMDUCA), 55
Animals, constant monitoring of, 92
ANSI. *see* American National Standards
 Institute (ANSI)
Antagonist opioids, 56
Antagonists, 55–56
Antibiotics, 58
 administration of, IV catheters, 62
 choice of, 58
Anticholinergics, 57–58
 administration of, 90–91
 deeper stages of, 94
Antimesenteric border, of intestine,
 139, 139f
Antimicrobial agents, 226
Antimicrobial rub agent, use of, 114
Antimicrobials, characteristics of, 111t
Antimicrobial scrub agent
 dispensation of, 111
 use of, 111–113
Antimicrobial skin-cleansing agents, 110